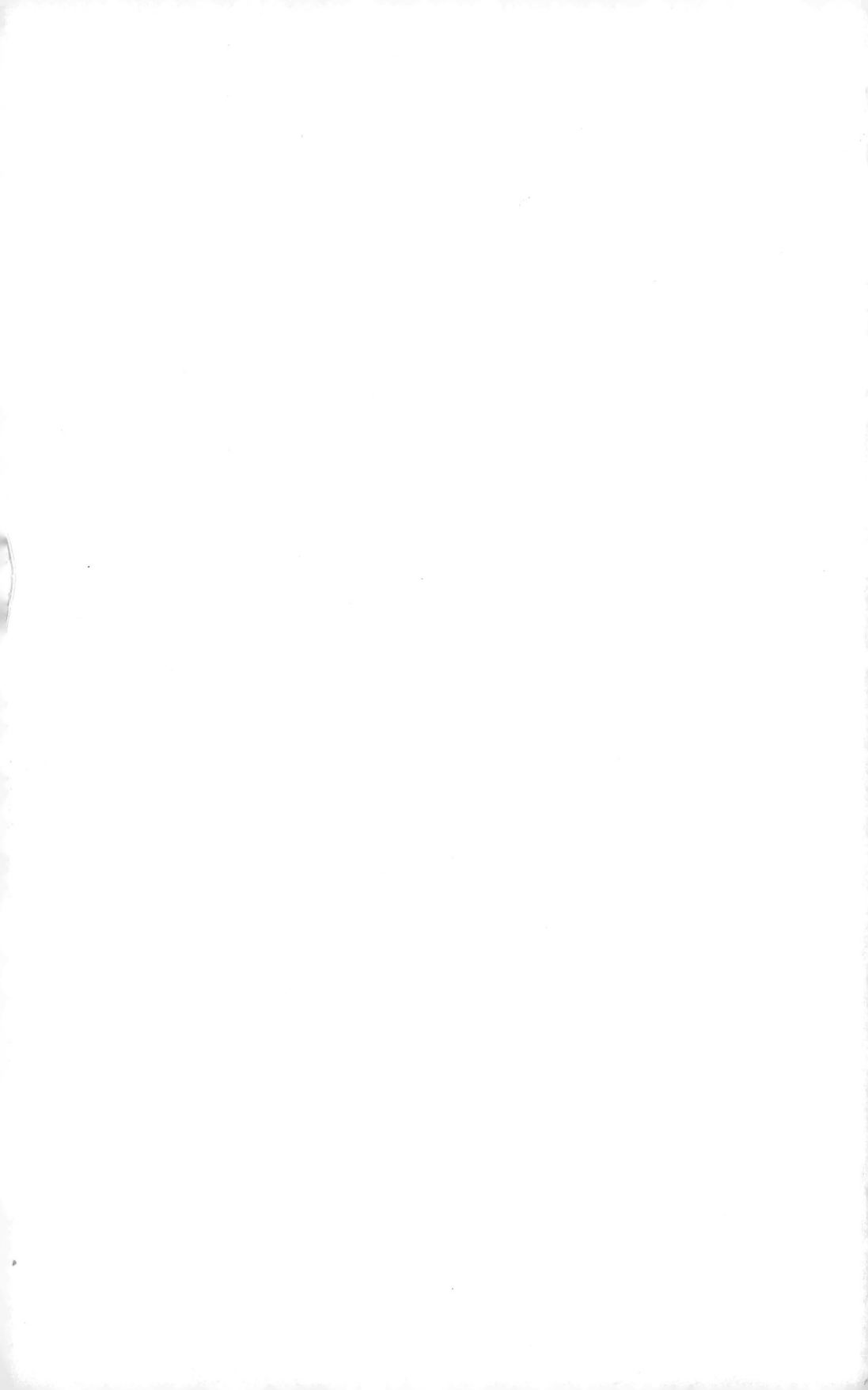

This Symposium was sponsored by the Scientific Council on Arteriosclerosis and Ischaemic Heart Disease of the International Society of Cardiology and arranged through the courtesy of the Edinburgh Post-Graduate Board for Medicine

Coronary Heart Disease in Young Women

Edited by **M.F. OLIVER**,
M.D., F.R.C.P., F.R.C.P.E., F.F.C.M., F.A.C.C.(Hon).

CHURCHILL LIVINGSTONE
EDINBURGH LONDON AND NEW YORK 1978

CHURCHILL LIVINGSTONE
Medical Division of Longman Group Limited

Distributed in the United States of America by
Longman Inc., 19 West 44th Street, New York,
N.Y.10036 and by associated companies,
branches and representatives throughout
the world.

First Edition 1978
  Reprinted 1979

ISBN 0 443 01625 9

British Library Cataloguing in Publication Data

Coronary heart disease in young women.
  1. Coronary heart disease — Congresses
  2. Young women — Diseases — Congresses
  I. Title   II. Oliver, Michael Francis
  616.1'23   RC685.C6   78-40188

Printed in Great Britain by Bell & Bain Ltd., Glasgow

Preface

It would appear that angina in a young woman was first described by Morgagni in 1769 in his celebrated *De Sedibus et Causis Morborum*. In October 1707 he examined the body of a woman 'the mother of a family, who was two-and-forty years of age, had liv'd long in a state of infirm health, and had long been subject to a kind of paroxysm, which appeared in the following manner: on using pretty quick exercise of body, a kind of violent uneasiness came on, within the upper part of the thorax, on the left side, join'd with a difficulty in breathing, and a numbness of the left arm: all of which symptoms soon remitted when those motions ceased'. On a journey to Venice in October, 1707 she had just such a paroxysm 'and saying that she should die; she actually died on the spot'. While no mention is made of the coronary arteries, extensive irregular hardening and ossification was found throughout the entire length of the aorta.

During the last twenty years or so, it has become increasingly evident that coronary heart disease occurring in women under the age of 45 is no longer a curiosity worthy of description as a single case report. Nor is it even a rarity, although clinical prejudices probably still operate in under-diagnosis of the condition. Because of changes occurring in the incidence of the disease and in the environment in which we live, I considered it timely to bring together a number of experts in different fields in order to examine in detail the extent of our knowledge concerning the epidemiology, pathological anatomy and endocrinology, aggravating causes, clinical characteristics, prognosis and management of coronary heart disease in young women.

I hope that the facts presented in this Symposium will form a firm basis for dissemination of knowledge on the subject and that the doubts and areas of ignorance will stimulate more basic research and further epidemiological and clinical studies.

MICHAEL OLIVER

Acknowledgements

Dr. Gavin Brown, Registrar in the Department of Cardiology, Royal Infirmary, Edinburgh acted as Scientific Secretary. The time he gave and his attention to detail made the Symposium a success. His participation in the editing of the tapes is also gratefully acknowledged. Miss Inez Johnston looked after many of the social details and is thanked for carrying the burden of all the correspondence. The Dean of the Post-Graduate Board for Medicine, University of Edinburgh, Major-General J.M. Matheson, OBE, kindly supported this venture and allowed use of the Pfizer Foundation for the meetings.

Financial support was received from:

The International Society of Cardiology
Chest, Heart and Stroke Association (Scotland)
The Tobacco Research Council
Astra Chemicals Limited
C.H. Boehringer Sohn
Bristol Laboratories
Ciba Foundation
Imperial Chemical Industries
May & Baker
Organon Laboratories
Ortho Pharmaceuticals
Pfizer Research
Schering Chemicals
G.D. Searle
Syntex Research Centre
Unilever Research
Wyeth Laboratories

List of Participants

BAIRD, Professor D.T., Department of Obstetrics and Gynaecology, University of Edinburgh.

BEAUMONT, Professor J.L., Institut National de la Sante de la Recherche Medicale, Hopital Henri Mondor, 51 Av. De Mal de Lattre de Tassigny, 94000 Creteil, France.

BEAUMONT, Dr V., Unite de Recherches sur l'Atherosclerose, Hopital Henri Mondor, 94010 Creteil, France.

BENGTSSON, Dr C., Department of Medicine ll, University of Goteborg, Sahlgrenska Hospital, S-413 45 Goteborg, Sweden.

BONNAR, Professor J., Department of Obstetrics and Gynaecology, University of Dublin, Rotunda Hospital, Dublin 1, Ireland.

BROWN, Dr G.J., Department of Cardiology, Royal Infirmary, Edinburgh EH3 9YW.

CHAKRABARTI, Dr R., Epidemiology and Medical Care Unit, Northwick Park Hospital, Watford Road, Harrow, Middlesex HA1 3UJ.

CLARKE, Dr Joan M., G.D. Searle & Co. Ltd., P.O. Box 53, Lane End Road, High Sycombe, Bucks HP12 4HL.

CLEMENS, Dr K., Schering Chemicals Ltd., The Brow, Burgess Hill, West Sussex RH15 9NE.

DOLL, Professor Sir Richard, Department of the Regius Professor of Medicine, University of Oxford, Radcliffe Infirmary, Oxford OX2 6HE.

DOUGLAS, Professor A.S., Department of Medicine, University of Aberdeen, Foresterhill, Aberdeen AB9 2ZD.

EPSTEIN, Professor F.H., Institute of Social and Preventive Medicine, University of Zurich, Zurich, Switzerland.

FAURE, Dr. D. MUNRO-, Director of Clinical Research, The Wellcome Research Laboratories, Langley Court, Beckenham, Kent BR3 3BS.

FAUX, Dr C., Wyeth Laboratories, Huntercombe Lane South, Taplow, Maidenhead, Berkshire SL6 0PH.

FORBES, Dr W., Scottish Home and Health Department, Chief Scientist Office, Trinity Park House, South Trinity Road, Edinburgh EH5 3SF.

FULLER, Dr J.H., Unit for Metabolic Medicine, Department of Medicine, Guy's Hospital Medical School, London Bridge, London, SE1 9RT.

FULTON, Dr Mary, Department of Community Medicine, Usher Institute, Warrender Park Road, Edinburgh EH9 1DW.

A*

FULTON, Dr W.F.M., Department of Materia Medica, University of Glasgow, Stobhill General Hospital, Glasgow G21 3UW.

GORDON, Mr T., Biometrics Research Branch, National Heart, Lung and Blood Institute, Bethesda, Md 20014, U.S.A.

GREENHALGH, Mr R.M., Department of Surgery, Charing Cross Hospital, Fulham Palace Road, London W6 8RF.

GRESHAM, Professor G.A., Department of Morbid Anatomy and Histopathology, The John Bonnett Clinical Laboratories, Addenbrooke's Hospital, Cambridge CB2 2QQ.

HAZZARD, Dr W., Northwest Lipid Research Clinic, 326 Ninth Avenue, Seattle, Washington 98104, U.S.A.

HORTON, Professor E.V., Department of Pharmacology, University of Edinburgh.

JARRETT, Dr R.J., Unit for Metabolic Medicine, Department of Medicine, Guy's Hospital Medical School, London Bridge, London SE1 9RT.

JULIAN, Professor D.G. Department of Cardiology, Freeman Hospital, Freeman Road, Newcastle-upon-Tyne NE7 7DN.

KITCHIN, Dr A.H., Cardiac Department, Western General Hospital, Edinburgh EH4 2XU.

LAWRIE, Professor T.D.V., Department of Medical Cardiology, Royal Infirmary, Glasgow G4 0SF.

LEWIS, Professor B., Department of Chemical Pathology, St Thomas' Hospital, London SE1 7EH.

LICHTLEN, Professor P.R., Medizinische Hochschule Hannover, Department fur Innere Medizin, Karl-Wiechert-Allee 9, 3 Hannover-Kleefeld, West Germany.

LOUDON, Dr Nancy, Family Planning Centre, 18 Dean Terrace, Edinburgh EH4 1NL

MACDONALD, Dr I.S., Scottish Home and Health Department, St Andrews House, Edinburgh EH1.

MACMAHON, Professor B., Department of Epidemiology, Harvard University School of Public Health, 677 Huntington Avenue, Boston, Mass 02115, U.S.A.

MAHLER, Professor R.F., Department of Medicine, University of Wales, Welsh National School of Medicine, Heath Park, Cardiff CF4 4XN.

MANN, Dr J.I., Department of Social and Community Medicine, University of Oxford, 8 Keble Road, Oxford OX1 3QN.

MARQUIS, Dr R.M., Department of Cardiology, Royal Infirmary, Edinburgh EH3 9YW.

MILLER, Dr H.C., Department of Cardiology, Royal Infirmary, Edinburgh EH3 9YW

MITCHELL, Professor J.R.A., Department of Medicine, University of Nottingham, General Hospital, Nottingham NG1 6HA.

MORRIS, Dr D.C., Emory University School of Medicine, 69 Butler Street S.E., Atlanta, Georgia 30303, U.S.A.

MUIR, Dr A.L., Department of Medicine, The Royal Infirmary, Edinburgh, Edinburgh EH3 9YW.

NORDIN, Professor B.E.C., MRC Mineral Metabolsim Unit, The General Infirmary, Great George Street, Leeds LS1 3EX.

OLIVER, Professor, M.F., Departments of Medicine and Cardiology, The Royal Infirmary, Edinburgh EH3 9YW.

POTTS, Dr M., International Planned Parenthood Federation, 18-20 Lower Regent Street, London SW1Y 4PW.

ROBERTSON, Dr J.I.S., MRC Blood Pressure Unit, Western Infirmary, Glasgow G11 6NT.

ROSE, Professor G.A., Epidemiology Department, St Mary's Hospital Medical School, London W2.

SAXTON, Dr C., Pfizer Central Research, Sandwich, Kent CT13 9NJ.

SHORT, Professor R.V., MRC Reproductive Biology Unit, 2 Forrest Road, Edinburgh EH1 2QW.

SINGH, Dr S., Dudley Road Hospital, Birmingham 18 7QH.

SLACK, Dr Joan, MRC Clinical Genetics Unit, Institute of Child Health, 30 Guildford Street, London WC1N 1EH.

SOMERVILLE, Dr W., Department of Cardiology, The Middlesex Hospital, Cleveland Street, London W1.

SPAIN, Dr D.M., Department of Pathology, The Brookdale Hospital Medical Center, Linden Boulevard at Brookdale Plaza, Brooklyn, N.Y. 11212, U.S.A.

VENNING, Dr R., G.D. Searle & Co. Ltd., P.O. Box 53, Lane End Road, High Sycombe, Bucks HP12 4HL.

VERMEULEN, Professor A., Dienst Voor Inwendige Ziekten, Akademisch Ziekenhuis, De Pintelaan 135, 9000 Ghent, Belgium.

VESSEY, Professor M.P., Department of Social and Community Medicine, University of Oxford, 8 Keble Road, Oxford OX1 3QN.

WALD, Dr N., Department of the Regius Professor of Medicine, University of Oxford, Radcliffe Infirmary, Oxford OX2 6HE.

WEIR, Dr R.J., Gartnavel General Hospital, 1053 Great Western Road, Glasgow G12 0YN.

WILHELMSEN, Dr L., Department of Medicine 1, University of Goteborg, Sahlgrenska Hospital, S-413 45 Goteborg, Sweden.

WYNN, Professor V., Alexander Simpson Laboratory for Metabolic Research, St Mary's Hospital Medical School, London W2.

Contents

xiv

SESSION 1 Epidemiology, Incidence and Genetic Influences

Chairman: Sir Richard Doll

Incidence

Genetic influences

Cigarette smoking

1. Epidemiology of coronary heart disease in young women

L. WILHELMSEN

The mortality from coronary heart disease (CHD) is lower in women than in men up to about 75 years of age in most industrialised countries. The incidence of CHD in women below the age of 50 is so low that statistics on incidence are rather uncertain and prospective population studies of risk factors are impossible.

Previous studies indicate that the sex differences in incidence and prevalence might be different for various manifestations of CHD. The risk factors might also be different. Thus, it is important to study the various manifestations of CHD separately.

The aim of the present paper is to compare the incidence of angina pectoris (AP), ECG-abnormalities at rest and during exercise, myocardial infarction (MI) and sudden coronary death (SD) in men and women in various countries as well as possible variations with time.

Angina pectoris

Cross-sectional population studies in Göteborg have shown about the same prevalence of chest pain on exertion indicating AP according to a standardised questionnaire, in middle aged women as in men. However, the prevalence of MI has definitely been higher in men than in women, Fig.1.1 (Bengtsson 1973).

Similar differences between the sexes with respect to the incidence of 'uncomplicated' AP (not following an MI) compared to MI and SD have been reported from the Framingham Study (Kannel and Feinleib, 1972). At younger ages uncomplicated AP was less frequent in women than in men but at older ages the sex ratio was reversed. Because of these circumstances, there is a distinct difference in the way CHD presents in women as compared to men, AP being the presenting symptom of CHD in women much more frequently than MI or SD. When women suffer an MI or SD they have more often had AP previously than is the case in men. The risk of MI or SD tended to be lower in women with AP than in men with AP (Kannel and Feinleib, 1972).

ECG abnormalities

The prevalence of ST-changes as well as other ECG abnormalities at rest and during exercise has been studied in male and female population samples in Göteborg (Wilhelmsen, Grimby, Bjure *et al*, to be publ; Vedin and Bengtsson, to be publ). Both at rest and after a maximal bicycle exercise, there was a slight tendency towards more ST-changes in women than in men at age 54 years. It has been argued that

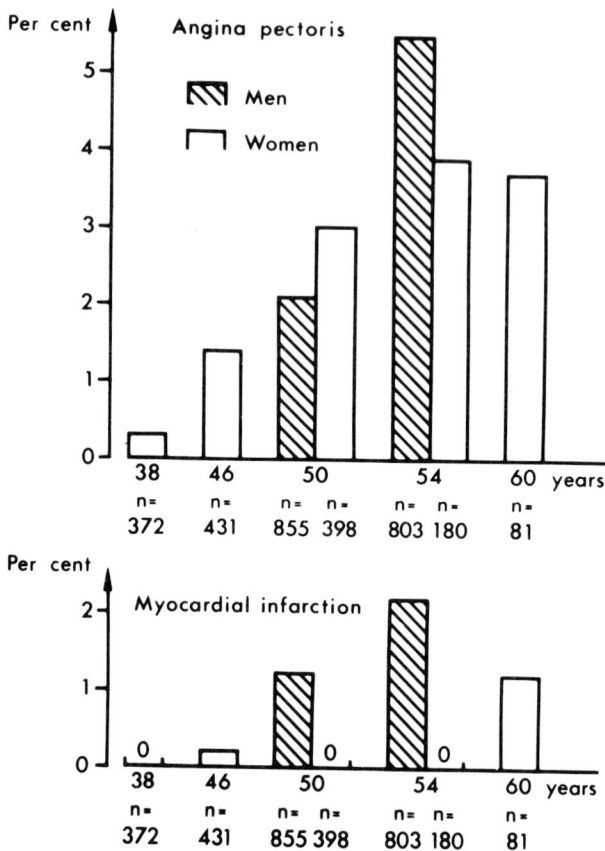

Fig. 1.1 Prevalence of angina pectoris and myocardial infarction in population samples of men and women in Göteborg, Sweden. According to Bengtsson (1973).

ST-changes during or after exercise might be unspecific in women and not mirror ischaemia. Recently it has been shown that oestrogens may affect the ST segments after exercise, but did not affect a normal post-exercise ECG in nine out of ten cases (Jaffe, 1977). It is not possible to say at present whether ECG changes have different meanings in men and women.

Incidence of myocardial infarction

Under the auspices of the European Region of the World Health Organisation, a comprehensive registration system for non-fatal and fatal MI + SD was in operation during 1971 (WHO 1976). A good correlation was found between CHD deaths and non-fatal and fatal cases of MI and SD (Fig. 1.2). For each fatal case of CHD there were about 1.5 non-fatal events. This relationship was similar in men and women and rather stable from place to place. Thus, mortality statistics might perhaps be used for assessing the total incidence of CHD (excepting AP) in other studies.

There was a fairly close association between the incidence of MI in men and

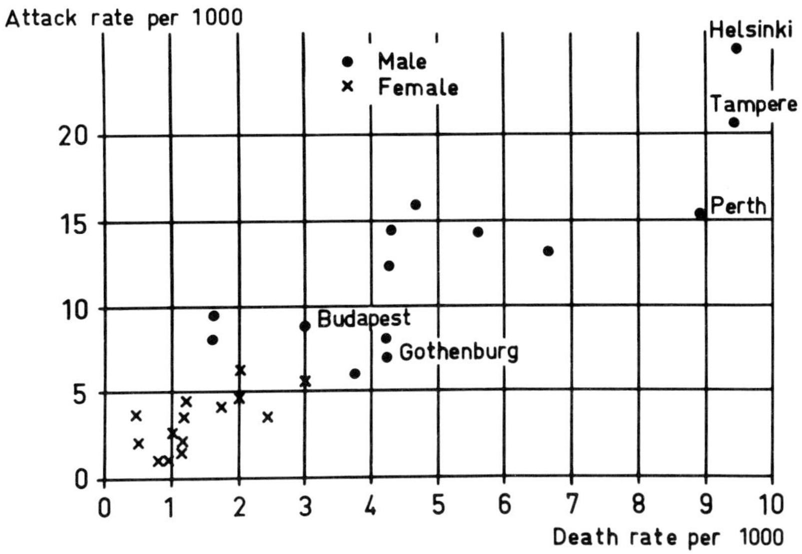

Fig. 1.2 Correlation between the attack rate of AMI computed from the registers and the death rate from category 410 of the ICD (8th revision) as given in the National Vital Statistics: age-group 55-64 years. According to WHO (1976).

women (Fig. 1.3). In areas with a high incidence in men it was generally high in women also. This finding suggests common genetic and environmental influences on MI in the two sexes. The female incidence did not reach the male incidence until at about 15 years higher age, 60 - 64-year-old women having the same incidence as 45 - 49-year-old men. At higher ages this difference in incidence diminished.

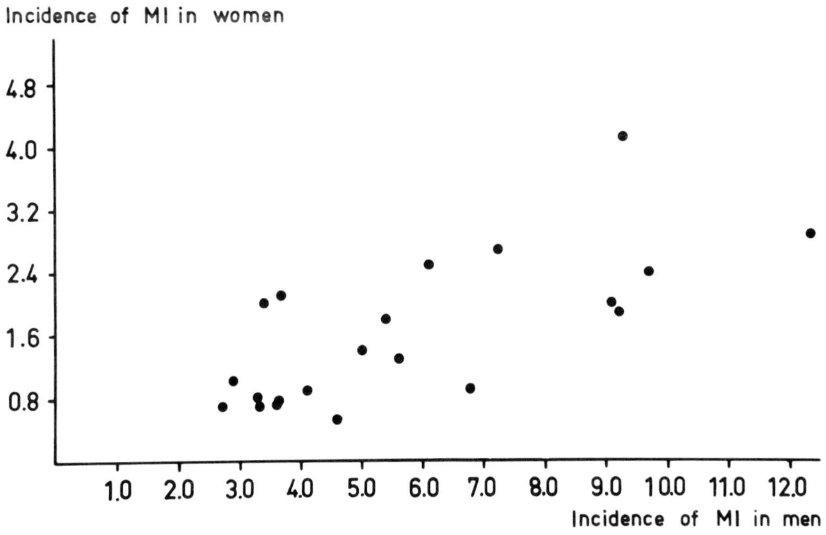

Fig. 1.3 Annual incidence rate of acute myocardial infarction (1st attack) per 1000 population (age 55 - 59 years). According to WHO (1976).

Postmortem findings

According to findings presented so far, the prevalence and incidence of AP and prevalence of ECG abnormalities seems to be similar in the two sexes but there is a marked difference in the incidence of MI. Thus, the female 'protection' against CHD seems to be much stronger for the two 'hard' end-points MI and SD than for AP. This difference implies differences in the pathogenesis of the various manifestations of CHD.

The answers to questionnaires on chest pain and ST-changes can be considered less specific than MI and SD. Thus, these manifestations have been taken as unspecific manifestations not necessarily due to ischaemia of the myocardium in connection with physical exertion. The degree of coronary atherosclerosis should be a better measure. No study of the coronary vessels by coronary angiography or by other means has been performed in population samples of men and women. However, Sternby (1968) studied 1.167 necropsies in men and 1.079 in women from a defined area (Malmo, Sweden). Women did not develop the same degree of atherosclerosis as men until at 10 - 15 years older age (Fig. 1.4). This was true for all age-groups between 20 and 85 years of age.

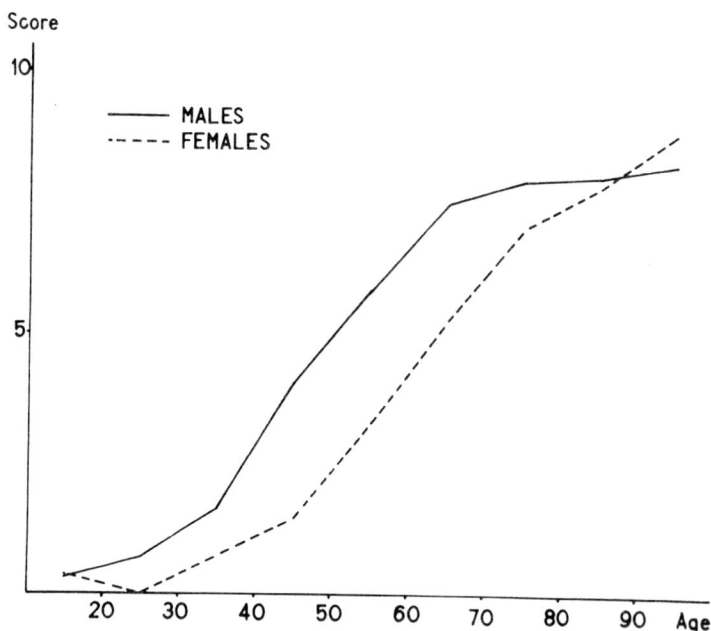

Fig. 1.4 Degree of atherosclerosis of three coronary arteries combined in males and females according to Sternby (1968).

This finding suggests a close relationship between the incidence of MI + SD and coronary atherosclerosis. However, a bias might have been introduced because the main causes of death were different in the two sexes. Young and middle-aged men died more often from CHD than women, who died from neoplasms more often than men. If women have a resistance to MI and SD (fatal and non-fatal), this postmortem finding is possible despite a fairly similar degree of atherosclerosis in the two sexes. There was, however, a tendency to less atherosclerosis in women than men of similar age even when groups dying from other causes than CHD were analysed. Thus, there is no complete agreement between results from clinical studies on various manifestations of CHD and postmortem studies on coronary atherosclerosis.

Secular trends in the incidence of CHD

Epstein (1968) reviewed the CHD mortality trend in 14 countries. There was a general trend towards higher age-standardised mortality for men aged 25 - 64 in 1961 - 1963 than in 1951 - 1953, but the mortality *decreased* in women for most countries studied. Over the decade the male/female sex ratio for every country increased. Since the death rates of males rose proportionately more in the countries with low rates than in those with high ones, the sex ratios also tended to rise more in these countries.

The revisions to the International Classification of Causes of Death in 1951 and 1968 necessitate caution with respect to changes in reported incidence over periods covering these years. However, between 1950 and 1968 Oliver (1974) reported a marked increase in the incidence of CHD in women aged 35 - 44 in England and Wales. de Haas (1969) found no similar trend between 1950 and 1968 in older Dutch women but the trend was the same in Dutch men. In Sweden we did not see any increased incidence in women or in men between 1951 and 1968 (Vedin *et al*, 1970).

During the most recent years there has been a slight decrease of incidence in women in USA, and an increasing tendency in England and Wales, Scotland and Sweden in the age-group 45 - 54 (years 1969 - 1974), but in Denmark, Finland and the Netherlands the figures have been rather stable. As stated previously it is important not to make too strong conclusions from these statistics because of various uncertainties in data, random fluctuations etc.

In Göteborg we have had a Myocardial Infarction Register since 1968. Exactly the same criteria for diagnosis of MI (non-fatal and fatal) and SD have been used. There has been a marked increase in the number of MIs in the age group 45 - 54 in women (Table 1.1). We have not seen a similar trend for other age groups of women or for men.

Prognosis after myocardial infarction

The immediate mortality from a coronary heart attack is similar in men and women (WHO, 1976). The same applies to the hospital mortality (Table 1.2) and to the long-term mortality as reported by Skall-Jensen (1967). Thus, a woman who has suffered an MI is no longer 'protected' from manifestations of CHD.

Comments

The prevalences and incidences of AP and ST-changes at rest and during exercise are similar in middle-aged women and in men, but MI + SD is considerably more

Table 1.1 Number of myocardial infarctions (MI) in women and the total female population in Göteborg. The Infarct Register in Göteborg

Year	Age			
	35 - 44		45 - 54	
	MI	Total	MI	Total
1968	1	26,430	4	31,964
1969	1	25,573	3	31,391
1970	0	24,699	9	31,285
1971	5	23,895	7	31,003
1972	1	23,172	19	30,030
1973	3	23,522	17	30,333
1974	3	23,155	16	29,477
1975	5	22,654	19	26,902

Table 1.2 Hospital mortality after myocardial infarction by age and sex. The Swedish CCU study. N = 2008   According to Henning & Lundman (1975)

Sex		Age					
		$\leq$39	40-49	50-59	60-69	70-79	80-89
Males Hospital	No	9	126	349	526	351	83
mortality	%	13	10	15	21	37	50
Females Hospital	No	1	11	55	203	212	75
mortality	%	-	27	15	25	43	47

common in men. These and other findings might indicate differences in the aetiology of these various manifestations of CHD. Female sex seems to protect against an acute myocardial catastrophe — MI or SD. The importance of myocardial factors as well as local (myocardial) and systemic catecholamine effects, and the modification of these effects by sex hormones must also be considered.

According to several reports, there is no increasing incidence of MI + SD in women, but according to some reports there has been an increasing incidence during the last decade in young women. An increase is to be expected as smoking is as strong a risk factor in women as in men, and the percentage of female smokers is increasing markedly at least in some countries for example Sweden. Dietary changes, with possible increases of serum lipids, and the effects of oral contraceptives might also influence the incidence of MI.

After an MI the female protection is lost. This seems to imply that other mechanisms are more important at this stage of the disease than before the primary event. This is in accordance with the different risk-factor pattern for a first and a second major CHD event (Wilhelmsen, Wedel and Tibblin, 1973; Vedin, Wilhelmsen, Wedel et al, 1977).

References

Bengtsson, C. (1973) Ischaemic Heart Disease in Women. *Acta Medica Scandinavica Suppl.* **549**:1 - 128.

Epstein, F. (1969) The changing incidence of coronary heart disease. In *Modern Trends in Cardiology*, ed. Jones, A.M. London: Butterworth. Ch.2, pp. 17 - 35.

de Haas, J.H. (1969) *Ischaemic Heart in the Netherlands. Facts and Figures.* Netherlands Heart Foundation, pp. 1 - 32.

Henning, R. & Lundman, T. (1975) The Swedish Co-operative CCU Study. Part I: A description of the early stage. *Acta Medica Scandinavica Suppl.* **586**:27 - 29.

Jaffe, M.D. (1977) Effects of oestrogens on post-exercise electrocardiogram. *British Heart Journal* **38**:1299 - 1303.

Kannel, W.B. & Feinleib, M. (1972) Natural history of angina pectoris in the Framingham Study. Prognosis and survival. *American Journal of Cardiology* **29**:154 - 163.

Oliver, M.F. (1974) Ischaemic heart disease in young women. *British Medical Journal* **II**:253 - 259.

Skall-Jensen, J. (1967) 601 *Myocardie infarcter.* Thesis. Århus, pp. 1 - 228.

Sternby, N.H. (1968) Atherosclerosis in a Defined Population. *Acta Pathologica et Microbiologica Scandinavica, Suppl.* **194**:1 - 216.

Vedin, J.A., Wilhelmsson, C.-E., Bolander, A.-M. & Werkö, L. (1970) Mortality Trends in Sweden 1951 - 1968 with Special Reference to Cardiovascular Causes of Death. *Acta Medica Scandinavica Suppl.* **515**:1 - 76.

Vedin, J.A., Wilhelmsen, L., Wedel, H., Pettersson, B., Wilhelmsson, C.-E., Elmfeldt, D. & Tibblin, G. (1977) Prediction of cardiovascular deaths and reinfarctions after myocardial infarction. *Acta Medica Scandinavica* **201**:309 - 316.

Vedin, J.A. & Bengtsson, C. *Value of exercise testing in a randomised population of women.* To be published.

Wilhelmsen, L., Wedel, H. & Tibblin, G. (1973) Multivariate analysis of risk factors for coronary heart disease in men aged 50 years in Göteborg, Sweden. *Circulation* **48**:950 - 958.

Wilhelmsen, L., Bjure, J., Ekström-Jodal, B., Aurell, M., Grimby, G. & Tibblin, G. *Value of exercise testing in predicting coronary heart disease.* The Study of Men Born in 1913. To be published.

World Health Organisation (1976) *Myocardial Infarction Community Registers.* WHO, Copenhagen, pp. 1 - 232.

Discussion 1A

Gresham (Cambridge) Can you account for the difference in the way CHD presents in women as compared to men?

Wilhelmsen It is possible that in the female the myocardial cell will tolerate more ischaemia than in the male, and in favour of this view, work recently reported from Japan, oestrogens reduce the metabolic activity of certain cells in the arterial wall when provoked, for example, by catecholamines. There may also be a better development of a collateral circulation in the female than in the male.

Singh (Birmingham)   What were your diagnostic criteria for angina?

Wilhelmsen   We used the London School of Hygiene questionnaire.

Rose (London)   You postulated a 'protective factor' in women to account for the apparent difference in incidence of CHD in men and women. Why do you assume that rather than an aggravating factor in men?

Wilhelmsen   The conservative approach is to postulate 'protective factors' but I quite agree that it could equally well be 'aggravating factors'. We have some animal data to suggest that male sex hormones might be aggravating factors.

Mitchell (Nottingham)   I would like to give some support to the comments you were making about pathological differences in the development of atheroma between the sexes. Schwartz and I studied several years ago 600/700 aortas and other great vessels in a widely based necropsy series, so we were able to take account of the problem of differential causes of death. Males had a 15 year lead over women in the development of atheromatous plaques in coronaries, carotids and aortas, whether calcification or ulceration was the index. This may not apply to individuals but for groups there is a 10-15 year difference between the two sexes.

Spain (Brooklyn)   In one of your charts you showed almost no angina pectoris in older men. The older age group was nearly entirely composed of women.

Wilhelmsen   We did not study men at the higher ages.

Spain (Brooklyn)   We should surely consider the survival of the fittest factor. Men having had their coronary artery disease earlier and longer and more severely would have died off with myocardial infarction or sudden death. This would tend to accentuate the proportion of women with angina pectoris in older populations. We studied atherosclerosis in every single accidental automobile and industrial death in a selected population for a 10 year period eliminating natural factors of disease, such as neoplasia. We found in every age group, considerable excess in the extent of atherosclerosis in the coronary arteries of men as opposed to women. The interesting thing was that this discrepancy between the two sexes was not as apparent in the aorta. This discrepancy has been borne out by similar autopsy studies in Sweden. In retrospective studies, we have reviewed autopsy material and the extent of coronary atherosclerosis in both males and females, trying to work back from our findings as to whether the patients had angina pectoris, with or without myocardial infarction, myocardial infarction alone, or sudden death. It was impossible to do this based upon the patterns of atherosclerosis in the coronary arteries.

Marquis (Edinburgh) With regard to the incidence or changing incidence of ischaemic heart disease in women, it is an interesting fact that in Scotland there has been no increase in instances of ischaemic heart disease in women undergoing pregnancy, for example, in the Simpson Maternity Pavilion. This also applies to the confidential reports on maternal mortality for England and Wales. There are, however, two other factors operative during the same 25 year period; first, there has been a tendency to have children younger and, second, families have tended to be smaller.

Wilhelmsen We should look upon angina pectoris as one part of the disease — myocardial infarction and sudden death as other parts of it — and not mix them together.

Oliver (Edinburgh) It should be remembered that changes in mortality rates observed in North America may have a completely different connotation to those which we see in Europe and certain European countries. The very striking and interesting fall in mortality rate in men in North America during the course of the last 8 years, which women also seem to be sharing, is not true here. There is an opposite picture, certainly in Scotland and to a lesser extent, in England and Wales, and several other countries in the Scandinavian areas. There is no clear explanation as to why we have three times the mortality rate in Scotland compared with Southern England. But if one can get a 3 to 1 gradient across a small island like this, then one must be extremely cautious in interpreting international secular changes.

2. Coronary heart disease in young women—
incidence and epidemiology

T. GORDON

Abstract

Under age 50 coronary heart disease is not only much less common in women than men but is more likely to be mild. Judging from the Framingham Study, CHD occurs in premenopausal women at about 1/3 the rate for menopausal women of the same age. In the age range 45-49 the bulk of CHD occurs in postmenopausal women. If surgical menopause is common in a population, a large part of CHD before age 45 may also come from postmenopausal women.

The protective factor − perhaps hormonal − found in menstruating women is further enhanced in early adult life by low levels of blood pressure and of cholesterol plasma in low and very low density lipoproteins. Furthermore, men have much lower levels of high density lipoproteins than women, a fact which puts them at greater risk. This protection can be overridden by other factors. Black women in the United States, who have a very high prevalence of hypertension, have much higher CHD death rates than white women. This is to be expected, since the usual CHD risk factors − blood pressure, blood lipids, glucose intolerance and cigarette smoking − seem to impinge on young women in the same way they do in young men.

Incidence and epidemiology

The chief feature about coronary heart disease (CHD) in young women is its rarity. In the Framingham Study not a single case of CHD arose in the age group 30-39, despite 6,726 person-years experience. Not until age 45-49 was there a respectable number of cases available for analysis (Table 2.1). The Göteberg study also reports a very low incidence òf CHD for women under age 50 (Bengtsson, 1973).

Table 2.1 Incidence of CHD in persons under age 50. Framingham Study, 20-year followup (Rate/1,000/year)

	WOMEN		MEN
	Premenopausal	Menopausal	
30 - 39	none	none	2.3(11)
40 - 44	0.2(1)	3.6(5)	5.3(29)
45 - 49	1.1(5)*	2.9(11)	7.2(51)

Parenthetical entries are the number of cases.

*One woman had a CHD event in the same interval that her menopause occurred. If that event is omitted the rate is 0.9. If it is added to the menopausal group their rate is 3.2.

If we consider only premenopausal women, the incidence of CHD is very low indeed. In the Framingham Study only one CHD case occurred in premenopausal women aged 40-44, despite 4,922 person-years experience (Kannel *et al*, 1976). In the age group 45-49, where experience is divided about equally between premenopausal and menopausal women, there were a third as many cases among premenopausal as menopausal women. Menopausal women, themselves, had a CHD incidence rate half that for men of the same age.

These facts have two important corollaries. The first is that we have precious little epidemiological information about CHD in premenopausal women. While we have reason to attribute a very low CHD incidence rate to this group, we do not have reliable estimates of the factors involved in that incidence. The second is that routine vital statistics data for CHD in young women, even very young women, probably do not reflect events in the premenopausal state as much as in the postmenopausal state. The extent to which this is true under age 45 will, of course, vary with the frequency of surgical menopause, since relatively few women have a natural menopause before age 45.

If we are in difficulties studying the relation of menopause to CHD at ages under 45 because of the paucity of CHD in premenopausal women we are in even more difficulties with women over age 45 because of the problem of dating a natural menopause. This problem is especially difficult when a fatal coronary event occurs to a woman who was still menstruating (or at least had not definitely stopped) when she was last interviewed. It is compounded when the interview occurs only every two years and, to be sure that menopause has definitely occurred, the requirement is made (as it was in the Framingham Study) that the woman should not have menstruated for a full year before the time of the interview for **her** to be considered menopausal. With such a rule we can be almost sure that a CHD event was post-menopausal but we cannot be sure it was premenopausal. The one exception, of course, is for surgical menopause, which is precisely dated.

More than half of the CHD cases under age 50 (16/27) presented in Framingham women as angina pectoris without any more severe manifestation of CHD. Thus, statistics on mortality or hospital admissions, to the degree that they are diagnostically accurate, will understate the incidence of total CHD in this group quite markedly. The understatement is much less for men. Less than a fourth of the CHD (21/91) occurring in Framingham men under age 50 presented solely as angina pectoris. It follows that the mortality sex ratio will tend to be greater than the incidence sex ratio for CHD. Another way of looking at this is to say that CHD tends to present in a milder form in young women than young men.

As stated, these conclusions presuppose reasonable diagnostic accuracy. It is always possible that a history of chest pain may be incorrectly evaluated as AP; that is, as due to CHD; and there is a feeling that this is more likely to occur in women than men. The Framingham experience does not bear this out. The risk of death or myocardial infarction (MI) in five years for persons with AP is, respectively, two times and four times that for persons without AP – equally for men and women. Furthermore, risk factors like hypertension and hypercholesterolaemia are as strongly associated, prospectively, with AP as with fully documented MI. Hence we feel comfortable treating the AP diagnosis as good evidence of underlying CHD.

Can we explain the relatively low CHD incidence in young women? Up to a point we can. What limits us from making quantitatively exact statements is the paucity of information not only for young women but also for young men.

So far as we can tell from the limited Framingham experience blood pressure, serum cholesterol, glucose intolerance and cigarette smoking are CHD risk factors of similar importance for young women as for young men; that is, they have logistic regression coefficients at least as large for women as for men (Table 2.2). However the level of all these characteristics is lower in women than men under age 45 (Table 2.3). Lower levels in women under age 45 would presumably correspond to a lower CHD risk at that age. Furthermore, if we assume that risk factors operate over time and that atherosclerosis is a response to a lifetime atherogenic dose, the lower levels in young women would continue to lead to lower risk at older ages, even after the risk factor levels have risen.

For example, at age 45-49 the average systolic blood pressure is the same in women as in men. From age 30 to age 44, however, it is much lower. We would therefore expect that risk for women at a given level of blood pressure at age 45-49 would in fact tend to be less than in men having the same blood pressure because it really correlates with a previous experience at a lower level. Unfortunately we cannot quantify this opinion.

Table 2.2   Standardised multivariate logistic regression coefficients for CHD in men and women aged 40-49 Framingham Study, 20-year followup

Characteristics	Men	Women
Age	0.237*	0.244
Systolic blood pressure	0.194*	0.307*
Serum cholesterol	0.371***	0.282***
Cigarette smoking	0.272**	0.363**
Number of CHD cases	78	22

*p <.05   **p <.01   ***p <.001
Note: Data insufficient for reliable estimates of coefficients for glucose intolerance.

Of the usual risk factors only one seems to be affected directly by the menopause (Hjortland et al, 1976). Blood cholesterol, particularly that portion in the low and very low density lipoproteins, rises abruptly with the menopause. There is even some suggestion from the Framingham Study that until that rise occurs total cholesterol is not predictive of CHD in young women. While this needs corroboration, it is logical since prior to the menopause the protective, or high density lipoprotein (HDL), portion of total cholesterol is relatively larger than it is after the menopause (Kannel et al, 1976).

It is possible, of course, for historical shifts to occur in all the various risk characteristics and such shifts ought to affect CHD risk. Cigarette smoking is of particular interest. In the United States, the proportion of young women smoking is greater these days than heretofore (Green and Nemzer, 1973). That should have an impact on the incidence of CHD (other than uncomplicated angina), tending to raise the relatively low CHD mortality in women as compared to that for men.

What other factors may account for the relatively low CHD incidence in young

Table 2.3 Average of some CHD risk characteristics in young men and women Framingham Study, Exam 2

Characteristic*	30 - 34 M	30 - 34 W	35 - 39 M	35 - 39 W	40 - 44 M	40 - 44 W	45 - 49 M	45 - 49 W
Systolic blood pressure (mmHg)	125.2	116.7	127.6	119.6	131.1	125.6	130.9	133.9
Diastolic blood pressure (mmHg)	79.3	73.5	81.6	76.0	84.0	79.7	84.2	83.2
Serum cholesterol (mg/dl)	218.0	198.0	223.8	204.8	228.6	219.2	229.7	230.4
Relative weight (%)	119.6	109.2	119.0	114.3	119.6	117.4	119.3	122.0
Cigarette smokers (%)	66.8	56.7	74.4	54.7	68.8	46.8	62.4	30.8
Diabetes (%)	0.6	1.0	0.9	0.4	1.4	0.8	3.2	1.6
S_f 0-20 lipoprotein (Svedberg)	402.7	246.4	405.0	374.2	424.4	421.6	437.9	432.0
S_f 20-400 lipoprotein (Svedberg)	179.8	85.2	178.0	97.8	204.1	113.3	193.1	134.6

* Except for data on lipoproteins (which were previously unpublished), all mean values may be found in Gordon T, Shurtleff D: Means at each examination and inter-examination variation of specified characteristics: Framingham Study, Exam 1 to Exam 10. (In Kannel W.B., Gordon T. (eds): *The Framingham Study*: Section 29). DHEW Pub. No. (NIH) 74-478, 1973. U.S. Gov't Printing Office, Washington, D.C. 20402.

women? We know of two. One is the much higher level of HDL cholesterol in women — in the age range 40-49 a level of 59 mg/dl as against a level of 45 mg/dl for men — a difference that may be associated with a differential CHD risk for men of nearly 2:1. The other is some protective factor — perhaps hormonal — found in menstruating women and lost with the menopause, surgical or natural. At age 40-44, where most menopause is surgically induced, the risk of CHD in menopausal Framingham women was three times that for premenopausal women. While this contrast is statistically significant, numbers of cases are quite small and we cannot closely bound the exact ratio.

Thus, the usual finding of a much lower CHD incidence in young women than young men is partly explicable on the basis of a few well-defined characteristics that distinguish the two sexes. On the other hand, there is scant explanation for the much higher proportion of more severe forms of CHD in men 40-49 relative to women, even postmenopausal women, of the same age. Furthermore, even after age 50 the CHD incidence rate in Framingham men remains 60 percent higher than that of women, even at comparable levels of HDL cholesterol and the proportion of more severe manifestations of CHD also remains higher in men. Moreover, it is equally conceivable that the gap can be narrowed by an alteration of these characteristics; for example, by an increased amount of cigarette smoking in young women. Whether for that reason, or some other, the male/female sex ratio for CHD mortality at age 35-44 in the U.S. white population decreased from 5.88 in 1965 to 5.23 in 1975.

That the relative immunity of young women is not immutable can be seen in the data for black women in the United States. In 1960-62 the prevalence of definite or suspect CHD at age 35-44 was 1.9 per cent for black women (almost the same as that for white men at that age). It was 0.9 per cent for white women (Gordon, 1964). U.S. death rates in 1975 for ischemic heart disease were 39.3 per 100,000 and 12.8 per 100,000, respectively, for black women and white women in this age group (Table 2.4). This ratio of 3 to 1 is less than the ratio of 3.6 to 1 reported for 1958, but not dramatically less. The comparable death rate for white men was 66.9/100,000-70 percent greater than for black women. Kuller in a careful study of deaths in Baltimore concluded that black women definitely had much higher arteriosclerotic heart disease death rates than white women (Kuller and Lilienfeld, 1966). Total mortality is also much greater; at age 35-44 the all-causes death rate in 1975 for black women was double that for white women.

Good epidemiological evidence relevant to this issue is hard to find but two facts are quite clear: Black women are much fatter and have much more hypertension than white women. In the age range 20-44, 29.2 percent of the black women were obese according to a national survey done in 1971-72, while only 18.9 of the white women were obese (Abraham *et al*, 1975). Moreover the 1960-62 U.S. Health Examination Survey found that 25.7 percent of black women aged 35-44 were definitely hypertensive, four times the rate for white women (Gordon, 1966). (Black men also had a higher prevalence rate for hypertension but were leaner than white men). On the other hand, the serum cholesterol level of black Southern women was the same as that for white women in the age group 35-44 (Moore and Gordon, 1967).

Table 2.4 Annual death rates for CHD by age and colour for young women United States, 1958-1975 (Rates per 100.000 population)

Age	1958	1959	1960	1961	1962	1963	1964	1965	1966	1967
					White					
25-34	2.2	2.2	1.9	1.8	2.2	2.4	2.1	2.1	2.0	2.0
35-44	12.7	12.6	12.7	12.4	13.1	14.7	13.6	13.9	14.1	14.3
45-54	64.2	63.7	61.9	64.2	65.9	65.8	66.7	66.8	66.7	65.2
					Non-white					
25-34	12.2	8.8	9.3	8.2	8.6	10.1	9.8	8.6	9.5	10.7
35-44	46.4	43.6	46.7	42.5	45.7	47.8	47.0	48.3	46.3	47.7
45-54	181.5	171.6	168.0	160.4	161.7	165.4	166.8	162.1	158.8	158.2

Age	1968	1969	1970	1971	1972	1973	1974	1975
				White				
25-34	2.2	1.9	2.2	2.1	1.7	1.9	1.7	1.4
35-44	16.3	16.1	15.1	15.5	15.2	14.6	13.1	12.8
45-54	72.8	69.8	70.0	69.5	65.5	65.8	65.8	60.7
				Non-white				
25-34	10.5	9.8	9.6	8.5	6.9	6.1	6.5	5.1
35-44	68.6	62.5	58.9	56.3	55.7	51.3	44.4	39.3
45-54	222.9	208.1	203.0	193.3	187.0	185.8	171.7	150.5

Note: For 1958-67 the 7th revision ICD classification was used (420-422). For 1968-75 the 8th revision ICD classification was used (410-413). The two classifications are not strictly comparable. Moreover 1968 was a year of exceptionally high mortality due to a flu epidemic. Data from Vital Statistics of the United States for the specified years.

B

Table 2.5 Annual death rates for CHD for women aged 35-44. Selected countries, 1958-1973 (Rates per 100,000 population)

	1958	1959	1960	1961	1962	1963	1964	1965	1966	1967
England & Wales	7.5	7.3	7.6	8.0	8.6	9.0	9.6	10.9	9.6	10.0
Scotland	18.5	15.8	15.2	13.5	14.9	18.5	17.6	16.9	17.0	19.7
Germany (FR)	15.1	15.4	15.9	15.2	15.8	16.8	15.2	15.5	15.9	14.2
Norway	5.0	3.5	2.7	5.1	4.4	5.3	7.0	5.0	4.8	4.4
Sweden	6.9	*	5.1	4.0	4.4	4.4	3.7	5.5	6.1	4.2
United States (white)	12.7	12.6	12.7	12.4	13.1	14.7	13.6	13.9	14.4	14.3

	1968	1969	1970	1971	1972	1973
England & Wales	10.7	10.9	10.1	9.4	10.1	10.6
Scotland	15.3	13.3	18.4	19.2	19.4	15.3
Germany (FR)	*	5.8	6.0	5.4	6.0	5.8
Norway	*	6.1	3.4	6.4	7.0	5.6
Sweden	*	5.2	4.4	4.2	3.1	3.8
United States (white)	16.3	16.1	15.1	15.5	15.2	14.6

See footnote to Table 2.4. Data from World Health Statistics Annual (Vol. 1) for specified years.
* Not available.

What are the trends in CHD incidence for young women? For this we must turn to routine vital statistics, suspect though they may be (Table 2.5). For England and Wales there was a rise in mortality from arteriosclerotic heart disease for women aged 35-44 from 7.5/100,000 in 1958 to 10.0/100,000 in 1967 (Oliver, 1974). Since 1968 there has been little change. Similar trends were not noted for other young age groups.

The trend in England and Wales does not seem to be duplicated elsewhere. Mortality for women 35-44 in other countries — at least those I've looked at — have held pretty steady during this decade. In Scotland — just to add a touch of local colour — only slight fluctuations were observed between 1958 and 1967 for the same age group. There was a slight rise in the United States among white women but during the following decade there was an even greater fall. There is little to distinguish the recent CHD mortality trends for young women from those of young men.

To conclude: young women have very low CHD incidence and mortality. This appears to be partly 'explicable' by known epidemiological evidence but much remains still to be explained. If any recent deterioration in their favoured status has occurred it is difficult to see it in available data.

References

Abraham, S., Lowenstein F.W., O'Connell, D.E. (1975) Preliminary findings of the first Health and Nutrition Survey: United States, 1971-72. *Anthropometric and clinical findings.* DHEW Publication Number (HRA) 75-1229. Washington, D.C.

Bengtsson, C. (1973) Ischemic heart disease in women. *Acta Medica Scandinavica,* Suppl. No. **549**, 1973.

Gordon, T. (1964) Heart disease in adults: United States, 1960-1962. *Public Health Service Publication* Number 1000-Series 11 — No.6. Washington, D.C.

Gordon, T., Devine, B. (1966) Hypertension and hypertensive heart disease in adults: United States, 1960-1962. *Public Health Service Publication* Number 1000-Series — No.10. Washington, D.C.

Green, D.E., Nemzer, D.E. (1973) Changes in cigarette smoking by women — an analysis, 1966 and 1970. *Health Services Reports,* **88**, 631-636.

Hjortland, M.C., McNamara, P.M., Kannel, W.B. (1976) Some atherogenic concomitants of menopause: The Framingham Study. *American Journal of Epidemiology,* **103**, 304-311.

Kannel, W.B., Hjortland, M.C., McNamara, P.M., Gordon, T. (1976) Menopause and risk of cardiovascular disease. *Annals of Internal Medicine,* **85**, 447-452.

Kuller, L., Lilienfeld, A. (1966) Epidemiological study of sudden and unexpected deaths due to arteriosclerotic heart disease. *Circulation,* **34**, 1056-1068.

Moore, F.E., Gordon, T. (1967) Serum cholesterol levels in adults. United States, 1960-1962. *Public Health Service Publication* Number 1000-Series 11-No.22. Washington, D.C.

Oliver, M.F. (1974) Ischemic heart disease in young women. *British Medical Journal,* **74**, 253-259.

Discussion 1B

Somerville (London)   Did I understand you to say that there was no clinical coronary heart disease in women aged 30-39 years?

Gordon   Yes

Somerville (London)   How can this possibly be? This cuts clean across what other people have said to me. Wilhelmsen has already shown the actual incidence in this age group.

Gordon   I do not imply that there is no risk in these age groups. It simply means that the incidence is very low in our experience, which, as I say, was 7000 person/years. There was no case of coronary heart disease — that would imply that the incidence is very low.

Spain (Brooklyn)   Did you use cigarette smoking in your statistics as a risk factor in coronary heart disease?

Gordon   Yes.

Spain (Brooklyn)   There are many causes of myocardial ischaemia besides having coronary atherosclerosis. Cigarette smoking may act through a multifactorial basis. There are a number of factors which act at different points in the manifestation of what we call coronary heart disease.

Gordon   Our data suggests that cigarette smoking is a weak factor, if at all, in the generation of angina pectoris. It is fairly strongly associated with the incidence of myocardial infarction and coronary heart disease death both in men and women.

Spain (Brooklyn)   I am also surprised at this lack of clinical coronary heart disease in women under the age of 39. I know in our studies of consecutive autopsies of every single sudden death in a population group of about 800,000 in Westchester County, there were a small number of women in this age group with CHD, although the ratio was 10/1 men to women.

Gordon   When there is a very low incidence, it is not improbable that there will be no cases at all unless a very large series of people are studied. While we had 6/7,000 person/year experience to record, that is not large enough when the incidence rate is very low. I just have to reiterate that there is a very low incidence disease in women under 40. The fact that we had no cases at all does not mean that such cases do not occur in the general population. It means that it is a very rare phenomenon.

Spain (Brooklyn) We did not find any differential in sudden deaths from coronary heart disease in black women as opposed to males. In fact, it was higher in black women and this has been attributed, I think, to greater elevation of blood pressure.

Hazzard (Seattle) It seems that there may be a differential sensitivity to angina pectoris at a given level of coronary atherosclerosis in males versus females. Does anybody know whether or not this differential in sensitivity in angina pectoris has been documented or investigations performed on a more basic level? Are women more sensitive to angina pectoris? Are they more likely to volunteer a positive answer on a questionnaire than men? Do women acknowledge pain more readily than men? What are we really dealing with here?

Wilhelmsen (Göteborg) There are population studies we have performed in Göteborg where I really think that women tend to answer more positively to questionnaires than men. As women do not suffer sudden death from myocardial infarction as often as men, ST changes on their exercise ECG's are often considered non-specific. This is probably wrong, and it might be that they are 'protected' against these ST changes.

Baird (Edinburgh) I think the word 'young' is being used totally at random in this population. I would suggest that we actually abandon the use of the word 'young' and define the ages in terms of pre-menarchal, reproductive or post-menopausal, or in terms of the actual ages quoted, that is the age groups 30-40 or 40-50.

Oliver (Edinburgh) Some years ago we made two studies of the relationship of a premature menopause to the premature development of coronary heart disease. What we did was to make a carefully controlled study of a group of women under the age of 35 who had had a bilateral oophorectomy and we compared these with a group of women of similar age who had had a unilateral oophorectomy but who continued to have periods. The second study, some years later was on a group of women who stopped menstruating spontaneously under the age of 35. The incidence of coronary heart disease increased after 15 years had elapsed. There was no higher mortality rate or incidence rate 5 years after a premature menopause. By 10 years there was a slight increase and by 15 years it was significant. This fits with what we know to be taking place around the normal menopause and with the high mortality rate that you have described at the age of 64. This is some 15 years after the expected age of the menopause.

Gordon Our experience is almost exactly the opposite in that soon after a surgical menopause there is an apparent increase in incidence of coronary heart disease. On the other hand, retrospectively analysis of older women did not show any association between the age of menopause and coronary heart disease incidence.

Lichtlen (Hannover)   I think one must be careful in defining angina in these women, because many studies have shown that a proportion of them have normal coronary arteries. It is known that many of these women have coronary artery spasm and I think the concept of spasm in provoking angina must probably be accepted today.

Wilhelmsen (Göteborg)   I think you are completely right, but you also have this type of angina in men. We are just performing a study on a random population sample of men with angina pectoris and there are many of them who have completely normal coronary arteries. We are left with the problem of defining angina pectoris either from the clinical viewpoint, by exercise testing, or by coronary angiography saying that only coronary arteriosclerosis is indicative of the disease.

Jarrett (London)   We should take into account that many women, post ovariectomy, are given hormone replacement therapy. My second point is whether the menopause is getting later in Western populations as this may possibly affect coronary heart disease deaths.

Gordon   The age of the natural menopause appears to be pretty close to a biological constant. There is one series which correlates age of menarche with age of menopause and they found no association at all.

Nordin (Leeds)   You are dealing with very small numbers of those with CHD, I think one case in the pre-menopausal group and 5 cases in the post-menopausal group of the same age. I doubt if there is any statistical significance, and I think you are basing rather a lot on those 1 and 5 cases. As far as the definition of the menopause is concerned, you said you had to allow a significant amount of time to elapse from the last period before you were certain, but you didn't define the amount of time. You really cannot be certain until 2 years have elapsed that the patient really is through the menopause in the sense that she has had her last menstrual period and has the associated hormonal changes.

Gordon   The difference was significant, as I remember in the youngest age group at a level of .001. The women were seen every two years and a history obtained. If she had not menstruated in the last year, she was considered to be post-menopausal. The date, therefore, was set back to the time of the last reported menstruation.

Beaumont (Paris)   Concerning surgical menopause and the problem of replacement therapy, was it taken into account what type of oestrogen was used?

Gordon   It was taken into account, but it was not a factor.

Doll (Oxford)   The lowest age of entry into the population in Mr Gordon's study was about 30. Thus, all observations in women aged 30-39 were finished by 1958. This refers to events that took place between 1948 and 1958, when incidences may be slightly different to what they are now. This is one point.

The second point refers to the relative incidence in post-menopausal and pre-menopausal women in an age group of 40-44 years when you have some proportion of both sorts of women. Now, this is a tricky statistical point that first came to my attention when comparing mortality rates in married and unmarried women ages 15-19 and finding that the mortality rate was higher in the married than the unmarried because the proportion of married and unmarried aged 15-19 changes quite dramatically as you go from 15 to 19, and so, the mortality rate rises. The same is happening with the menopause at ages 40-44. The post-menopausal women in that age group will be concentrated in the 43 and 44 year-olds and the pre-menopausal women will be in relatively higher proportion in the 40 to 42 ages. As the incidence of coronary heart disease rises very rapidly over those age groups, you will get a higher incidence as a statistical artefact in post-menopausal women than in pre-menopausal women in those ages. I am not wanting to suggest that is the whole explanation, but it is a point that needs to be borne in mind when we talk about pre and post-menopausal women in a particular age group where the menopause is actually occurring.

Gordon   It ought to be pointed out that the CHD incidence in post-menopausal women in each of these age groups, whatever the probabilities associated with them, is greater than the incidence in pre-menopausal women. In the oldest age group in our studies some of the women cited as pre-menopausal and were, in fact, post-menopausal.

3. Genetic influences on coronary heart disease in young women

JOAN SLACK

Risks in the population

Differences in risk of coronary death in men and women

The Registrar General's statistics for England and Wales (1973) show that the risks of coronary death are greater for men than for women throughout the whole life span, and the difference has been consistent at least since 1932.

Figure 3.1 (a) shows the difference in coronary mortality rates in men and women Registered in England and Wales in 1973 under the International Classificatic 410. The risks to men are greater than the risks to women at all ages, and there is no sudden change after the menopause. If the wider classification of arteriosclerotic heart disease is used in order to include any possible misclassified deaths, the same pattern holds good.

Figure 3.1 (b) shows the male/female ratio of coronary mortality at different ages in 1973. At the present time there is a nearly 6-fold increase of coronary deaths among men under 55 years, compared with women at the same age with 10,764 men and 1,958 women under 55 registered as coronary deaths in England and Wales in 1973.

There are, of course, still some differences in life style between men and women which might account for a difference in coronary risk, but the main unarguable difference between the sexes is a genetic one, and in order to test whether genetic differences make any contribution to the variation in coronary risk we must turn to twin studies.

Inheritance of liability

Evidence for genetic contribution to liability to coronary heart disease

The Danish twin study, Harvald and Hauge (1970), showed that there is a greater similarity for coronary heart disease among monozygotic than among dizygotic twins.

Among like-sex twins there was a significant difference in concordance rates between monozygotic and dizygotic twins.

Among unlike-sex, dizygotic twins there was an indication that the risks were greater to the male twins when the female was the index patient, (see Table 3.1). These findings confirm the idea that genetic factors do contribute to the liability to coronary heart disease, and suggest that the genetic contribution may be greater in women than in men.

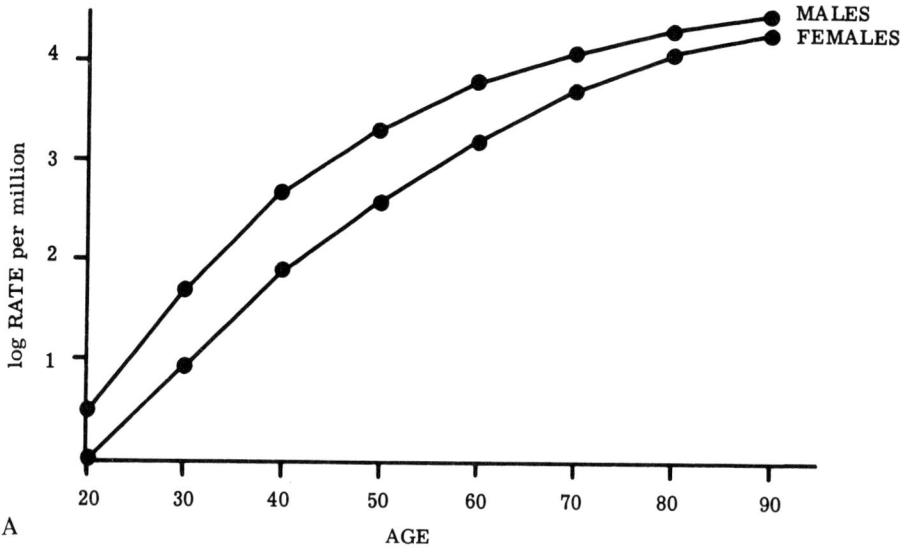

A

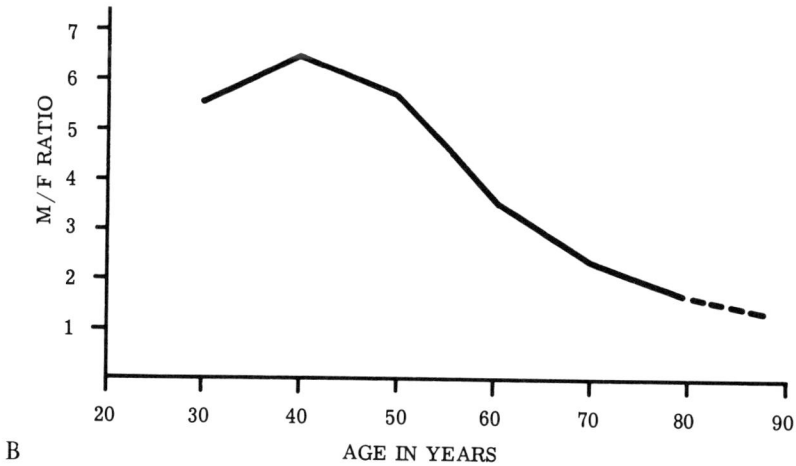

B

Fig. 3.1 (a) Deaths from acute myocardial infarction in England and Wales.
Classification 410. Registrar General 1973.
        (b) Male/female ratio of deaths from acute myocardial infarction.
Registrar General's statistics, England and Wales, 1973. Classification 410.

B*

Table 3.1   Concordance rates for coronary heart disease in twins

Sex	Zygosity	Concordance rate Numbers		Significance of difference in concordance rate
♂ ♂	MZ	30/77	0.39	p = <0.05
	DZ	32/122	0.26	
♀ ♀	MZ	12/27	0.44	p = <0.01
	DZ	8/54	0.14	
♂ ♀	DZ♂ probands	7/53	0.13	
	DZ♀ probands	8/19	0.43	

Model for inheritance of liability to coronary heart disease

Clearly the condition is not sex linked in any simple Mendelian fashion, but a model for a multifactorial condition which included polygenic inheritance will account for the variation between sexes as well as accounting for a sensitive response to environmental change.

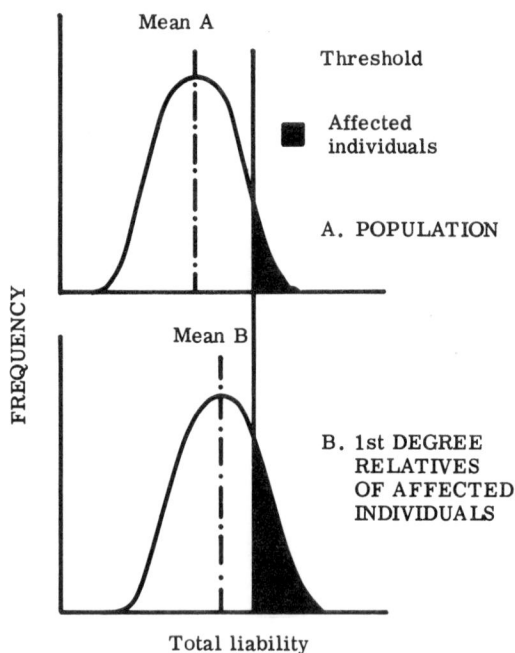

Fig. 3.2   Falconer's model for polygenic inheritance of liabilitv to disease.

A simple diagram based on Falconer's model for polygenic inheritance is shown in Fig. 3.2 (Falconer, 1965). Along the horizontal axis are increasing increments of liability to early coronary death which includes all the environmental as well as the genetic factors contributing to the condition. It is assumed that there is a normal distribution of total liability — this is shown in the upper part of the diagram with a mean marked at **A**. There is a threshold for liability beyond which all are affected. For coronary death this can be drawn accurately for either sex and at any age, since the death rate is known. If there is random mating for coronary heart disease, no significant dominant inheritance and no epistasis and if the liability to coronary death were entirely genetically determined, first degree relatives of coronary patients (having half their genes in common), would have a mean liability to coronary death mid-way between the mean of the index patients' and the mean in the general population. This is shown at B in the lower part of the diagram. The liability in first degree relatives would be normally distributed about that mean, and consequently there is an increased number of relatives beyond the threshold for coronary death. It follows from this model that if coronary death in the population is rarer in women than in men, the female threshold will be further to the right of the distribution and the shift of the distribution of liability in the relatives of female patients, and as we saw in the Danish twin study, a specially high risk among the male relatives of the female patients.

Any change in environment, either increasing or decreasing liability will cause a shift of the whole distribution, and because of the shape of the Gaussian curve, this will cause a substantial difference in the number appearing above or below the threshold. The discrepancy between the observed number of affected first degree relatives and the expected number represents the extent of the environmental contribution to the total variation in liability. The proportion of the total variation contributed by genetic factors is called the heritability.

Risks of coronary death in first degree relatives of coronary patients

Family studies of first degree relatives can be used to make a quantitative estimate of the proportion of the genetic to the environmental contribution to the total liability.

Table 3.2 Increased risk of early coronary death in first degree relatives of index patients with coronary heart disease under 55 years. (Slack and Evans, 1966).

	Male patients under 55
Male relatives under 55	5.16 ***
Female relatives under 65	2.75
	Female patients under 55
Male relatives under 55	9.01 ***
Female relatives under 65	4.62 **

sig. ** = $p < 0.01 > 0.001$.   *** = $p < 0.001$.

In a comparison of the risks of coronary death to the first degree relatives of the male and female coronary patients under 55 years of age, Slack and Evans (1966) found that there was an increased risk of coronary death in the male relatives under 55, and the female relatives under 65 years of age.

Heritability of early coronary death in men and women

If Falconer's model is used to estimate the heritability of early coronary death from these observations it seems that genetic factors may be contributing as much as 60 per cent of the total liability to early coronary death in men and as much as 80 per cent in women. Common family environment could be causing an over-estimate in these family studies, but its contribution is likely to be small in a condition which occurs at an age when families have usually split up for some length of time.

Inheritance of risk factors

So far we have only considered the total liability to early coronary death, assuming this liability to be continuously distributed. The liability includes risk factors such as smoking habits, serum cholesterol concentration and blood pressure as well as other less well known risk factors contributing to the total liability and the genetic contribution to this liability is by definition polygenic. Dominantly inherited risk factors such as monogenically determined Familial Hypercholesterolaemia have been specifically excluded from the polygenic model and must be discussed separately.

Smoking habits

There is probably little useful known about the influences of genetics or common family environment upon smoking habits, but there have been several substantial family studies of blood pressure and of serum cholesterol levels from which some conclusions can be drawn about the genetic contributions to the variations observed in the population.

In order to establish whether genetic factors play any part at all it is necessary to look at the available twin studies.

Heritability of blood pressure

Table 3.3 shows the results of using Falconer's model and Charles Smith's method (personal communication) to calculate standard errors of heritability of blood pressure from Percy Stocks (1930) study of Welsh twins.

Table 3.3 Heritability of systolic blood pressure from Welsh twin study from Percy Stocks (1930)

	% Heritability $\pm$ 1 standard error
r_{MZ}	69 $\pm$ 5
$2r_{DZ}$	64 $\pm$ 20
$2(r_{MZ} - r_{DZ})$	74 $\pm$ 22.4

Among monozygotic twins Stock found a correlation for systolic blood pressure of 0.69, suggesting that 69 per cent of the variation in blood pressure observed in the Welsh twins was genetic. This calculation has a small standard error but makes no attempt to exclude common family environment. Dizygotic twins showed a correlation of 0.32 giving an estimated heritability of 64 per cent. The last estimate which is used in order to minimize the effects of common family environment gives an estimated heritability for blood pressure of 74 per cent. This estimate has a large standard error, but by comparison with the other 2 estimates suggests that common family environment plays little part in causing family resemblances in blood pressure. A little more information can be obtained by studying resemblances in first degree relatives of different generations and different sexes. Table 3.4 shows the result of Miall's family studies of blood pressure.

Table 3.4 Parent/child correlations for age adjusted systolic blood pressure (Miall *et al* (1967))

	n	r
Father/son	132	0.14
Father/daughter	137	0.22
Mother/son	129	0.20
Mother/daughter	140	0.41
Spouse	130	0.009

There was no significant correlation between man and wife, the correlation between father and son were negligible and the highest correlation was observed between mother and daughter.

For blood pressure estimates suggest that heritability is in the region of 70 per cent with little contribution from common family environment.

Heritability of serum cholesterol concentration

Table 3.5 shows the estimate of heritability calculated from Pikkarainen's study of male Finnish twins.

Table 3.5 Heritability of serum cholesterol from Finnish Twin study calculated from Pikkarainen (1966)

	% Heritability $\pm$ 1 standard error
r_{MZ}	56 ± 9
$2r_{DZ}$	74 ± 24
$2(r_{MZ} - r_{DZ})$	38 ± 30

The estimate of heritability from the difference observed between monozygotic and dizygotic twins was less than direct estimates from the observed correlations indicating that for serum cholesterol concentration common family environment may play a more important part in determining family likeness than for blood pressure.

Table 3.6 shows the results of Adlersberg's study of serum cholesterol concentrations.

Table 3.6   Parent/child correlations for age adjusted serum cholesterol concentration

	n	r
Father/son	181	0.16
Father/daughter	192	0.26
Mother/son	181	0.34
Mother/daughter	192	0.39
Spouse	201	0.006

There was no significant correlation between husband and wife and as for the family similarities for blood pressure the highest correlation was observed between mother and child. Perhaps the best explanation for the differences and similarities between the inheritance of blood pressure and cholesterol is that intrafamilial correlations in blood depend upon the inheritance of characteristics that are modified by sex while family similarities in cholesterol concentration are more dependent upon common family environment with mother sharing more meals with her children than the father. Whatever the explanation for the differences it seems that for these 2 risk factors the mother has greater similarities to her offspring than the father. For serum cholesterol estimates suggest that heritability is in the region of 40 per cent with a substantial contribution from common family environment increasing similarities between first degree relatives.

The effects of the heritability of blood pressure and serum cholesterol concentration

A heritability of 70 per cent for blood pressure means that first degree relatives of a patient with blood pressure elevated 2 standard deviations above the mean could be expected to have their mean blood pressures elevated 70 per cent of 1 standard deviation above the level expected for their age and sex. Similarly first degree relatives of patients with serum cholesterol levels elevated 2 standard deviations above the mean could be expected to have serum cholesterol levels distributed around a mean cholesterol level 40 per cent of 1 standard deviation above the expected level.

Table 3.7   Mean diastolic blood pressure and serum cholesterol concentration in first degree relatives of index patients at 50 years.

	Diastolic BP mm. Hg.	Serum cholesterol mg./100ml.
Female patient	112.8 (2 SD)	334.2 (2 SD)
Male 1st° Rel.	94.5	255.5
Inc. Risk	X 1.2	X 1.3
Female 1st° Rel.	93.7	253.5

Table 3.7 shows the elevations of serum cholesterol and blood pressure expected in first degree relatives of patients with these risk factors elevated 2 standard

deviations above the population mean. The calculations are based on a study of coronary risk factors we are currently making in collaboration with Dr. Meade's Unit on an Industrial Population in N.W. London. The mean diastolic blood pressure between 40-64 was 84.2 and for women 84.7 with standard deviations of 14.6 and 13.1 respectively. The male first degree relatives of a female patient with diastolic blood pressure of 97.8 would be expected to have a mean diastolic pressure of 89.2 and her female relatives 89.1. While male first degree relatives of a female patient with diastolic blood pressure of 112.8 would be expected to have a mean diastolic blood pressure of 94.5 and the females 93.7. Calculations using data from the same population study have been used to calculate the expected deviation in serum cholesterol with a heritability of around 40 per cent and the results are shown in Table 3.7. For relatives of female patients with serum cholesterol raised 1 standard deviation males would be expected to have mean serum cholesterol of 245.8 and females 244.9 and for relatives of women whose cholesterol was elevated by 2 standard deviations males could expect a mean serum cholesterol level of 255.4 and females a mean of 253.5.

Data from the National Pooling Project (Stamler *et al*, 1970) from the United States has been used to calculate the expected effect of these increases on coronary mortality rates in men. Unfortunately there is no data on which to make similar deductions for women. For blood pressure, middle aged men with a diastolic blood pressure of 94.5 mm. Hg. the risk is 1.3 times the risk in the general population. These are the increased risks expected for first degree relatives of those whose blood pressure or serum cholesterol are elevated 2 standard deviations above the population mean and it would seem that the inheritance of neither hypertension nor hypercholesterolaemia alone as risk factors for coronary heart disease is sufficient to account for the 9-fold increase observed in male relatives of female patients in the general population.

I would suggest that there are other inherited characteristics which contribute substantially to the family aggregates, such as diabetes or disorders of clotting factors immunological characteristics or even unknown risk factors, and that the study of these high risk families of female patients could reveal some unexpected mechanisms and additional risk factors. However, risk factors which produce coronary heart disease in women may not be the same as the risk factors for men. We must not be too hasty in extrapolating our findings in women to conclusions about risk factors in men.

Familial hypercholesterolaemia

The difference in risks of coronary death in men and women heterozygous for familial hypercholesterolaemia

Models for the inheritance of liability to coronary heart disease assume a normal distribution and that the genetic contribution is polygenic. Dominantly inherited conditions are excluded from the calculations, and indeed are likely to make only a very small contribution to the problem in the general population.

However dominantly inherited Familial Hypercholesterolaemia characterised by high serum cholesterol concentrations is associated with a high risk of coronary heart disease and the risks are different in men and women.

In the homozygous form of Familial Hypercholesterolaemia the extreme condition seems to affect men and women equally but in the heterozygous form the prognosis in women is markedly better than the prognosis in men.

Table 3.8 Percentage cumulative incidence of ischaemic heart disease in patients with familial hypercholesterolaemia

Ages	Years at risk	42 Affected Men		Percentage deaths from IHD
		Percentage incidence of IHD		
< 30	1090	5.4	(2)	0.0 (0)
30 - 39	280	23.7	(6)	6.5 (3)
40 - 49	175	51.4	(9)	23.5 (4)
50 - 59	70	85.4	(7)	54.1 (4)
60 - 69	10	100.0	(2)	77.5 (1)
		39 Affected Women		
< 30	1005	0.0	(0)	0.0 (0)
30 - 39	225	0.0	(0)	0.0 (0)
40 - 49	230	12.2	(3)	0.0 (0)
50 - 59	145	57.5	(10)	15.4 (3)
60 - 69	40	74.4	(2)	15.4 (0)

Table 3.8 shows the percentage cumulative risk of coronary heart disease in men and women with Familial Hypercholesterolaemia. 25 per cent of the men had died from coronary heart disease by 50, the risk of coronary death was 54 per cent by 60 and about 75 per cent by 70. For coronary death, however, the experience among women was much better. Among the female heterozygotes there was an 85 per cent chance of survival until 60 years of age. It seemed that though symptoms of ischaemic heart disease were not uncommon, indeed present in over 50 per cent of the female heterozygotes by the age of 60, their risks of coronary death were disproportionately better than among affected men. The genetic influences found among females in the general population seems to afford a substantial protection against early coronary death in the female heterozygotes for Familial Hypercholesterolaemia. In the heterozygous form women show an increased survival rate over affected men of about 9½ years.

The time lag in the expression of coronary heart disease in the female heterozygotes was similar to the time lag found among women in the general population. Presumably the same factors are effective in preventing coronary death in women with Familial Hypercholesterolaemia.

Family similarities in age at coronary death in familial hypercholesterolaemia

Table 3.9 SIB/SIB correlations for age at coronary death in heterozygotes for familial hypercholesterolaemia (Heiberg and Slack, 1977)

Norwegian series (31)	r = 0.60 $\pm$ 0.12
London series (12)	r = 0.64 $\pm$ 0.24
Combined (43)	r = 0.70 $\pm$ 0.06

A recent examination of the age at coronary death in families with Familial Hypercholesterolaemia (Heiberg and Slack, 1977) showed a highly significant intrafamilial correlation between the age at coronary death in sibs after allowance for the age difference in the age of death between the sexes. The similarities could not be accounted for by intrafamilial correlations in serum cholesterol concentrations, furthermore there was no correlation between the age at death and the serum cholesterol level found in the patients at the time of diagnosis. The findings could be explained by heterogeneity of the gene mutations found in the families, each with its own expected age at death, but it seems more likely that many factors are contributing to death from coronary heart disease, even in the presence of Familial Hypercholesterolaemia and that in addition to the rare single mutant genes there is a strong genetic contribution which is likely to be polygenic but which acts differently in men and women.

Summary

The risks of death from coronary heart disease in the population of England and Wales are less for women than for men throughout adult life and the difference is especially marked below 55 years of age. Family studies and twin studies together indicate that family aggregates for coronary heart disease are best explained by a multifactorial model, in which both genetic and environmental factors contribute to the variation in liability to early coronary death, and that genetic liability is greatest in female patients.

The mode of inheritance of a few risk factors for coronary heart disease is known, but then estimated contribution to liability does not seem to account for the apparently large genetic liability in women. Among women with dominantly inherited Familial Hypercholesterolaemia, where the risks of early coronary death are high, there is a substantially higher risk of early coronary death among men than among women. There is a significant sib/sib correlation for age at coronary death within families with Familial Hypercholesterolaemia, which cannot be explained by serum cholesterol concentrations alone.

It is suggested that some risk factors for coronary heart disease are, as yet, unknown or poorly understood, and they may be making an important contribution to the genetic liability to coronary heart disease in young women.

References

Registrar General (1973) *Statistical Review of England and Wales,* Part I Tables Medical, London. HMSO.

Adlersberg, D., Schaefer, L.E. & Steinberg, A.G. (1957) Studies on genetic and environmental control of serum cholesterol level. *Circulation,* 16, 487-488.

Falconer, D.S. (1965) The inheritance of liability to certain diseases, estimated from the incidence among relatives. *Annals of Human Genetics,* 29, 51-76.

Harvald, B. & Hauge, M. (1970) Coronary occlusion in twins. *Acta Geneticae et Geinellologiae,* 19, 248-250.

Heiberg, A. and Slack, J. (1977) Familial similarities in the age at coronary death in familial hypercholesterolaemia. (1977) *Brit. Med. J.* 2, 493.

Pikkarainen, J., Takkunen, T. & Kulonen, E. (1966) Serum cholesterol in Finnish twins. *Amer. J. Hum. Genet.,* **18**, 115-126.

Slack, J. & Evans, K.A. (1966) The increased risk of death from ischaemic heart disease in first degree relatives of 121 men and 96 women with ischaemic heart disease. *Journal of Medical Genetics,* **3**, 239-257.

Slack, J. (1969) Risks of ischaemic heart disease in familial hyperlipoproteinaemic states. *Lancet,* **ii**, 1380-1382.

Stamler, J., Beard, R.R., Connor, W.E., de Wolfe, V.G., Stones, J. & Wills, P.W. (1970) Primary prevention of the atherosclerotic diseases. *Circulation,* **42**, A55.

Stocks, P. (1930/31) A Biometric investigation of twins and their brothers and sisters. *Annals of Eugenics,* **4**, 49-108.

Discussion 1C

Mahler (Cardiff)   There has been a report recently that the death rate from coronary heart disease is very high among diabetic, obese women. Did you specifically exclude them from your series?

Slack   The only individuals excluded from any discussion about the distribution of liability were those where it is dominantly inherited, because they do not fall into a normal distribution. Obese, diabetic women are included.

Hazzard (Seattle)   In your sib/sib correlations among those with familial hypercholesterolaemia, did you restrict your correlations only to the affected?

Slack   Yes.

Rose (London)   In your estimates of the expected familial aggregation of CHD based on cholesterol and blood pressure, you made the assumption that these two risk factors were equally heritable in coronary disease families as in the general population studies. Do you think that is likely?

Slack   The contribution made by the families who were known to have familial hypercholesterolaemia was very small indeed and when we took them out of the study they made essentially no difference to the increases in risk. They were few in number.

Hazzard (Seattle)   One would expect that there might also be a correlation in risk factors between spouses particularly to serum cholesterol concentrations. A recent study in Seattle suggests that there is an increased chance that the spouse of a survivor will have the same constellation of risk factors as the affected individual. If this is so, one would have to go to the general population for absolute controls for studies of this sort.

Slack   The correlations in the spoused pairs in the two studies that I quoted were negligible. I think this is surprising but maybe the husbands did not eat at home much.

Vessey (Oxford)   Do you think that the possible explanation of the weaker correlation between father and child as compared with mother and child with regard to blood pressure and cholesterol might be due to the fact that the father is often not the father? As many as 15 or 20 per cent of children believed to have been born within a marriage have a father from outside.

Slack   Neither study gives us any data on which to calculate illegitimacy.

McMahon (Boston)   I don't think that we should conclude that familial environment is unlikely to be an explanation of familial occurrence, because the family is dispersed by the time the disease appears. The spouse correlations of risk may be an underestimate of the importance of this familial environment and require more study.

Wynn (London)   Women with hypercholesterolaemia are particularly susceptible to the effect of oral contraceptives in raising serum cholesterol and in such studies as you are doing it will be necessary to elicit their contraceptive usage.

Slack   The women with familial hypercholesterolaemia who died in our study were without exception over an age which one would expect them to be using the pill, so I don't think this alters the conclusions that I would draw about the difference in age of death, between the men and women.

4. Smoking

G. A. ROSE

Cigarette smoking is widely believed to be a major cause of coronary heart disease (CHD). This view is based on the general consistency of evidence from a variety of sources, each of which is indirect and fallible. Most studies have either been confined to men or have included insufficient nunbers of women. Some results of studies in younger women will be reviewed and assessed, both as independent evidence and as indicating whether conclusions from the extensive evidence available on men are likely also to apply to women.

Longitudinal population surveys

The American Cancer Society study (Hammond and Garfinkel, 1969) applied a questionnaire on smoking habits to 804,409 men and women aged 40 to 79 years, with a subsequent follow-up based on death certificates. For the younger decade the results (Table 4.1) show a strong dose-related association between smoking and CHD mortality, but the risk gradient is a little shallower in women than in men. A large Japanese study came to a similar conclusion, with standardised mortality ratios for smokers of 1.56 in men and 1.44 in women.

Table 4.1 Cigarette smoking and the risk of death from CHD in the American Cancer Society study

Cigs./Day	CHD: Mortality ratio	
	Men	Women
0	1.0	1.0
1-9	1.6	1.3
10-19	2.6	2.1
20-39	3.8	3.6
$\geqslant 40$	5.5	(3.3)

In studies which include personal examinations the numbers are inevitably much smaller, and low incidence rates make it difficult to interpret results in younger people, particularly women. In the Framingham Study (Table 4.2) the pattern for men was fairly clear and it could be demonstrated that the predictive power of a smoking history was largely independent of the other major risk factors; but the apparently negative result for women is meaningless, since it may simply reflect sampling variation due to small numbers.

Table 4.2 Cigarette smoking and the incidence of CHD in the Framingham Study

| Cigs./Day | CHD: Relative risk | | | |
| | 35-44 yr | | 45-54 yr | |
	Men (854)	Women (1083)	Men (698)	Women (864)
0	1.0	1.0	1.0	1.0
<20	1.5	0.6	1.6	0.9
>20	2.0	1.7	1.4	0.8

Table 4.3 Smoking and CHD mortality in the Whitehall Study of men aged 40-64 (Reid, Hamilton, McCartney, Rose, Jarrett and Keen, 1976)

| Smoking Category | 5-year deaths from CHD | |
	No.	Relative risk
Never smoked	34	1.0
Ex-smokers	79	1.0
Pipe/cigar smokers	10	1.3
Cigarettes:		
< 20/day	92	1.6
> 20/day	62	1.8
'non-inhalers'	27	1.2
'inhalers'	127	1.8

In our own studies of male civil servants aged 40 to 64 years there is a significant overall association between cigarette smoking and 5-year CHD mortality (Table 4.3). The difference between light smokers and heavy smokers is smaller than when men are classified according to how they answered a question on inhalation. This is perhaps particularly surprising in view of the report that such statements correlate poorly with variations in carboxyhaemoglobin level. In this study numbers were large enough to enable us to cross-classify subjects simultaneously according to their levels of blood pressure, plasma cholesterol and smoking and to report actual rates for men in these various sub-groups (Fig. 4.1): in other studies only indirect estimates have been obtained. At each level of blood pressure, and whether cholesterol level is in the lowest or the highest quintile, the age-adjusted CHD mortality rate is higher in those who smoke cigarettes. (In contrast, for the other two risk factors there is a suggestion of a 'ceiling' effect; for example, in high-cholesterol men who smoke, risk seems to be unaffected by blood pressure.) Corresponding data for young women do not exist, and it is unlikely that they ever will; one can only say that there seems no reason to suppose that the smoking effect in this group would be any less independent of the other risk factors.

Cross-sectional and case control studies

Smoking and chest pain

In a large cross-sectional population survey among participants in the New York Health Insurance Plan (Shapiro, Weinblatt, Frank and Sager, 1969) the increase in angina among smokers at ages 35 to 44 was 3.4-fold in men but only 1.6-fold

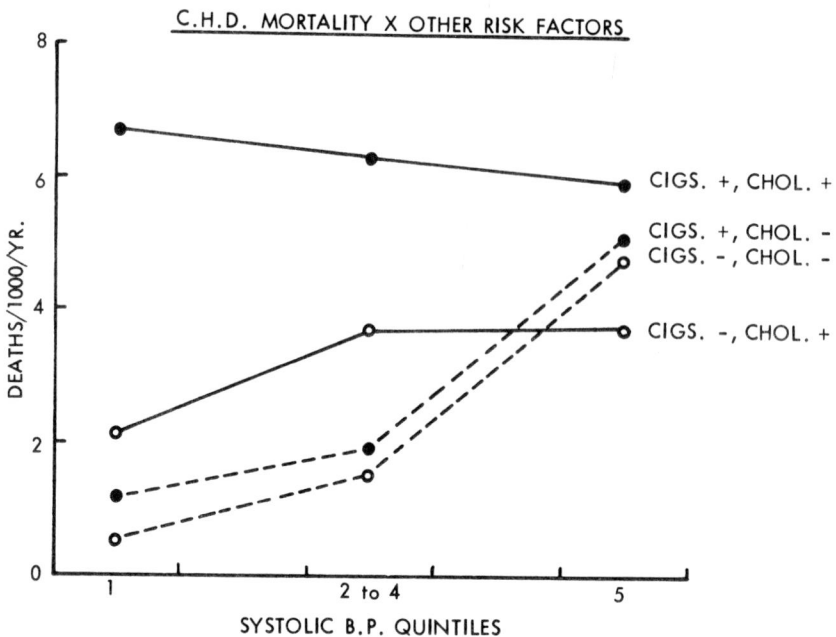

Fig. 4.1   CHD mortality according to cigarette smoking habit, blood pressure and plasma cholesterol level (top quintile versus bottom quintile) in men aged 40-59 (Whitehall Study)

in women. In an angiographic study of 1000 women with chest pain under the age of 50 it was reported that there was significant coronary artery disease in 35 per cent of those smoking 10 or more cigarettes daily, compared with only 19 per cent in the remainder (Welch, 1975).

In a study of 64 women in whom a diagnosis of angina had been made before the age of 45, Oliver (1974) found the same proportion of smokers as in the general population. This contrasted with his finding in 81 women in the same age group with myocardial infarction, when he found more than twice the expected number of heavy smokers.

Smoking in survivors of myocardial infarction

The case/control method is sometimes the only method of measuring the association between an uncommon condition and its suspected causes. Its simplicity and cheapness are attractive, but the interpretation of results is much more hazardous than in population-based studies. The clinical diagnosis of myocardial infarction is often missed, and the probability of its recognition may be different in smokers. If smoking is particularly associated with sudden death (and the evidence in men on this point is conflicting) then it could be misleading to study only those patients who survive long enough to reach hospital. Smoking habits in women who have heart attacks are immediately modified, and the women may also be biased in their recollection of earlier habits. Finally it is impossible to be sure that an appropriate control group has been assembled. For all these reasons it is necessary to be cautious in generalising risk estimates from case/control studies to the general population, and in inferring causality. With these caveats, it may be said that the results (Table 4.4) of the careful study by Mann and his colleagues (1976) indicate a strong association between smoking and myocardial infarction in these young women. The relative risk estimate for heavy smokers is remarkably high. The relative risk of smoking in this study seemed to be largely independent of the effects both of hypertension and of oral contraceptives.

Table 4.4   Risk estimates from a case/control study of 77 women under the age of 45 who had survived a myocardial infarction (Mann, Doll, Thorogood, Vessey and Waters, 1976)

Smoking habit	Estimated relative risk of MI
Non-smokers	1.0
1-15 cigs./day	1.8
15-24 ''	4.3
25 ''	18.5
All smokers	5.7
'' '' (standardised for B.P. and O.C.)	4.0

National statistics

International patterns

Even within Europe there is wide variation both in reported CHD mortality rates and in their changes over time. For 16 countries the change in mortality (1961-1967) from 'arteriosclerotic and degenerative heart disease' in women aged 45 to 54 ranged from a decrease of 6 per cent p.a. to an increase of 7 per cent p.a. Over the previous 20 years there had also been tremendous variations in national cigarette consumption, ranging from a fall of 17 per cent to an increase of more than 700 per cent. There was however no discernible association between these trends, which showed a non-significant negative correlation (r - 0.23). With a disease of multifactorial aetiology, and with social and environmental changes of such complexity, it would perhaps have been surprising if international differences could have been assigned clearly to any single explanation.

National trends

Within one country the changes may be rather less complex. Table 4.5 shows the changes in life-time consumption of cigarettes among younger women, esti-mated from Tobacco Research Council data (Lee, 1976). It is evident that there has been a tremendous increase, but that the rate of increase has been slowing down. In the youngest age-group (16-19 years), however, the rate of increase has recently shown some alarming signs of acceleration. It is believed by some that the effect of smoking depends on the current rather than on the cumulative dose, and in that case it can be noted that current cigarette consumption among

U.K. women aged 40-44 has also shown a declining rate of increase over the period since 1950.

Table 4.5 Estimated increases over successive quinquennia in life-time cigarette consumption by U.K. women up to their 45th birthday

Period	Increase in total cigs. smoked to age 45
1950-1955	+ 42%
1955-1960	+ 38%
1960-1965	+ 32%
1965-1970	+ 15%
1970-1975	+ 11%
Total (1950-1975)	+ 330%

It is difficult to relate these changes in cigarette consumption to changes in CHD mortality, partly because we do not know what would be the appropriate latent interval, but also because of changes in diagnostic habit and nomenclature. Table 4.6 sets out some figures, based on a recent report by Clayton, Taylor and Shaper (1977). The apparent increase is less if deaths attributed to hypertensive heart disease are included; but either way, there is clearly an acceleration in the rate of proportionate increase. This would make it difficult to conclude that changes in cigarette consumption have been the major determinant, since their rate of increase has been declining. The results do not, however, exclude the possibility that smoking may have played some important role, albeit not the dominant one, in this alarming increase. Wald (1976) made a similarly cautious statement, saying simply that 'some of the increase may be related to cigarette smoking'.

Table 4.6 Changes in cardiovascular mortality for women aged 40-44 years over two successive 10-year periods in England and Wales (from Clayton *et al*, 1977)

Categories of death	Mortality change %	
	1950/2-1960/2	1960/2-1970/2
Arteriosclerotic + degenerative	+13	+38
Arteriosclerotic + degenerative + hypertensive	- 4	+24

Conclusions

There is solid evidence that young women who smoke cigarettes are much more likely to suffer myocardial infarction or to die from CHD than are their non-smoking contemporaries. Smoking undoubtedly serves to identify a high-risk group, and it seems likely that, as in men, this predictive effect is more or less independent of the level of other major risk factors: thus risk is probably compounded when smoking and other risk factors occur together in the same woman.

Mechanisms exist which might account for this association being one of cause and effect. Experimentally in animals atherogenesis can be accelerated by exposure to carbon monoxide; and nicotine lowers the ventricular fibrillation threshold, increases plasma free fatty acids and activates thrombotic mechanisms, as well as having powerful acute haemodynamic effects. An unexplained association has recently been reported between cigarette smoking and earlier menopause (Jick, Porter and Morrison, 1977). But all the evidence in humans is indirect and currently only observational, and so it is capable of various interpretations. (The experimental findings from our randomised controlled trial of smoking cessation will not be available until next year.) Furthermore, observational studies large enough to permit detailed analysis and sub-classifications are largely confined to males.

The central problem in interpreting these observational data is that smokers are a self-selected group with their own psychological, environmental and life-style characteristics: it is not only smoking which makes them a distinctive group. When 'A' is found to be associated with 'B', it is always possible that the real explanation lies with a factor 'C' which has not been considered or could not be measured. This important point can be illustrated from our study of smoking in civil servants. As shown in Table 4.3, mortality from CHD among smokers was 50 per cent higher among those who said that they inhaled, the rate in 'non-inhalers' being little higher than that for non-smokers. The simplest interpretation would be that cigarettes cause CHD, but only if the smoke is inhaled. However, further analysis has shown that inhalation habit is strongly correlated with employment grade, and that this in turn is powerfully and independently related to the risk of death from CHD. The association in the crude data between in-halation and disease was largely spurious, and within individual employment grades it is small (Table 4.7).

Table 4.7 Relationship between 5-year CHD mortality, 'inhalation' of cigarette smoke, and employment grade in male civil servants (Whitehall Study)

Employment grade	'Inhalers'	CHD mortality per 1000	Mortality excess in 'inhalers' above 'non-inhalers'
Whole study group	33%	15.1	+50%
Administrative	10%	4.7	+ 6%
Professional & executive	20%	13.4	+ 7%
Clerical	42%	18.3	+12%

An apparently powerful argument for the causal hypothesis comes from the experience of male ex-smokers, whose excess risk of CHD diminishes progressively according to the number of years since they stopped smoking. Nevertheless, even this association is capable of an alternative explanation, since ex-smokers again are a self-selected group, biased in respect of social class and perhaps other, unidentified factors; and with each succeeding year this bias will increase, as those with (presumably) less distinctive features resume the smoking habit. Like is not being compared with like.

Within wide limits, then, the interpretation of the strong association between smoking and CHD is uncertain. At the one extreme it is possible that it is nearly all one of cause and effect. In that case it can be estimated that cigarette smoking might be responsible for as much as two-thirds of mortality from CHD in women under the age of 45 (based on Tobacco Research Council data on smoking in the U.K., and risk estimates from Mann *et al.*, 1976). At the other extreme it must be admitted that until we know more about the social class-related factors in smoking and in this disease, it may be impossible to refute the hypothesis that the association is largely spurious. Nevertheless, the strength and general consistency of the association in men and women make it likely that at least a substantial part of the explanation is causal; and this is particularly true at younger ages. Despite the uncertainty, it seems for most purposes at present that the best working hypothesis is one of causality.

References

Clayton, D.G., Taylor, D. & Shaper, A.G. (1977) Trends in heart disease in England and Wales, 1950 to 1973. *Health Trends,* **9,** 1-6.

Hammond, E.C. & Garfinkel, L. (1969) Coronary heart disease, stroke, and aortic aneurysm. Factors in the aetiology. *Archives of Environmental Health,* **19,** 167-182.

Jick, H., Porter, J. & Morrison, A.S. (1977) Relation between smoking and age of natural menopause. *Lancet,* **1,** 1354-1355.

Kannel, W.B. & Gordon, T. (1970) The Framingham Study. An epidemiological investigation of cardiovascular diseases. Section 26, 16-year follow-up. U.S. Govt. Printing Office, Washington, D.C.

Lee, P.N. (1976) Statistics of smoking in the United Kingdom. *Tobacco Research Council, Research Paper I,* Seventh Edition. Tobacco Research Council: London.

Mann, G.I., Doll, R., Thorogood, M., Vessey, M.P. & Waters, W.E. (1976) Risk factors for myocardial infarction in young women. *British Journal of Preventive & Social Medicine,* **30,** 94-100.

Oliver, M.F. (1974) Ischaemic heart disease in young women. *British Medical Journal,* **4,** 253-259.

Reid, D.D., Hamilton, P.J.S., McCartney, P., Rose, G., Jarrett, R.J. & Keen, H. (1976) Smoking and other risk factors for coronary heart-disease in British civil servants. *Lancet,* **2,** 979-984.

Shapiro, S., Weinblatt, E., Frank, C.W. & Sager, R.V. (1969) Incidence of coronary heart disease in a population insured for medical care (HIP). *American Journal of Public Health,* **59** (Suppl.).

Wald, N.J. (1976) Mortality from lung cancer and coronary heart-disease in relation to changes in smoking habits. *Lancet,* **1,** 136-138.

Welch, C.C. (1975) Coronary artery disease in young women. *Cardiovascular Clinics,* **7,** 5-18.

5. Cigarette smoking and coronary heart disease in young women

N. J. WALD

Introduction

This paper describes patterns of cigarette consumption among women in the U.K. and summarises the results of studies investigating the relationship between smoking and coronary heart disease (CHD) in women. Recent data relating to the influence of smoking on the age of menopause are referred to, since it has been suggested that the risk of CHD in women may be altered by the menopause. Finally, trends in cigarette consumption and CHD mortality in England and Wales are examined.

Cigarette smoking among women in the U.K.

Consumption of manufactured cigarettes among women in the U.K. has been increasing since the time when women began to take up the habit in about 1920.

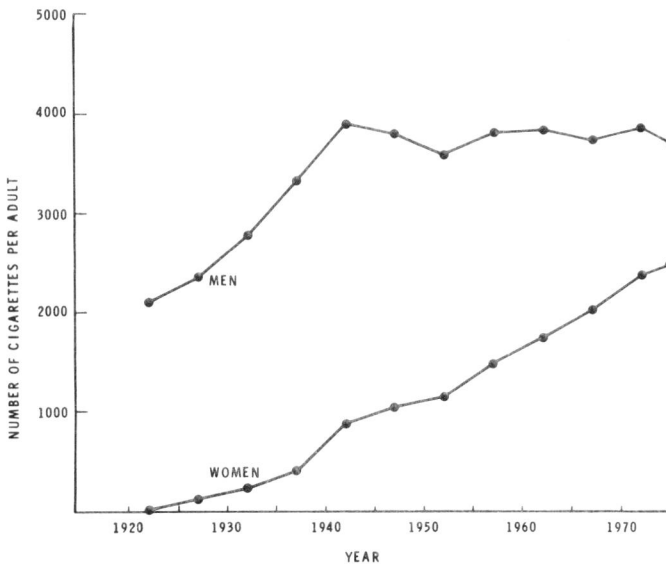

Fig. 5.1 Annual consumption of manufactured cigarettes per person aged 15 years or more in the U.K. Each point on the graph is the average for consecutive five-year periods, except for the last point which is the value for 1975.

Figure 5.1 shows the cigarette consumption per adult male and female aged over 14 years in the United Kingdom from 1920 to 1975. In spite of the continuous increase, women were smoking no more in 1970 than men were smoking in the 1920s. Although the rise in consumption has continued in recent years, the proportion of adult women who smoked manufactured cigarettes hardly changed from 1961-1973, reflecting the fact that the average number smoked per smoker has risen. Among women aged 16 to 24, 25 to 34, 35 to 59 and 60 or more years of age, the percentages of manufactured cigarette smokers were 49, 50, 50 and 24 percent respectively in 1961, and the corresponding percentages in 1971 were 52, 48, 53 and 25 percent. Girls are taking up smoking at an earlier age now than they did in former years. The proportion of girls aged 14 years who smoked at least 1 cigarette a day rose from 0 percent in 1961 to 7 percent in 1971.

Over the last 15 years the percentage of adult female cigarette smokers among the different social classes has remained similar (ranging from 42 to 49 percent) in all but social class I (professional occupations). In 1961, 46 percent of women in social class I smoked manufactured cigarettes, but by 1973 this had almost halved, to 26 percent. In 1958 women in different social classes smoked similar numbers of manufactured cigarettes ranging from 30 to 36 per week per adult female. From then on, cigarette consumption by women in social class I remained steady until about 1970, and declined thereafter. Women in social class V increased their consumption from 32 cigarettes per week in 1958 to 50 per week in 1974.

Apart from differences in the numbers of cigarettes smoked by men and women in the U.K. there is an additional important difference in their smoking habits. Men who smoked cigarettes during the first half of the century smoked mainly plain cigarettes without filters; but filter cigarettes have contributed proportionately more to female consumption, and many women smoking today have probably never regularly smoked plain cigarettes in their life. The substantial switch in cigarette sales from the plain to the filter variety, which occurred mainly between 1955 and 1970, is likely to have important medical implications. Associated with their switch, the tar and nicotine yields have declined by nearly 50 percent. The Tobacco Research Council has proposed a method of adjusting cigarette consumption since 1965 to take account of this change, and it has published such adjusted figures for cigarette consumption after 1965. Women in 1965 smoked, on average, 5.1 cigarettes a day per adult female, and by 1972 this had risen by 24 percent to 6.3 cigarettes a day. But if adjustment is made for the reduction in tar yields which has occurred since 1965, the 1972 level of consumption would only have been 4.1 cigarettes per day, a *fall* of 24 percent. Applying similar tar adjustments to the cigarette consumption of women in the different social classes, women in classes III to V smoked slightly less in 1974 than in 1958; women in class II smoked about three quarters as much, and women in class I about half as much. It is now generally agreed that the tar yields of cigarettes are related to the risk of lung cancer, but the constituent or constituents of tobacco smoke which might lead to the development of CHD is unknown, although both nicotine and carbon monoxide may be involved. It is, therefore, difficult to predict what effects the changing composition of cigarettes will have on the mortality from this disease.

Cigarette smoking and coronary heart disease in women

There is now little doubt that cigarette smoking is associated with CHD in women, particularly in women under about 60 years of age. In the prospective study organised by the American Cancer Society, the age-standardised mortality from CHD among women aged 45-64 years was 0.83 per 1,000 among those who had never smoked cigarettes regularly, and the rate was 1.48 per 1,000 among current smokers (Hammond, 1966). Women who smoked 20 or more cigarettes per day or, 10 or more cigarettes and had started to smoke before the age of 25 years, had an even higher mortality of 1.75 per 1,000. The number of deaths in each group was large, namely 857, 523 and 272 deaths respectively. A more recent paper using results from the same study showed that the mortality ratio among women aged 40-49 was 1.31, 2.08, 3.62 and 3.31 for smokers of 1-9, 10-19, 20-39 and 40 or more cigarettes daily respectively (Hammond, 1971). A Danish epidemiological survey of 523 women demonstrated a statistically significant association between smoking and the pevalence of CHD (mainly angina pectoris) and intermittent claudication (Wald *et al*, 1973). Twenty six women had CHD or intermittent claudication, and the prevalence was 0.8 percent among non-smokers, 1.3 percent among light smokers, 5.7 percent among moderate smokers and 14.3 percent among heavy smokers. The proportion of affected women were also classified by carboxyhaemoglobin (COHb) level; among those with COHb levels less than 2, 2-3.9, 4-5.9, 6-7.9, 8-9.9 and 10 percent or greater, the proportions of affected women were 1.0, 3.6, 7.6, 10.3, 13.3 and 24.1 percent. A multiple regression analysis indicated that the association between COHb level and the vascular disorders was independent of age and serum cholesterol, and the effect was similar in men and women. Bengtsson has studied women aged 38-60 years who lived in Gothenberg, Sweden, and survived an acute myocardial infarct which occurred during the period 1968-1970 (Bengtsson, 1973). Thirty seven out of 46 (80 percent) of the women were current cigarette smokers, while only 218 out of the 578 age-matched controls (38 percent) smoked cigarettes. This difference was statistically significant, and the relative risk was 6.8. Among women with angina pectoris, 15 had never smoked cigarettes (52 percent), a similar proportion to that found among controls, suggesting that smoking was not related to angina pectoris. Oliver, in Edinburgh, obtained similar results; among women aged 30-45 the proportion of non-smokers in 81 patients who had had a myocardial infarction and in 64 patients with angina was respectively 4.2 times and 1.3 times greater than in women of the same age in the general population (Oliver, 1974). Mann and his colleagues in Oxford found a statistically highly significant association between current cigarette consumption and myocardial infarction (Mann *et al*, 1976). The study was based on 77 women discharged from hospital with a diagnosis of myocardial infarction, and 207 controls, who were matched with the cases for age, marital status, hospital and year of admission. In comparison with non-smokers the relative risk was 1.8:1, 4.3:1 and 18.5:1 in women smoking less than 15, 15-24 and 25 or more cigarettes a day respectively. Among women smoking 15 or more cigarettes a day the relative risk was 5.7. This was only reduced to a 4-fold risk after allowance was made for the presence or absence of three other risk factors for CHD, namely, hypertension, history of pre-eclamptic toxaemia or oral contraceptive use. The small numbers of subjects in this study made it impossible to standardise completely for the separate effects of the various variables studied. Nonetheless, the presence of a dose-response relationship between amount smoked and the prevalence of myocardial infarction, and the small reduction in relative risk after the standardisation that was used, suggests that the association between smoking and myocardial infarction was a direct one. A result from this study which is of particular grave concern is the indication that smoking interacts with other risk factors for myocardial infarction in young women in a multiplicative manner, so the effect of, say, hypertension, oral contraceptive use, and a history of smoking more than 15 cigarettes a day, acted together to increase the risk of myocardial infarction 128 times.

A recent American case-control study of acute non-fatal myocardial infarction (MI) involving 653 subjects aged 40-69 years showed that smokers of one and two packets of cigarettes a day experienced 1.5 and 1.7 times the risk of a non-fatal MI compared to non-smokers (Miettinen *et al*, 1976). Among subjects aged 40-49 the relative risks were 3.2 and 4.5 respectively. These estimates of risk were calculated after allowing for the possible confounding influence of the hospital where the patients were admitted (33 were involved), age (in decades), sex, religion (Jewish or other), coffee consumption (none, 1-5, or 6 or more cups daily), season (four), angina, diabetes, hypertension. The risk associated with smoking after allowing for the other factors was similar in women and men. In contrast to the results of Mann, patients with diabetes who smoked did not have a higher risk of MI than non-smokers.

Several surveys of women have, therefore, demonstrated that CHD, particularly myocardial infarction, is more common in cigarette smokers than in non-smokers. Moreover, the relative risk is greater among young women than old, and the risk increases with amount smoked although the precise dose-response relationship is unclear. The association between smoking and CHD appears to be similar in men and women. The risk is independent of confounding factors such as serum cholesterol level, diabetes, hypertension or oral contraceptive use. The interaction of certain risk-factors appears to be multiplicative, although the data are scanty and inconsistent. Almost all the data are based on cross-sectional or case-control studies, and it is clearly important to investigate prospectively the effect of smoking and its interaction with other risk factors on the incidence of CHD, and to see if the effect can be reversed by giving up smoking.

Cigarette smoking and the menopause

The effect of the menopause on the incidence of CHD is still uncertain. There are data to suggest that the disease is more common among post-menopausal women than it is in pre-menopausal women of the same age. A recent report of the Framingham Study (Kannel *et al*, 1976) presents data relating to 59 cases of CHD, and the difference in incidence between pre- and post-menopausal women was statistically significant in the 40-44 year age group. However, this was based on only 6 coronary events? the differences found in the 45-49 year and 50-54 age groups were each not statistically significant, although the rates were somewhat higher in the post-menopausal women. The menstrual histories of women with CHD and from a random sample of the female population were also recorded in the Gothenberg study (Bengtsson, 1973). Twenty eight out of 37 patients (76 percent) admitted to hospital with myocardial infarction had already had the menopause by the age of 50, compared with 280 out of 578 (48 percent) controls, a statistically significant result. There is, however, one piece of evidence that weighs against the suggestion that the menopause affects the risk of CHD. Examination of national mortality statistics shows that death rates from CHD do not rise more steeply with increasing age after the age of the menopause than it does before (Fig. 5.2).

Although the effects of the menopause on the incidence of CHD need clarification, it is nonetheless of interest to note a recent observation published by the Boston Collaborative Drug Surveillance Program (Jick *et al*, 1977) that women who smoke cigarettes have an earlier menopause than women who do not. The study investigated the smoking habits and menopausal history of two large groups of women (one involving 2,143 subjects, and the other 1,391 subjects), who were admitted to hospital with a variety of diagnoses. In the first group studied, among women aged 48-49 years in the following categories: those who had never smoked cigarettes, who smoked less than one packet of cigarettes per day, who smoked a packet or more a day, the proportions who had passed the menopause were 26, 33 and 46 percent respectively; in the second group the corresponding figures were 47, 54 and 61 percent. While it is not clear why the proportion of post-menopausal women of the same age and in the same smoking categories were different in the two studies, there is nonetheless a striking association between the smoking of cigarettes and age of menopause. Kinlen collected information on the age of menopause among smokers and life-long non-smokers as part of a case-control study concerned with the relationship between hair dye use and cancer, and I am grateful to him for allowing me to use these unpublished data. The mean age of menopause among 72 women aged 55-69 years who had never smoked cigarettes was 47.6 years (SE 0.57). The mean age of menopause among 53 cigarette smokers in the same age group was 46.2 (SE 0.79), 1.43 years less than that found among the non-smokers. These data are therefore consistent with those described by the Boston group, but the difference was statistically not significant (P=0.07). The mean age of menopause among 44 ex-smokers was, however, 48.2 years (SE 0.9) higher than in both smokers and life-long non-smokers.

If the associations between early menopause and smoking and CHD are both confirmed, the data would suggest that cigarette smoking might cause both an early menopause and CHD.

Trends in coronary heart disease among women

Figures 5.3, 5.4 and 5.5 show the age-specific mortality from CHD among men and women from 1950 to 1974 in the U.K. together with the corresponding annual consumption of cigarettes over the same period. In general CHD has risen more rapidly among young women than it has among young men, and this has also been the pattern in the cigarette consumption of the two sexes. These trends, therefore, are consistent with the observation that cigarette smoking is related to

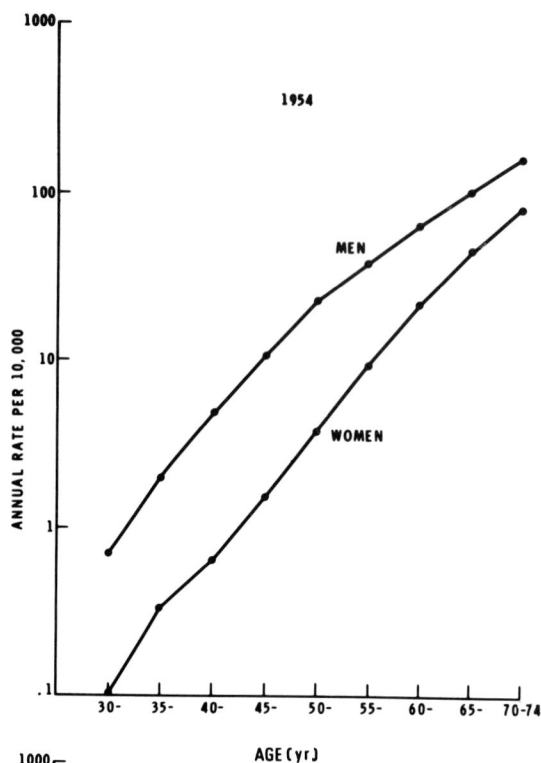

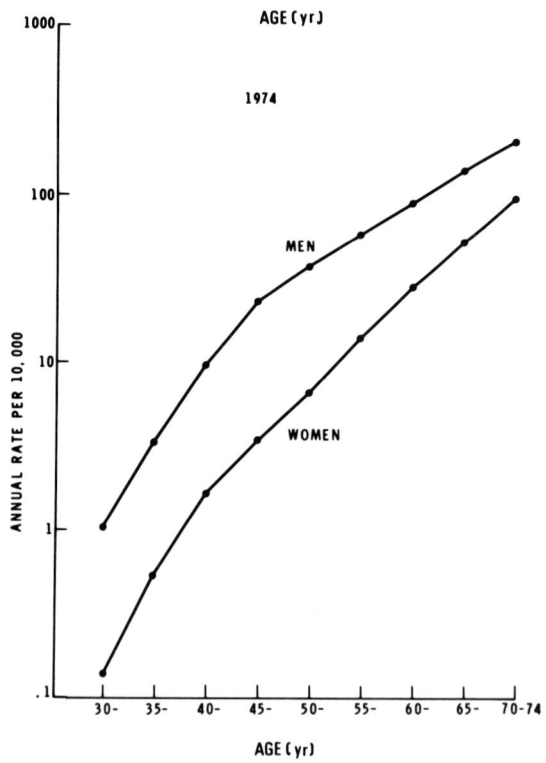

Fig. 5.2 Coronary heart disease mortality in England and Wales among persons aged 30-74 in 1954 and 1974.

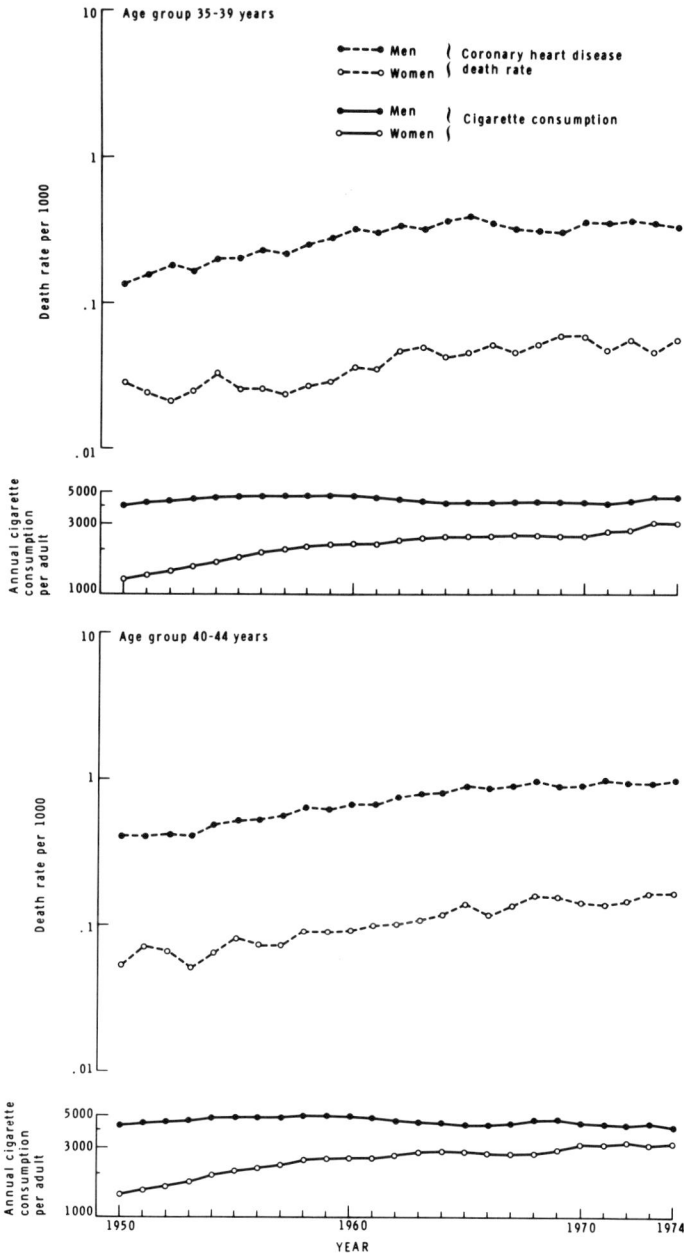

Fig. 5.3 Coronary heart disease mortality in England and Wales from 1950 to 1974 and U.K. *per capita* adult (15 years and over) annual cigarette consumption from 1950 to 1974 (three year moving average) in men and women aged 35-39 and 40-44 years.

c

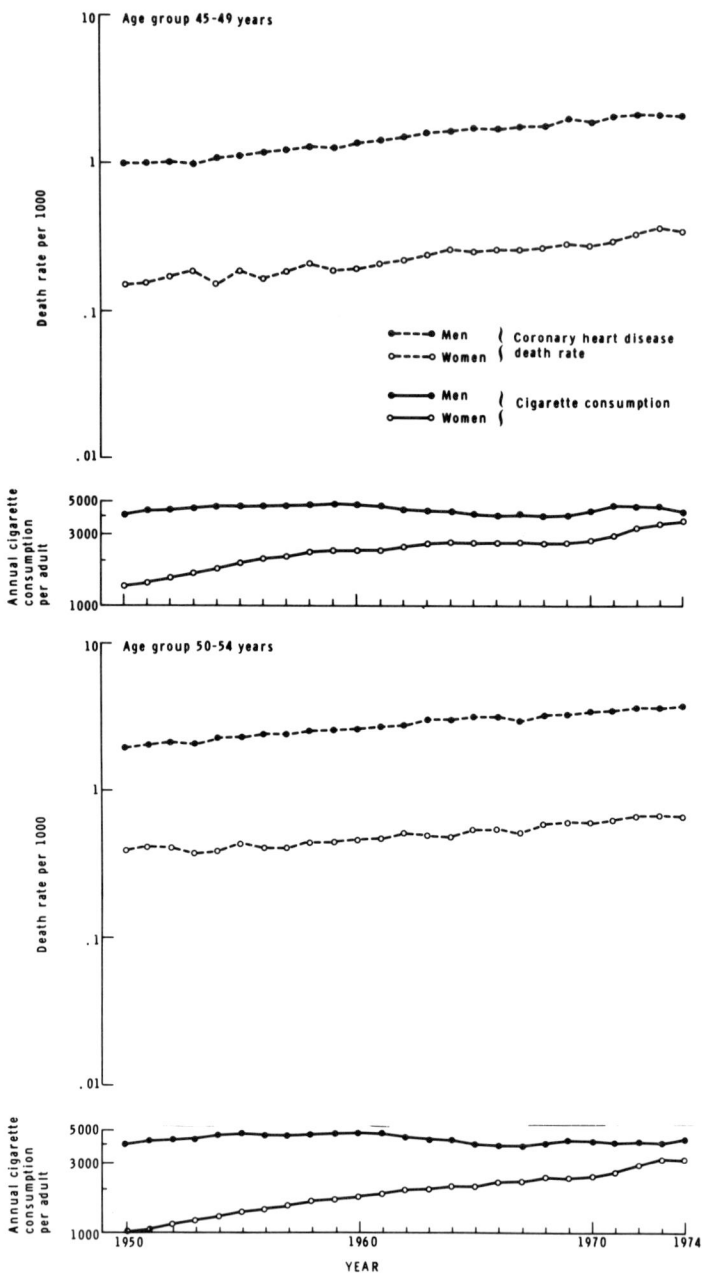

Fig. 5.4 Coronary heart disease mortality in England and Wales from 1950 to 1974 and U.K. *per capita* adult (15 years and over) annual cigarette consumption from 1950 to 1974 (three year moving average) in men and women aged 45-49 and 50-54 years.

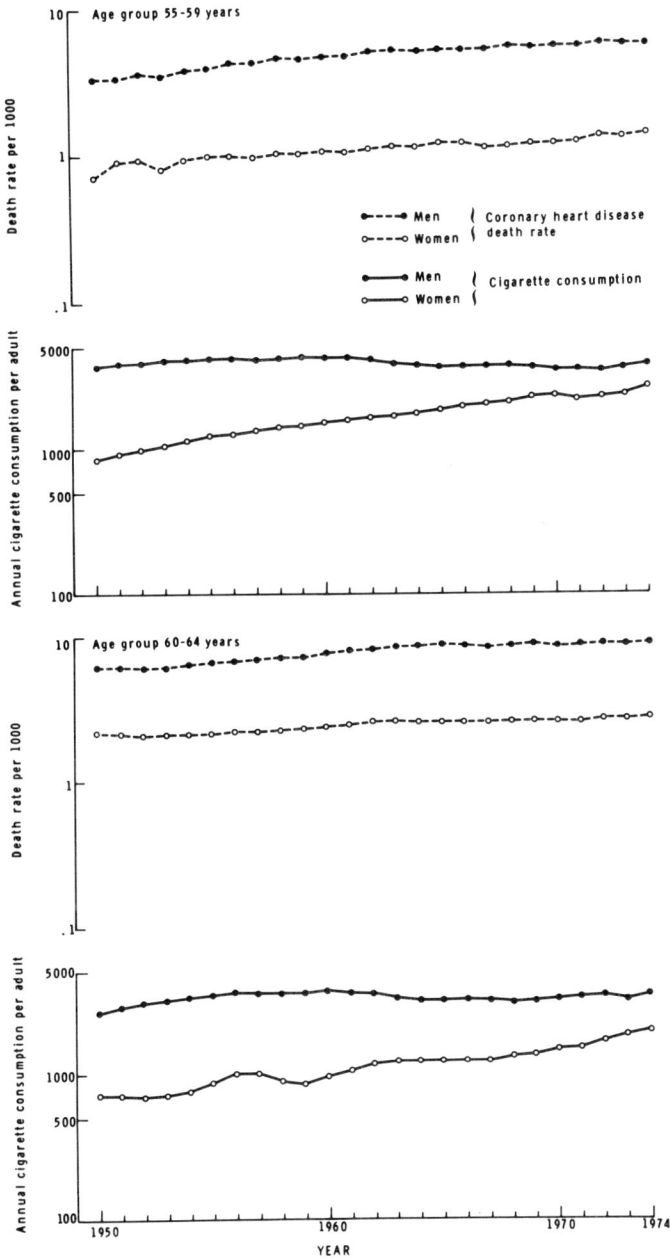

Fig. 5.5 Coronary heart disease mortality in England and Wales from 1950 to 1974 and U.K. *per capita* adult (15 years and over) annual cigarette consumption from 1950 to 1974 (three year moving average) in men and women aged 55-59 and 60-64 years.

CHD mortality in young women. On a constant tar basis, cigarette consumption has declined in women aged 20-59 years over the period 1965-1974. For example, among women aged 40-44 years the annual consumption of cigarettes per adult was 2,750 in 1965, and 1,850 in 1975, a reduction of 33 percent. It would appear, therefore, that the trends in CHD in women are better correlated with current cigarette consumption than with adjusted cigarette consumption calculated on a 1965 constant tar basis. In the U.K., CHD mortality among women of different social classes is less well correlated with their consumption. In 1961 there was little difference in the cigarette consumption among women from the different social classes, but, by this time a social class mortality gradient had already emerged; the standardised mortality ratios for CHD in married women were 69, 81, 103, 107 and 143 in classes I-V respectively. It would appear, therefore, that women in social class I had experienced a relative reduction in their mortality from CHD compared to women in the other social classes before a divergence in their smoking habits had emerged. A similar anomaly has been noted with respect to trends in the social class pattern of lung cancer and cigarette smoking (Wald and Doll, 1976).

Comparisons of trends in coronary heart disease mortality with changes in cigarette consumption is fraught with difficulty and needs to be interpreted cautiously. The trend in mortality among non-smokers needs to be known and the interaction between smoking and other risk factors better understood before national trends can be satisfactorily interpreted. In general, the value of examining such trends is restricted to the generation of hypotheses which can subsequently be investigated by more detailed specific epidemiological investigations, or as a check to see whether epidemiologically identified risks are consistent with the changes in the pattern or exposure and the pattern of mortality.

Conclusion

There is considerably less information on the effects of cigarette smoking in women than there is for men. Extensive prospective epidemiological data are only available from one study, and data are not yet available on the effects of giving up smoking in women. However, information on the prevalence of CHD in women suggests that smoking is associated with the disease, that the risk is similar to that found in men, and there is a dose-response relationship between amount smoked and the incidence of the disease. There is evidence that smoking is associated with an early menopause, and this may account for the observation that an early menopause is associated with an increased risk of CHD. The interaction between smoking and other risk factors is inconclusive, but one investigation suggests that they act multiplicatively, so that the risk in women with three or more risk factors may be very high indeed.

Note

Details of cigarette consumption in the U.K. described in this paper were obtained from Todd, G.F., Occasional Papers 1, 1975, and 2, 1976, Tobacco Research Council, London, and Lee, P.N., Research Paper 1, Seventh Edition, 1976, Tobacco

Research Council, London. Mortality Statistics for coronary heart disease in England and Wales were obtained from the Registrar General's Statistical Reviews of England and Wales, (1950-74), Part 1, tables, medical, H.M. Stationery Office, using I.C.D. codes 420 and 422.1 until 1967, and I.C.D. codes 410-414 thereafter.

References

Bengtsson, C. (1973) Ischaemic Heart Disease in Women. A study based on a randomised population sample of women and women with myocardial infarction in Goteborg, Sweden. Elanders Bodtryckeri Aktiebolag, Kungsbacka.

Hammond, E.C. (1966) Smoking in relation to the death rates of one million men and women. Epidemiological Study of Cancer and Other Chronic Diseases. *National Cancer Inst. Mono.,* **19**, U.S. Dept. of Health, Education and Welfare.

Hammond, E.C. (1971) Smoking in relation to diseases other than cancer. Total death rates. *The Second World Conference on Smoking and Health.* Pitman.

Jick, H., Porter, J., Morrison, A.S. (1977) Relation between smoking and age of natural menopause. *Lancet,* i, 1354-55.

Kannel, W.B., Hjortland, M.C., McNamara, P.M. and Gordon, T. (1976) Menopause and risk of cardiovascular disease. The Framingham Study. *Annals of Internal Medicine,* **85**, 447-452.

Mann, J.I., Doll, R., Thorogood, M., Vessey, M.P. and Waters, W.E. (1976) Risk factors for myocardial infarction in young women. *British J. of Preventive and Social Medicine,* **30**, 94-100.

Miettinen, O.S., Neff, R.K. and Jick, H. (1976) Cigarette smoking and non-fatal myocardial infarction: rate ratio in relation to age, sex and predisposing condition. *American J. of Epidemiology,* **103**, 30-36.

Oliver, M.F. (1974) Ischaemic heart disease in young women. *British Medical J.,* **4**, 253-259.

Wald, N., Howard, S., Smith, P.G. and Kjeldsen, K. (1973) Association between atherosclerotic diseases and carboxyhaemoglobin levels in tobacco smokers. *British Medical J.,* **1**, 761-765.

Wald, N.J. and Doll, R. (1976) Chapter II: Epidemiology. In: *Lung Cancer, UICC Technical Report Series,* Vol. **25**, (edited by E.L. Wynder and S. Hecht), Geneva.

Discussion 1D

Somerville (London) Professor Rose, you challenge us by casting doubt on the causal role of cigarette smoking and CHD but end by saying that you personally believe them to be strong. Would you mind expanding this a little?

Rose As researchers we live in two worlds. One where we are sceptical, collectors of information and avoid jumping to conclusions. In this world, and as an epidemiologist, I regard the case for cigarettes causing CHD as very suggestive but by no means proven. But then there is also the world of action and what you advise the public to do. Here one takes into account other factors than just the scientific evidence. The consequences of alternative policies have to be considered. In that world and wearing that hat, as it were, I think the best working hypothesis, for the moment, is that cigarettes are a major cause of coronary heart disease in younger people. I am quite open-minded to the possibility that in 5 years time we might think differently.

McMahon (Boston)   While you commented on the slightly lower relative risks for CHD mortality in the American Cancer Society Study for women than males, I am impressed by their similarity. The data on non-smokers shows that the risk of CHD death is much lower for women than for men. Yet given a similar relative risk for a given amount of smoking, it seems that the attributable risk caused by smoking must be much lower for women than for men. I think this can only be explained in terms of interaction with some other risk factor which is also sex related.

Bengttson (Goteborg)   I want to comment on the relationship between smoking, early menopause and myocardial infarction. I think it can explain part, but not all, of the difference between the higher incidence of myocardial infarction in post-menopausal than in pre-menopausal women of the same age.

The data from our case controlled study showed that there is a higher incidence of smoking in women with myocardial infarction than in women with angina pectoris. The prevalence however was different since there were fewer smokers among the women with angina pectoris than in the control group. In the control group, about 40 percent were smokers, in the myocardial infarction group 80 percent and in the angina pectoris group 28 percent. It is important that we separate women with myocardial infarction from women with angina pectoris for they are not the same. The incidence in female smokers is about the same as in male non-smokers. The difference between the extreme groups is very marked comparing female non-smokers than in smokers. It seems that there is a relative risk in smoking women and proportionately higher than in smoking men.

Epstein (Zurich)   Dr. Slack emphasised that familial resemblances for CHD cannot be wholly explained on the basis of inheritance of cholesterol and blood pressure levels. Years ago I showed that it seemed as if blood pressure and smoking could not account for familial aggregations. While the relationships between parents and children are statistically significant in regard to cholesterol and blood pressure, the resemblance in smoking habits between parents and children are perhaps more striking. The greater influence, or the seemingly greater influence of the mother in the habits of the child, with regard to nutrition is probably also true with regard to smoking. Young women who smoke have a particularly strong influence on the smoking habits of their children. In particular, a young mother who subsequently develops coronary heart disease may have a different influence on the smoking habits of her children. What do we know about the restraints in smoking habits between parents and children or other relatives at different ages, by sex? It is an important question, both from the point of view of prevention and from the point of view of explaining at least part of the familial aggregations of CHD.

McMahon (Boston)   We have some data on high school children aged 15-17 years. The percentage of smokers among the children where both parents smoked was of the order of 80 percent; where one parent smoked it was about 60 percent and when neither parent smoked it was about 40 percent. There was no difference with regard to which parent smoked or whether only one smoked and the other did not. The sex of the child did not influence the very strong correlation with either, or particularly both, parents smoking.

Epstein (Zurich)   Was there any difference with regard to age? Did younger parents affect their children more strikingly than older parents?

McMahon (Boston)   We did not check that.

Venning (High Wycombe)   It seems to me, particularly after Dr. Slack's presentation, that evidence of a relationship between cigarette smoking and CHD would have to be based on independence simultaneously of all known risk factors. Your list specifically excluded social class and genetic factors. So I would like to ask whether any of the evidence presented contributes actual evidence of relationship between smoking and heart disease.

Rose   The only evidence that would get close to proof of causality would be a trial in which a randomised half of a defined group were given cigarettes and compared with the other half who had never smoked. This is not possible. A randomised trial of withdrawal of cigarettes is possible, but a trial of withdrawal is only indirect evidence. A cause may be a cause, but it's effect is not necessarily reversible. So, I don't think that one should refuse to draw a conclusion because proof is not available. If one were to show that within defined social classes, there are still differences in risk between smokers and non-smokers independent of other risk factors, the possibility still exists that there are class or environmentally related factors that are not sufficiently standardised. The Registrar General's classification of five social classes is an extraordinarily crude method of standardising for social class. I think that there is a consistency from a lot of evidence that much of the smoking association is causal although it is unlikely that it all is.

Bonnar (Dublin)   There is in these islands considerable variation in the age of menopause. In the Scottish Hebrides, the mean age approaches 53-55. The figure that you gave in your data in a smoking population was 46-47. It is higher than this in the North of Scotland and probably in Scandinavia.

Doll (Oxford)   We must be careful not to confuse means and medians.

Wald   The mean age was around 47. The median is about 2 years more.

Vessey (Oxford) I think data based on recalled 'age of menopause' is the only sound method of assessment to classifying a woman by her status at a given point in time.

Wald I did the analysis both ways and the results were very similar.

Wynn (London) By how much would the CHD incidence have to change due to the menopause before it would show on a semilogarithmic plot? If the contribution of the menopause is an increase in coronary heart mortality of 20 percent, would that be identifiable?

Wald There would be a change in the slope if the rate of change were 20 percent.

Gordon (Bethesda) This has bothered us. I have assumed that one group of women had a risk double that of the other. When the two curves were merged very little change occurred. One can actually take two different distributions and merge them and find that the evidence of merging is varied in terms of a trend. There was very little evidence of any upward turn, well illustrated in the cross-sectional data.

Charkrabarti (London) We are engaged in a prospective study of 3000 people concerning the prediction of CHD. In addition to the usual risk factors — blood pressure, serum cholesterol, smoking etc — we are studying coagulation factors. Fibrinolytic activity is depressed by smoking. This activity is the ability to dissolve fibrin and so the higher the activity the better for the person so far as prevention of thrombosis is concerned.

Mitchell (Nottingham) While it is theoretically better for the fibrinolytic level to be higher there is no actual evidence that it is. To say that it is better to have a high value is going ahead of the evidence which you are going to collate.

Spain (Brooklyn) In our study of autopsies on sudden deaths, in which retrospective studies on smoking history was obtained, realising all the difficulties, we do not see smoking as a factor which increased the rate of sudden death. In 1000 autopsies, or so, with sudden death, defined as a first witnessed event dying within half an hour we found thrombi in 15 percent of the group as a whole and in 15 percent of smokers, non-smokers, women and men.

Gordon (Bethesda) In general serum cholesterol and blood pressure are lower in cigarette smokers than non-smokers. These two other risk factors are enhancing the risk of not smoking. In other words multi-variate analysis *are* necessary to take other risk factors into account. Generally speaking, the association between cigarette smoking and myocardial infarction or other forms of CHD death is greater in the multi-variate analysis.

Muir (Edinburgh) Presumably the relationship between smoking and CHD must depend on the inhaled dose, but there is no difference between those who inhale and those who don't inhale. Is this just because we are liars about smoking habits? We have been studying patients with chronic bronchitis who are on long term oxygen therapy and we have been totally convinced that they were telling us the truth, but when we measured carboxyhaemoglobin (COHb) levels, there was no relation between what they said about their smoking habits and blood carbon monoxide levels.

Doll (Oxford) We should be careful of the meaning of the words we use. To accuse people of being liars when they say they inhale or don't inhale on the basis of their blood carbon monoxide is not quite fair because by inhaling the person may either mean that they inhale into the small bronchi or only into the upper trachea.

Wald We classified subjects according to the number of cigarettes they smoked before blood was taken for COHb estimation. We also classified them by their self-described inhaling category into those who said they did not inhale at all, inhaled slightly, moderately, and deeply. The mean COHb level in each of these categories increased with the amount smoked before the test. Although there was not a lot of overlap between these categories, in general people who said they did not inhale had lower COHb levels and those who said that they inhaled deeply had higher COHb levels. The magnitude of the relationship was small, and in small numbers one would be very unlikely to detect a correlation between self-described inhaling categories and COHb levels. In very large numbers, one would expect to find a positive association between self-described inhalation and disease.

Spain (Brooklyn) Our study was originally designed to study bronchial changes in relation to smokers with metaplasia as the end point and we found that in 100 percent of the cases with sudden death there was metaplasia of the bronchial tree, whereas in the population as a whole only 50 percent had such pathological changes − probably due to pollution or other factors.

Gordon (Bethesda) In the multiple risk factor prevention trial, very clear dose response relationship was evident in the data between the number of cigarettes smoked and COHb levels, similar to what you have shown. In general, they were telling the truth. The question of inhaling or not inhaling may be a question of perception.

Doll (Oxford) I would like to give you the results I've been able to get out recently on the mortality of women doctors in relation to their smoking habits. We have not been able, as yet, to calculate the women years at risk in the 22 years of observation on 5000 women doctors. There were 163 deaths attributed to coronary thrombosis in women by smoking habits, compared with 494 women who died from diseases which from the male study could be defined as not being associated with smoking. Analysis of these results after standardising for age gives a relative risk value for the light smoker (1-14 a day) compared with a non-smoker of 1; for the moderate smoker (15-24 a day) 1.8; and for those smoking 25 or more a day, 2.5. These are very similar results to those obtained in men. We had only 6 deaths attributed to coronary thrombosis in women under 55 and therefore, it is not worth making an analysis below this age.

Another point I would like to make refers to this difficult question of how you interpret all these relationships and I entirely agree with what Professor Rose has said. There is a general consistency in a large amount of data throughout the world, any sample of which can be explained in several different ways, but which when taken all together is extremely difficult to explain other than on the basis that cigarette smoking is a causal factor. One example relating to women of this consistency is that the highest rate of CHD mortality in the world in women is found in women who smoke the most in the world — namely, the Maori women in New Zealand. Another evidence of consistency is one found within doctors. It may well be that doctors in different specialities have entirely different eating habits and different personalities, but general practitioners in this country have had about a 40 percent higher mortality from coronary thrombosis between 1951 and 1971, compared with hospital consultant physicians and the amount they have smoked has, on average, been just about 40 percent more than the hospital consultant. This is another example of the type of data which becomes increasingly difficult to explain by common factors associated both with smoking and production of CHD.

SESSION 2 Arterial wall

Chairman: G.A. Gresham

Pathology

Arteriography

6. Concerning the pathology of acute coronary heart disease in young women

DAVID M. SPAIN

Three acute events are characteristic of coronary heart disease — angina pectoris, myocardial infarction and sudden death. Statistical studies indicate that acute myocardial infarction is on the increase in pre-menopausal women and this has been attributed to oral contraceptive use (Mann *et al*, 1975). Other studies suggest that in individuals with coronary heart disease, the chances for sudden death are greater in heavy cigarette smokers. This may account for the seeming recent increase in sudden death in young women (Spain *et al*, 1973). The mechanisms whereby oral contraceptives and cigarette smoking operates in these situations has never been clearly defined. In any case their roles appear to be different and what these might be is the subject of this report.

Oral contraceptives and myocardial infarction

The statistical association between acute myocardial infarction and oral contraceptive use was generally unanticipated because of the strong evidence supporting the view that the higher physiological levels of estrogens in women was regarded as a major reason for the relatively greater immunity to coronary heart disease enjoyed by pre-menopausal women (Stamler, 1971). Therefore any concept of the pathogenesis whereby oral contraceptives precipitate acute myocardial infarction must account for this and reconcile this seeming contradiction. Assigning a specific role to oestrogens in this problem is complicated by the varied ways oestrogen may exert an influence on different aspects of the process leading to acute myocardial infarction. Oestrogen affects the atherogenic process, the level of serum lipids, lipoproteins and their transport, the local morphology of the vascular intima, the structure and function of platelets and the thrombogenic process. This report will focus on those morphologic alterations which may affect the atheromatous lesion in the coronary arteries. This in turn may play a key role in the chain of events leading to myocardial infarction.

Sources of information

The findings upon which the comments and conclusions in this report are based are derived from the following sources:—
1. A review of published reports of the autopsy observations in fatal cases and of the angiographic findings in non-fatal cases of young oral contraceptive users who developed acute myocardial infarction;

2. A review of the morphologic alteration in the arteries of pre-menopausal women which have been attributed to higher than usual levels of sex steroids as seen in the last trimester of pregnancy, in the post-partum period or with oral contraceptive use;
3. A review of the pertinent experimental studies in animals concerning the influence of oestrogens, progestagens and oral contraceptives on atherogenesis and on the role of oestrogens in the removal of cholesterol at a local tissue level;
4. Detailed autopsy observations on the lesions in the coronary arteries in three young contraceptive pill users who were free of most risk factors (except for cigarette smoking) for coronary heart disease and who also died shortly after the onset of acute myocardial infarction.

This is the crucial portion of this study because an essential first step in the resolution of this problem requires a determination of the nature of the basic coronary arterial lesion responsible for the acute ischaemia leading to myocardial infarction. For this purpose it was essential to study only the younger women with limited or no coronary heart disease risk factors and who died shortly after the onset of the acute event. This was necessary in order to avoid the significant lesion from being obscured by widespread and advanced atherosclerosis, and also to prevent the passage of time with healing from masking the essential ingredients in the early lesion. These preconditions severely reduced for study the availability of an already limited number of cases. Fortunately, we were able to locate and gain access to three carefully performed autopsies which filled these preconditions.

Morphological findings in women

Published reports of cases with autopsies or with coronary angiograms revealed with few exceptions, in each instance an isolated segment of major coronary artery occlusion, most often located in the proximal left anterior descending branch. Elsewhere in that vessel and in the other major coronary arteries there was little or no evidence of more than focal or minimal atherosclerosis. In two cases there was more than one major occlusion. All of the occlusive lesions were described as having the characteristics of thrombi. Unfortunately, significant details of the morphology in the coronary artery forming the nidus for the thrombus were lacking.

In the coronary arteriograms the extent of the luminal obstruction was directly related to the length of the interval between the onset of the acute infarction and the performance of the coronary arteriography, the longer the interval the less the degree of stenosis. This has been explained by the partial resolution of the original thrombus with progression of time.

The morphologic alterations in pregnancy, in the post-partum period and with oral contraceptives, in the absence of atherosclerosis, consisted of local changes in the intima of such arteries as the pulmonary, mesenteric and an occasional coronary artery. These were regarded by the investigators as specific and consisted of endothelial proliferation and intimal thickening without any alterations in the media or adventitia. A second change consisted of focal nodular thickening of the intima, media or adventitia. The nodularity was probably related to medial cell proliferation. A third and most frequent change consisted of a three layered thrombus related to areas of focal intimal thickening. Thrombosis was found in the mesenteric and pulmonary arteries but not in the coronary artery. No athero-sclerosis was described in association with these changes (Irey *et al*, 1970). The three layered thrombus showed variation in degrees of organisation.

Experimental studies.   It has been demonstrated that the administration of oestrone in rabbits and mice stimulates macrophage activity and facilitates the removal of cholesterol from local subcutaneous implants of gelfoam sponges previously impregnated with cholesterol. Examination after 35 days of oestrone administration revealed marked infiltration with macrophages, many of which have become laden with lipids. Macrophages were much fewer in the implants of the placebo treated control group. In the oestrone treated animals cholesterol implants were much smaller than in the placebo treated control. Only scant lipid remained in the implants of the oestrone treated animals. Repetition of the experi-ment with rabbits maintained on an atherogenic diet revealed the same results despite the high serum cholesterol levels (Spain *et al*, 1959). When norethnodrel with mestranol was given to rabbits simultaneously with the administration of an atherogenic diet the development of atherosclerosis was inhibited (Spain and Mestel, 1965).

Most pertinent was the experimental production of ulceration in atheroma in cockerels by first placing these birds on an atherogenic diet for 5-8 weeks, allowing time for atheroma to develop. The birds were then treated with conjugated equine oestrogens for a period of 1-5 weeks (Pick *et al*, 1962). Sequential sacrifice revealed with time an increasing frequency of ulcerated atheroma in the aorta and coronary arteries. This reached a pead of 40 percent ulceration in three to four weeks. Also with time the healing changes in the atheroma superceded the destructive lesions. Only an occasional ulceration occurred in the control group of chicks maintained only on a high atherogenic diet. These investigators stated that ulceration with oestrogen treatment was predictably limited to those lesions containing a core of lipid pools covered with rigid fibro-hyaline caps. It was suggested that the oestrogens caused the atheroma to ulcerate by first stimulating the removal of lipid from the atheromatous core. General dissolution with softening of the lesion followed causing the rigid cap to collapse and fracture under the influence of hemodynamic forces.

Findings in the specially selected autopsies.   The women were 24, 31 and 33 years old and had been using oral contraceptives for a period ranging from 10 months to 5 years up to the point of the acute fatal event. Except for cigarette smoking they had no known coronary heart disease risk factors. All 3 died in a short period after the onset of the acute event. The 3 cases contained four recent occlusive thrombi. Three were located in the proximal LAD branch and one in the right coronary artery. The morphologic findings were similar in the three cases. Atheroma formed the nidus upon which the coronary thrombi were formed. These were minimal to moderate in size and their cores consisted of atheromatous debris in a state of dissolution with extensive extracellular pools of lipid. There was focal infiltration with lipid laden macrophages. Modified medial cells, a few with atypical and enlarged nuclei were actively proliferating into the base and sides of the atheroma. The activity was such that the cells appeared to be growing in a tissue culture. Of interest, similar change in the smooth muscle cells in uterine leiomyoma under the influence of oral contraceptives has been reported (Fechner, 1967). Surrounding and involving the periphery of the atheromatous core was an intensive inflammatory reaction. Overlying the softened cores were fibro-hyaline caps which in places were fractured leaving a denuded and hemorr-hagic surface with adherent recent thrombi (Figs. 6.1, 6.2 and 6.3). A stenotic lesion, proximal to the occlusive thrombus in one case revealed an almost acellular intimal thickening with collagen deposition, some medial cell proliferation and no visible lipid (Fig. 6.4). The few other lesions scattered throughout the major branches were minimal, fibrotic and almost entirely devoid of visible lipid.

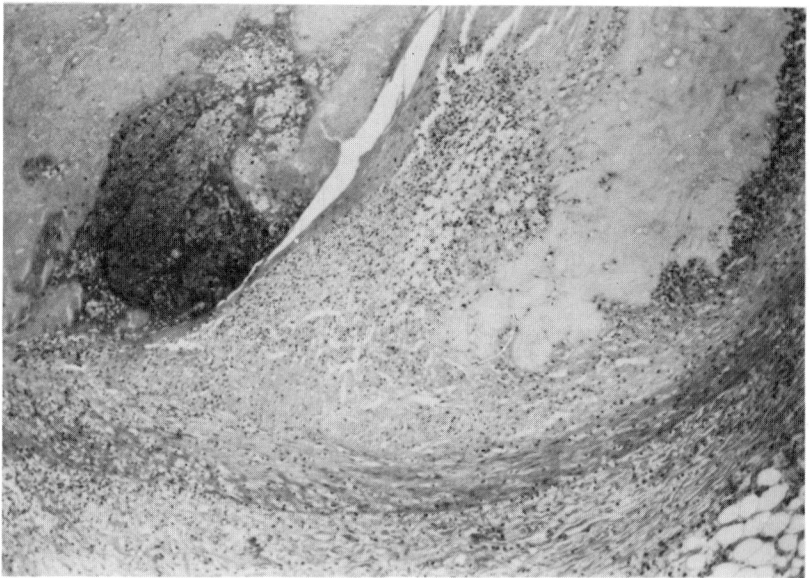

Fig. 6.1 Photomicrograph (H & E x40) showing disrupted atheroma with lipid pools, medial cell proliferation, many foam cells and inflammation. Fibro-hyaline cap is fractured with an adherent recent thrombus.

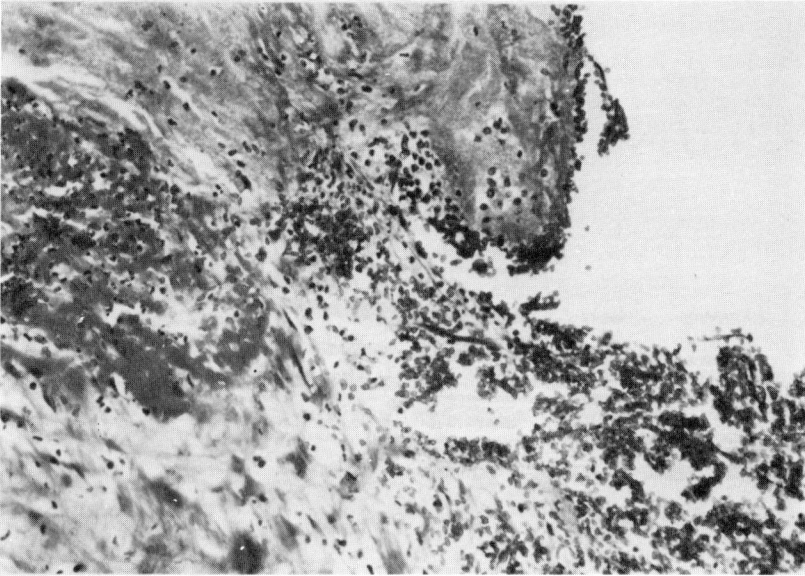

Fig. 6.2 Photomicrograph (H & E x40) showing edge of atheromatous ulcer with focal haemorrhage.

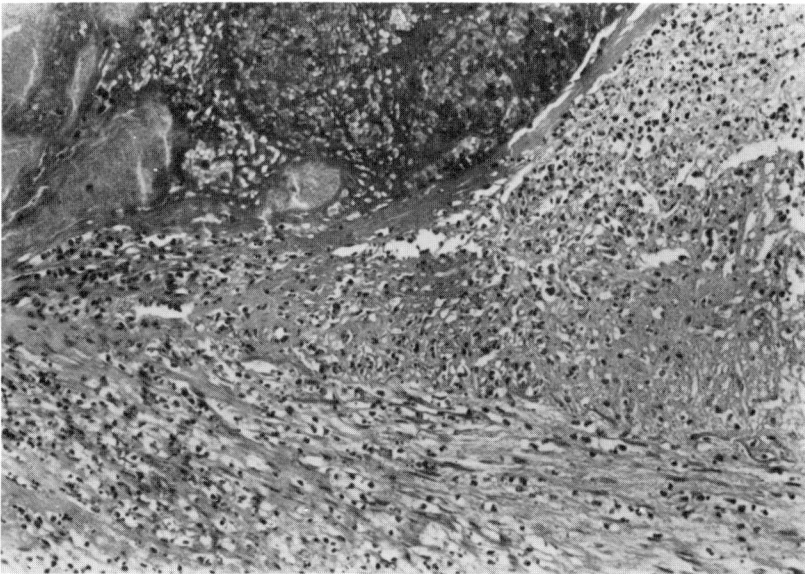

Fig. 6.3 Photomicrograph (H & E x100) showing a close-up view of Figure 1 focusing on the break in the continuity of the thin cap adherent to which is a recent thrombus.

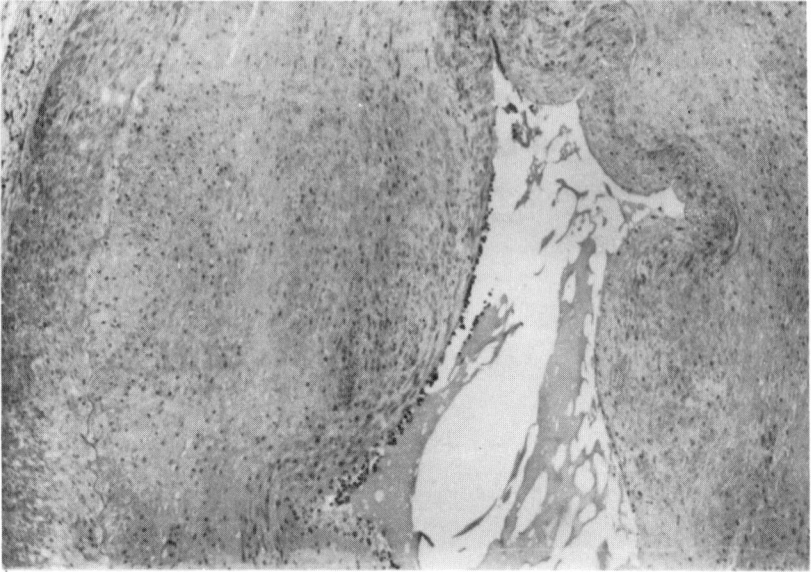

Fig. 6.4 Photomicrograph (H & E x40) showing partially stenosed healed lesion.

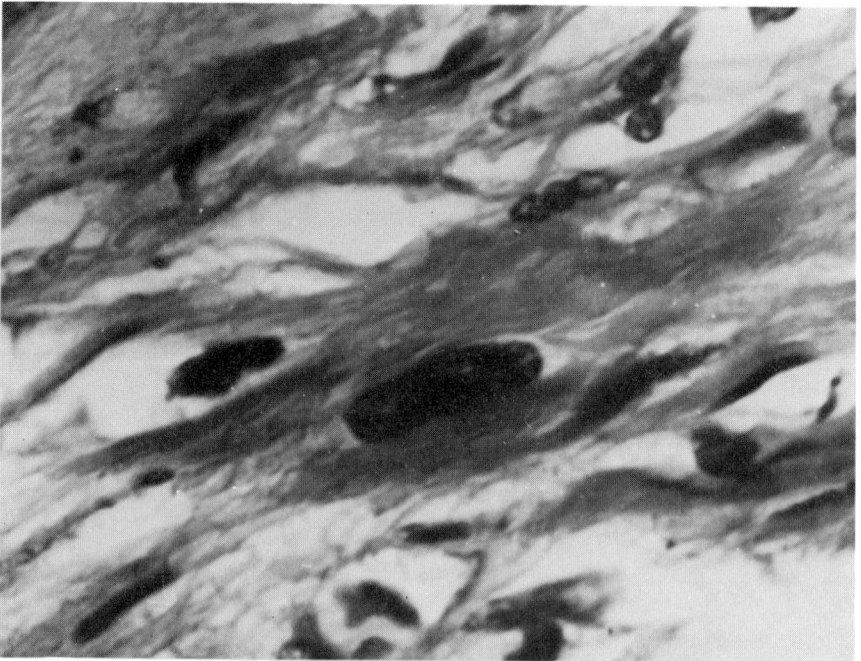

Fig. 6.5 Photomicrograph (H & E x320) showing enlarged view of medial cells containing enlarged and hyperchromatic nuclei.

Comments

Substantial clinical, post-mortem and experimental observations support the established view that a systemic influence of oestrogen on lipids and lipid transport tend to inhibit the atherogenic process. This fact plus the lack of any close correlation between the length of exposure to oral contraceptives with the risk of developing acute myocardial infarction; the increased risk for myocardial infarction at higher oestrogen dose levels where the effect on serum lipid levels is greatest; and the rapid return to a low-risk state for developing myocardial infarction after short intervals of discontinuation of oral contraceptives argue against a direct acceleration of atherogenesis as the underlying reason for the increased risk in oral contraceptive users. The influence of oestrogen on thrombogenesis cannot be invoked as a primary reason because coronary thrombosis is rare in the absence of an underlying atheromatous ulcer.

The striking similarity between the circumstances and the nature of the coronary artery lesion leading to myocardial infarction in the autopsied cases and that seen in the chicks is highly significant. In both there was intense cellular infiltration, acute inflammation and medial cell proliferation (the medial cell is believed by many to be crucial in the local development of the atheroma). Unfortunately, there is no single pathognomonic feature which unequivocally distinguishes spontaneous atheromatous ulceration from that induced by oestrogens. There are certain features however in the currently presented cases which are quantitatively greater than usually seen in the spontaneous ulcerations. For example there is the very active proliferation of medial cells with highly atypical nuclear changes. To our knowledge this does not occur in spontaneous ulceration. In spontaneous ulceration the atheroma are larger, encroach more on the lumen and are inevitably associated with more advanced and widespread atherosclerosis in the remainder of the major coronary arteries. Ulcers are believed to form as a result of accretion of the underlying atheroma producing attenuation of the overlying cap. In contrast to this the oestrogen induced atheroma is a result of softening and reduction in the size of the atheroma. This in turn mobilises the cap making it vulnerable to dislocation and fracture under the stress of coronary flow pulse pressure. The pulse pressure in the coronary arteries is unique because of cardia contractility and ranges from a maximum pressure to zero pressure.

There is a close correlation between the risk for developing atheroma vulnerable to ulceration under the influence of oestrogens and the risk for developing acute myocardial infarction from oestrogens or oral contraceptive use. The risk is greater in those exhibiting the major coronary heart disease risk factors as diabetes mellitus, hypertension and hyperlipidemia. The risk is greater in the older pre-menopausal women than in the younger and a risk is greater in men than in women as for example as seen in the Coronary Drug Project where men who were known to have advanced coronary disease were treated with a 5.0 mg. daily dose of natural oestrogen experienced approximately twice the number of acute coronary events than did the placebo treated control group. The point is that for oestrogens to cause ulceration, vulnerable atheroma must be present which can become disrupted and softened causing the thin but rigid fibro-hyaline cap to collapse and fracture.

In the experimental studies where oestrogens had been introduced simultaneously with a high atherogenic diet, ulcer-prone atheroma had no chance to develop and hence no ulcerations were seen. Where an atherogenic diet preceded the treatment with oestrogens, the passage of time allowed for vulnerable atheroma to develop. The later introduction of oestrogens produced ulcerations in these lesions.

Certain conclusions can be drawn from the previous observations. The occurrence of acute myocardial infarction in contraceptive pill users may to a great extent be dependent, if not entirely so, on the presence of atheroma vulnerable to ulceration. The precipitation of ulceration appears to be dose dependent. Excess levels of oestrogen are required whether their origin is endogenous or exogenous. The duration of contraceptive use does not appear to correlate closely with the frequency of acute myocardial infarction.

The role of oestrogen induced alterations in the vascular intima, independent of atherosclerosis, and its effect on platelets and the thrombotic process in the pathogenesis of myocardial infarction is unclear and requires further investigation. The pathogenesis of myocardial infarction in oral contraceptive pill users, as suggested in this report, has the added feature of resolving the seeming contradiction between the relative immunity granted to pre-menopausal women against atherosclerosis because of their naturally higher oestrogen levels and the increased risk for the precipitation of acute myocardial infarction in contraceptive pill users and in men receiving relatively high doses of oestrogen for coronary heart disease or prostatic cancer.

Women smokers and sudden death from coronary disease

Although there is some autopsy evidence that cigarette smokers have more coronary atherosclerosis at comparable ages than do non-smokers (Strang *et al*, 1966) the effect of cigarette smoking on atherogenesis does not seem to be an important factor in increased morbidity and mortality. The exact time or site in the life history of coronary heart disease where cigarette smoking might exert its harmful effect has not been definitely pinpointed. Numerous studies suggest that cigarette smoking might play its key role in the precipitation of acute coronary events especially of sudden and unexpected death in individuals already harboring advanced coronary atherosclerosis.

Heavy cigarette smoking has increased considerably in women in the past decade. To determine the relationship of this change in women's smoking habits a retrospective autopsy study was made of the smoking habits of women who died suddenly and unexpectedly of a first clinical episode of coronary heart disease. A close correlation between heavy cigarette smoking and sudden deaths was found. In the sudden deaths from causes other than coronary heart disease, only 28 percent of the women were heavy smokers, whereas in the coronary heart disease sudden deaths there were 62 percent. The mean age at the time of sudden death was 19 years less for those who smoked cigarettes heavily than for non-smokers, while the mean age of death for lighter smokers was intermediate. During the period of 1949-1959, in the population group studied, there were 12 coronary heart disease sudden deaths in men for every similar death in women. In contrast, there were only four of these sudden deaths in men for every similar death in

1967 through 1971 among women. The shift has been associated with an increase in heavy cigarette smoking among women.

Although as yet there are no definitive answers, several mechanisms have been suggested for the precipitation of an acute episode of ischemia which would lead to sudden death in individuals already exhibiting widespread stenotic coronary atherosclerosis. Studies of catecholamine secretion and free fatty acid mobilisation stimulated by an inhalation of cigarette smoke may provide a partial rational explanation for some of these adverse effects of cigarettes in individuals already at a precarious state of balance between the ability of the coronary circulation to supply the myocardial needs and any rise in these myocardial needs (Kershbaum et al, 1967). Some claim that chronic elevation of carbon monoxide levels in the blood may be an important factor in the precipitation of sudden death. The important point is that in these sudden death cases no new or recent changes are found in the coronary arteries to explain the sudden development of an acute fatal ischemic event. Both in men and in women as well as in smokers and non-smokers who die suddenly from coronary heart disease the proportion of cases exhibiting recent changes such as a fresh thrombus rarely exceeds 15 percent. This has not changed in the women smokers who have died suddenly. This would indicate that cigarette smoking does not increase the risk for sudden death through any effect on thrombogenesis. The influence of cigarette smoking appears to be functional and not related to any specific morphologic alteration.

References

Fechner, R. (1967) Atypical leiomyomas and synthetic progestin therapy. *Am. J. Clin. Path.* **49**, 697-703.

Irey, N.S., Manion, W.C., Taylor, H.B. (1970) Vascular lesions in women taking oral contraceptives. *Arch. Path.* **89**, 1-9.

Kershbaum, A. *et al.* (1967) Regular, filter tip, and modified cigarettes: Nicotine excretion, free fatty acid mobilisation, and catecholamine excretion. *JAMA*, **201**, 545-546.

Mann, J.I., Vessey, M.P., Thorogood, M., Doll, R. (1975) Myocardial infarction in young women with special reference to oral contraceptive practice. *Brit. Med. J.* **2**, 241-245.

Pick, R., Katz, T.N., Century, D., Johnson, P.J. (1962) Production of ulcerated atherosclerotic lesions in cockerels. *Circ. Res.* **11**, 811-819.

Spain, D.M., Aristozabal, N., Ores, R. (1959) Effect of oestrogens on resolution of local cholesterol implants. *Arch. Path.* **68**, 30-33.

Spain, D.M., Mestel, A.L. (1965) Influence of norethnodrel and mestranol in atherogenesis rabbits. *Circulation II*, **31 & 32: 32.**

Spain, D.M., Siegel, H. and Bradess, V.A. (1973) Women Smokers and sudden death — the relationship of cigarette smoking to coronary disease. *JAMA*, **224**, 1005-1007.

Stamler, J. (1971) Current status of knowledge on oestrogen treatment of hyperlipidemia and atherosclerotic disease in Casdorph HR: Treatment of hyperlipidemia states, Charles C. Thomas, *Springfield, Ill,* 310-322.

Strong, J.P. *et al.* (1966) Relationships between cigarette smoking habits and coronary atherosclerosis on autopsied males, abstracted. *Circulation,* **31**, 33-34.

7. Coronary arteriosclerosis in women

G. A. GRESHAM

The concept of an 'epidemic' of coronary heart disease in white males in America and Europe has been supported, over the years, by a vast amount of work from various centres. Many aspects of the problem have been studied, the main facets being epidemiological, clinical and pathological. Much of the work has been done on male subjects; it is only in relatively recent times that similar reports have dealt with the problem in women. Whilst it is true that the incidence of ischaemic heart disease is lower in the premenopausal female than in the male there is nevertheless a growing appreciation of the fact that ischaemic heart disease in younger women is increasing in incidence. Parrish et al (1966), investigated the epidemiology of coronary heart disease in white women aged 40 and over. This was done by examining the autopsy records of about 6,000 women and grading the degree of coronary artery disease at various ages.

They found a significant increase in the incidence of coronary artery disease in women with and without diabetes mellitus in the 25 years starting in 1935. They also found that pre-existent hypertension aggravated the degree of coronary artery disease in every age group that they studied. There was no association between body weight at the time of death and the degree of coronary artery disease. It must be remembered however that the weight at death may not be an accurate representation of the weight of the subject in life. They also found an increase in the incidence of the disease in the coronary arteries of women whom they regarded as reasonably representative of the general population. Such persons died as a result of accidents of one sort or another. This increase could hardly be accounted for by a change in genetic predisposition and could be much better explained by multiple, additive aetiological factors which were occurring in the environment during the period from 1935 to 1959.

These results contradicted the work of Moriyama et al (1958) and Stamler (1959). The first authors suggest that there had been an increase in deaths amongst males from cardiovascular and renal disease whereas the rates for females had, in fact decreased. Stamler suggested that there had been no change in the rates for women whereas that for males had increased. It is clear, however, that Moriyama and Stamler were measuring different parameters from those observed by Parrish et al. The former were studying death rates, the latter were measuring the degree of coronary artery disease. It could well be that similar degrees of coronary artery narrowing were more compatible with longer survival in the female than in the male and this might have explained the discrepancy in the results.

71

One of the major problems in appraising the evidence for an increase in the incidence of coronary heart disease in women is presented by differences in the definition of atherosclerosis and considerable variations in the methods used to examine the cardiac vessels. An agreed specification of the initial stages of the atherosclerotic process is an essential prerequisite for an understanding of the results of animal experiments: particularly those concerned with the effects of oestrogens and progestrogens on the arterial wall.

A wide range of possible initial events have been proposed for the atherogenic process. These range from deposition of platelets and fibrin on damaged or intact endothelium, deposition of lipids, in particular cholesterol esters such as the oleate or lipoproteins in the intima, increased endothelial permeability, fragmentation and fraying of the internal elastic lamella, to deposition of proteoglycans. All of these suggested possibilities have one common feature which is an association with smooth muscle cell proliferation in the altered intima.

Some workers doubt whether any of the proposed processes for initial atherogenesis are the precursors of the advanced ulcerated atheromatous plaque which leads to occlusion of the artery either by the size of the lesion itself or because of superimposed thrombosis. There has for example, been considerable debate about the significance of the fatty streak or spot which is found in the arteries of young persons in their teens. They are found mainly in the thoracic aorta near to the intercostal orifices and also in a line above the aortic valve cusps in the ascending part of the aortic arch. Because these sites are less commonly the seat of advanced atherosclerotic disease, complicated by ulceration and often by thrombosis, it has been argued that fatty streaks are unlikely to be the first steps in the atherogenic process. The fatty streak is largely composed of smooth muscle with lipid in and between the cells. There is no doubt that animal experiments have shown them to be reversible lesions disappearing when the atherogenic stimulus such as dietary cholesterol or hypertension are reversed. This being so it is possible that thoracic aortic lesions disappear from those vessels to reappear elsewhere in the aorta at a later age and to progress to advanced atherosclerosis. Alterations in pressure and flow that occur in the arteries of growing animals would account for the varying stimulus to different parts of the intimal surface as the individual gets older.

Studies of the incidence of coronary artery disease are also complicated by considerable variations in techniques used to investigate the vessels. The degree of atherosclerotic narrowing is an example of one aspect that shows considerable differences in incidence in reports of various workers. There are some who prefer to examine the arteries by opening them along their lengths, others cut them transversely at intervals of a millimetere or so. The former method gives a better assessment of the extent of atherosclerosis along the course of the artery. The latter method provides a more accurate measure of the degree of narrowing at various points and can be made more precise by the use of callipers. Both methods are useless, if there is extensive calcification of the diseased artery, unless there is prior decalcification of the vessel. This is not often done and provides the explanation of much of the confusion about the incidence of coronary artery disease. For example the reported association of thrombosis with severe atheroma varies from as little as 20 to 90 percent. The latter figure was reported by Harland and Holburn (1966) following decalcification of the vessels and detailed serial block sectioning.

In recent years there has been a radical change of view about the early stages of the atherosclerotic process (Gresham (1975)) and this has to some extent produced varied figures about the incidence of the disease. It has also affected the interpretation of experimental studies in animals. Lesions which were hitherto regarded as early atherosclerosis have been rejected and others have become acceptable. Few would doubt, nowadays, that the fatty streak or spot is a stage of atherosclerosis but many would agree that more fundamental changes precede it and that fatty streaks are only one aspect of the early disease in which lipid accumulation preponderates.

Vlodaver *et al* (1969) studied changes in the intima of the coronary arteries of three ethnic groups: Ashkenazy, Yemenites and Bedouins. The basic structural change in the arteries of children from these three groups, under the age of 10, was essentially the same but they varied in degree. The changes consisted of fragmentation and duplications of the internal elastic lamella with proliferation of subendothelial fibroblasts, collagen formation and subsequent intimal thickening. They considered that such changes represented an early step in the atherosclerotic process because the degree of intimal thickening, which was greatest in the Ashkenazy and Yemenite males, related well with the degree of coronary athero- sclerosis found in these ethnic groups, in later life.

Recent research has been concerned with even earlier changes than those described by Vlodaver *et al* (1969). These changes were produced by experimentally denuding a patch of endothelial cells and then studying the subsequent changes in the following days and weeks. The surface endothelium was removed from parts of the aorta by means of a balloon catheter inserted into the vessel through the femoral artery; other mechanical methods of injury have also been employed. Following endothelial injury there is a rapid proliferation of intimal smooth muscle cells. This occurs within a day or so of the experimental damage. Most workers now regard endothelial injury and smooth muscle proliferation as the earliest atherogenic event. The cause of endothelial injury in man is not yet determined. There may be more than one cause; some that have been postulated include haemodynamic stresses as they occur in hypertension, hypoxia associated with cigarette smoking, hyperlipidaemia and so on.

The factor concerned with smooth muscle cell proliferation after endothelial injury is more clearly defined. Harker *et al* (1974) noted the high incidence of thrombotic vascular occlusions in patients with the rare disorder of homocysteinuria and attempted to reproduce the same situation in baboons by infusing l. homo- cystine. The effect was to increase turnover of blood platelets and to produce endothelial cells that circulated freely in the blood. When the vessels were examined by the Hautchen method they found that areas of the endothelium had been de- nuded. Subsequent experiments showed a reactive proliferation of smooth muscle cells in areas of denudation and a factor causing this cell growth was identified from the blood platelets. It was found to be a protein of low molecular weight which caused smooth muscle cells to proliferate when tested on such cells which had been grown in tissue culture.

Smooth muscle cell proliferations have been described in the intima of arteries in women by Ivey and Norris (1973). Such changes are associated with variable amounts of proteglycan deposition and are associated with changes in the hormonal status. It is seen for example in vessels of postmenopausal women, it also occurs in pregnancy and has been well documented particularly in the uterine vessels of man and animals such as the guinea pig. Waves of proliferation occur with each pregnancy in many ways reminiscent of growth rings in a tree. Changes occur not only in arteries but also in veins and recent interest has centred upon the possible effects of oestrogenic substances in their production.

Rats treated with synthetic sex hormones such as ethinyl oestradiol develop intimal thickenings in the aorta, carotid, mesenteric and renal arteries in 30 days (Gammal (1976)). Gammal injected ethinyl oestradiol and the progestogen, chlormadinone acetate daily into rats for either 30 or 90 days. Using light and scanning electron microscopy he found subendothelial smooth muscle cell proliferation to be the most constant finding. At 30 days the effects of the combined treatment was not different from that produced with the oestrogen alone. But at 90 days it was significantly less in arteries other than the aorta in the combined group, suggesting that the progestogen inhibited the enhancing effect on the proliferation process in these arteries. These experiments also emphasise an important point in atherosclerosis research which is that studies of atherosclerotic changes in the aorta do not necessarily reflect changes in arteries elsewhere in the body.

The arterial lesions produced by oestrogens are similar to those produced in experimental animals by feeding atherogenic diets (Gresham 1973). This is a perplexing story because many other workers have shown reduction of induced hyperlipidemia, lowering of cholesterol-phospholipid ratios and even regression of induced lesions when oestrogens are given (Robinson (1965)).

There is little doubt that the use of ethinyloestradiol when myocardial infarction is established does no good. Indeed the effects might prove deleterious as oestrogen tends to increase the incidence of thromboembolic episodes (Oliver and Boyd (1961)).

The cause of the increasing incidence of coronary heart disease in women is clearly a complex problem. The variable interplay of sex hormones on the vascular tree and upon blood coagulation may be of major importance particularly as it now seems that intimal damage and platelet activity may combine together to initiate atherogenesis.

References

Gammal, E.B. (1976) Intimal Thickening in Arteries of Rats Treated with Synthetic Sex Hormones. *Br. J. exp. Path.* **57**, 248-254.

Gresham, G.A. (1973) The Use of Primates in Cardiovascular Research. In *Non-Human Primates in Medical Research*, 225-244 ed. G.H. Bourne. Academic Press. New York and London.

Gresham, G.A. (1975) Early Events in Atherogenesis. *Lancet,* **i**, 614-617.

Harker, L.A., Slichter, S.J., Scott, C.R. and Ross, R. (1974) Homocystinemia — Vascular Injury and Arterial Thrombosis. *New England Journal of Med.* **291**, 537-543.

Harland, W.A. and Holburn, A.M. (1966) Coronary Thrombosis and Myocardial Infarction. *Lancet,* **ii**, 1158-1160.

Ivey, N.S. and Norris, H.J. (1973) Intimal Vascular Lesions Associated with Female Reproductive Steroids. *Arch. Path.,* **96**, 227-234.

Moriyama, I.M., Woolsey, T.D. and Stamler, J. (1958) Observations on Possible Factors Responsible for the Sex and Race Trends in Cardiovascular — Renal Mortality in the United States. *J. Chronic. Dis.,* **7**, 401-412.

Oliver, M.F. and Boyd, G.S. (1961) Influence of Reduction of Serum Lipids on Prognosis of Coronary Heart Disease. *Lancet,* **ii**, 499-505.

Parrish, H.M., Carr, C.A., Silberg, S.A. and Goldner, J.C. (1966) Increasing Autopsy Incidence of Coronary Heart Disease in Women. *Arch. Int. Med.,* **118**, 436-445.

Robinson, R.W. (1965) Use of Estrogen Therapy in the Treatment of Coronary Heart Disease. *Geriatrics,* **20**, 87-91.

Stamler, J. (1959) The Epidemiology of Atherosclerotic Coronary Artery Disease. *Postgrad. Med.,* **25**, 610-622, 685-701.

Vlodaver, Z., Kahn, H.A. and Neufeld, H.N. (1969) The Coronary Arteries in Early Life in Three Different Ethnic Groups. *Circulation,* **XXXIX**, 541-550.

Discussion 2A

Marquis (Edinburgh)   Why is it, of all the millions of young women on oestrogens, very few of them get such lesions?

Spain   Atherogenesis is not a continuous gradual process. Experimental and human evidence indicates that it occurs in episodes. There may therefore occasionally be a concurrence between the harmful effects of oestrogens and the presence of vulnerable lesions. Many people develop atheromatous lesions with ulcerations but not all of them develop thrombosis.

Somerville (London)   Am I correct in saying that such lesions can happen in the foetus or, if not in the foetus in the first few weeks or months of life, giving rise to something which may lead to a fatty streak?

Gresham   There is no doubt that people have described fatty streaks in stillborns. I have seen only one — they are not very common. Focal intimal oedema can be found in newborns. Focal smooth muscle proliferation can occur at a much later age, 10-12 years, but it is also uncommon and involves a lot of screening of the vessels to identify. Progressive, diffuse uniform thickening of the intima is a human characteristic — not seen, for example in other primates — perhaps because we generally have higher blood pressure.

Mitchell (Nottingham)   How do you know what you have been describing are the initial lesions? The difficulty about the fatty streak argument is that fatty streaks are fairly universally distributed in animal, primates and humans and occur in different areas of the arterial tree from those that are sites of election for raised and complicated lesions. Even if some fatty streaks turn into complicated lesions, the influences that make them do so must be different from those that initiated them. There is no universal progression.

Gresham   The arterial wall is probably in a continuous state of minor injury and repair. The imposition of turbulence, for example, may delay resolution in some areas. The still-born aorta has an internal diameter of about less than half a centimetre and the adult aorta of a man aged 40 has an internal diameter of about 3 centimetres. Such a change on haemodynamics is bound to alter the sheers or pressures on the vessel wall. Some fatty streaks may go, some fatty streaks may stay. How do I know what the first lesion is? Of course, I don't and a lot is circumstantial. For example, intimal oedema occurs with hypoxia by making animals smoke or reducing the oxygen. In the rabbit and monkey, smoking can be followed by smooth muscle proliferation. Intimal oedema also occurs in isolated leg arteries from rats perfused with catecholamines or 5-hydroxy-tryptamine.

Mitchell (Nottingham)   Another problem is that in many injury situations only a monolayer of platelets occurs and this does not actually go on to thrombus formation unless stasis coexists. We are back to Virchow's triad, it seems. Which is the most important? Is it the vessel wall? Is it flow? Is it the blood itself?

Gresham   In the microcirculation in the mesentery of rats, electrical injury immediately causes a clump of platelets to form. This is a substantial clump and will block the lumen temporarily, detach embolise and not recur. Flow must also be impaired. All these are probably essential.

Spain   In the human, thrombosis in the coronary arteries, with rare exceptions, is always superimposed upon ulcerated atheroma. So, we know it is related to that. The importance of stasis of flow as an initial event is not known but in conjunction with ulcerative and fibrotic lesions, which act as a partial obstruction stasis will contribute. There is also tremendous proliferation of thrombogenic substances. It is not simply a monolayer of platelets. In addition, in young women, oestrogens may add to the whole problem as a secondary factor enhancing thrombo-genesis.

Slack (London)   Some of the lesions illustrated by Dr. Spain in women on the pill resemble those seen in familial hypercholesterolaemia.

Beaumont (Paris)   I agree with you. They also looked like the lesions found in homocysteinaemic hypercholesterolaemia. Yet the lesions found in women dying from vascular disease induced by oral contraceptives are usually described as intimal lesions without lipid accumulation. Another point is that in the diseases induced by oral contraceptives, there is not only arterial disease but also venous thrombosis. This is one big difference compared with other arterial diseases, which are usually not associated with venous thrombosis. The risk of oral contraceptives may be different. You emphasised the cellular reaction and an inflammatory reaction. I do not think it is common in atherosclerosis to have such an inflammatory reaction.

Spain   Yes it is!

Oliver (Edinburgh)   Is it clearly established that women, aged 30, killed accidentally, have less total coronary disease than men of that age and also less obstructive disease, which may not be the same thing? Are we clear as to whether the oral contraceptive increases either the fibrotic or ulcerative lesions, or is the effect mostly on thrombus formation?

Spain   The original study that we did on healthy people with accidental death at various age groups clearly showed less atherosclerosis, less obstructive disease at every age level in women as compared to men.

Gresham   Obstructive disease needs careful definition. Every now and then one finds one isolated large obstructive lesion, particularly in the anterior descending left coronary artery in young women. This is not frequent but is different from diffuse obstructive disease.

Spain   In men these isolated lesions occur, as you say, at the origin of the left anterior descending coronary artery, where the artery is very small. It is not part of a widespread atherosclerosis.

Mitchell (Nottingham)   Coronary and other vascular diseases are not diffuse. It is focal lesions, which are most vulnerable.

Gresham   I don't know the answer to Dr. Oliver's second question concerning evidence that women who are on the oral contraceptive have more disseminated focal disease.

Mitchell (Nottingham)   Professor Beaumont, do children with homocysteinaemia have those very early, very characteristic lesions that Dr. Spain described?

Beaumont (Paris)   I have never seen one. The reports about them are that they do tend to get premature occlusive atherosclerosis of the coronary arteries. Infusion of homocystein leads to smooth muscle cell proliferation.

Wald (Oxford)   Astrup has described experiments in which carbon monoxide leads to arterial change in animals. Is it your opinion that these changes are atherosclerotic changes, or is that not the case?

Gresham   Well, they are early lesions seen by electromicroscopy
and are not well quantified. I would hesitate to extrapolate from electronmicro-
graphs.

Fulton (Glasgow)   So far little has been said about the part played by thrombus
in the pathogenesis of atherosclerosis. My experience has shown that many plaques
are pigmented with brown or orange coloured areas and it would be hard to deny
that there was a blood element in the formation of such plaques. This may start
in a small way and more complex lesions show layers suggestive of an origin in
layers of thrombus. These plaques are friable. A large majority of thrombotic
occlusions showed this sort of underlying structure in the diseased intimal. Thus,
lesions which ultimately become the seat of complete thrombotic occlusion
commonly bear evidence of earlier episodes of thrombosis in the genesis of the
atherosclerotic material. We have heard today about the influence of oestrogens
on coagulation factors and it may be that in young women disturbance of haemostatic mechanisms − in relation to other local influences − give a clue as to why
they tend to produce these very localised lesions. If this is indeed a special
tendency in young women, it may follow that they develop acute thrombotic
occlusion at such sites.

Greenhalgh (London)   I specialise in seeing arterial disease in the living person
during operations on various arteries, and I would like to draw a comparison
between the carotid arteries and the coronary arteries. In cases of so-called
carotid artery stenosis, one often sees something which is far from a stenosis
but an atheromatous ulcer in the origin of the internal carotid artery. The lesion
is segmental and short. In the middle of an atheromatous area is an ulcer − exactly
like these illustrations of the coronary arteries. We also know from a number of
series that aspirin and persantin, both antithrombotic drugs, tend to reduce the
number of transient ischaemic attacks, though we do not know whether the
incidence of strokes will alter over 5 years. In other words, the control of the
thrombotic part is one thing but the continuation of the atheroma may be
another. Now in the coronary artery, is it possible, therefore, with a minimum
amount of atheroma and a small ulcer in the presence of increased oestrogen
levels that microembolisation will take place into the periphery, triggering off
a cardiac event?

Gresham   It is certainly true that some people have described
multiple platelet emboli as a cause of sudden cardiac death in the absence of
severe stenotic atherosclerosis.

Somerville (London)   By the very nature of the word, ulceration is a secondary
event. Something must cause some of these plaques to ulcerate and others to
remain intact. What causes this and specifically, is it caused by intimal haemorrhage?
Is intimal haemorrhage into the plaque an invariable, common or uncommon
situation?

Spain Haemorrhages are found in about 80-90 percent of the plaques on post-mortem examination but the relationship to ulcer formation is unclear. Haemorrhage may cause dissection and ulceration, but the finding of haemorrhage does not *per se* mean that it caused ulcerated plaques. These plaques may not even have haemorrhage or the haemorrhage may be a consequence of the ulceration.

Greenhalgh (London) When we operate on these lesions, there is no haemorrhage to the naked eye but there is increased inflammation around the artery. The artery is stuck where the ulcer is.

8. Angiographic aspects of coronary heart disease in young women

PAUL R. LICHTLEN AND HANS-JUERGEN ENGEL

From previous studies (Maleki, 1973; Engel, 1974, 1976, 1977) it was shown that coronary artery disease (CAD) in young women is a rare phenomenon and might differ from the typical aspects of CAD in many regards (Bretholz, 1974). The following presentation deals mainly with the angiographic aspects based on our own patients' material.

Patients and methods

All cases were studied by selective coronary and left ventricular (LV) angiography using either the Judkins or the Sones techniques. Multiple projections were used, including half-axial ones, in order to provide an optimal exposure of critical areas. Left ventricular (LV) angiograms were performed either in RAO-projection of 40^0 or biplane. Regional LV wall motion was evaluated from RAO-LV angiograms by recording percentage systolic shortening of six halfaxes drawn perpendicularly to the long axis (extending from the aortic-mitral valve junction to the apex) at 25 percent of its length. Systolic shortening above 25 percent was called normal, between 25 percent and 10 percent hypo-, and below 10 percent akinetic.

Angiographic incidence of CAD in young women (Table 8.1)

From January 1974 to June 1977, 2781 patients underwent cardiac catheterisation at the Hannover Medical University. In 2074 of these cases (74.6 percent) a coronary angiogram was performed. The studies included only 110 women with CAD (3.9 percent), CAD being characterised either by the presence of an abnormal coronary angiogram and an abnormal or normal VL angiogram, or a normal coronary angiogram with an abnormal LV angiogram [regional LV wall lesions]. The average age of these women was 50.2 years and thus did not differ from the average age of 51 years of the total population of patients with abnormal coronary angiograms. 24 of these women (0.86 percent of all patients undergoing coronary angiography) were below the age of 45. These will represent the group of 'young women with CAD'. Table 8.1 demonstrates the age distribution of all women with positive coronary angiograms, that is, CAD, 78 percent being above the age of 45, 10.8 percent below the age of 40.

Table 8.1 Angiographic aspects of CAD in women (Hannover Medical University) Age distribution (No. of cases: 110)

Average age: 50.2 $\pm$ 8.2 years (range 29 - 68)

Years	No. of Pat.		Percentage	
>60	12 ⎫		10.9%	
55 - 59	19 ⎬ 86		17.3%	78.2%
50 - 54	28 ⎬		25.5%	
45 - 49	27 ⎭		24.5%	
40 - 44	12 ⎫		11.0%	⎫
35 - 39	7 ⎬ 24		6.4%	10.8% ⎬ 21.8%
30 - 34	4 ⎬		3.5%	⎬
<30 (29)	1 ⎭		0.8%	⎭

Angiographic severity and extent of CAD in young women (Tables 8.2 and 8.3)

Table 8.2 reveals the high incidence of normal or only mildly diseased coronary arteries in this group of patients, 57 percent of the vessels being completely normal at the time of angiography, 7 percent only minimally diseased, and only 18 percent showing subtotal or total obstructions. Furthermore, regarding the three major arteries, left anterior descending (LAD), left circumflex (LCX) and right (RCA), only 1.29 vessels were involved per patient. Thus, 20.8 percent of the patients exhibited normal coronary arteries, and in 41.7 percent only one vessel, mainly the LAD was involved. Double vessel disease was present in 25 percent and triple vessel disease in 12.5 percent only (Table 8.3). Most often affected was the LAD (55 percent) which was completely occluded in seven instances.

Table 8.2 Angiographic aspects of CAD in women age below 45 (Hannover Medical University, 1/1974 - 6/1977)

Degree of Obstructions		
24 Patients, 72 Vessels (LAD, RCA, LCX)		
Obstruction	No.	Percentage
Normal vessels	41 (19)	56.9% ⎫ 63.8%
<50% or minimal	5 (1)	6.9% ⎭
50 - 75%	13 (3)	18.9% ⎫
76 - 99%	2	2.7% ⎬ 36.2%
100%	11 (1)	15.5% ⎭

1.29 Vessels/Patient
(   ) Patients on oral contraceptives

Angiographic severity of LV lesions (Table 8.3)

13 patients (54.2 percent) showed akinetic areas either of the anterior (11) or postero-inferior (2) wall; in nine patients, left ventricular wall motion was hypo-kinetic, and only in two cases (8.3 percent) was the left ventricle angiographically

D

Table 8.3 Angiographic aspects of CAD in women age below 45 (Hannover Medical University, 1/1974 - 6/1977)

No of vessels involved	No of patients	%	Avg Age (years)	Cor. arteries			LV Wall Motion			Oral Contraceptive
				LAD	LCX	RCA	Normal	Hypokinetic	Akinetic	
All normal	5	20.8%	35.8	-	-	-	0	1	4	4/5
One	10	41.7%	38.9	9	1	-	0	4	6	3/10
Two	6	25.0%	39.7	5	2	5	0	3	3	1/6
Three	3	12.5%	41.7	3	3	3	2	1	0	0/3
Total	24	100%	38.8	17 55%	6 19%	8 26%	2 8%	9 38%	13 54%	8/24

normal. It is interesting to note that four of the five patients with normal coronary arteries showed large akinetic areas, whereas the two normal left ventricular angiograms were encountered in patients with triple vessel disease. In addition, the age of the five patients with normal coronary arteries, yet abnormal left ventricular wall motion was markedly lower (average 35.8 years) than of the three subjects with triple vessel disease (average 41.7 years).

Possible influence of oral contraceptives on the angiographic aspects of CAD in young women (Table 8.4)

Due to the peculiarities of the angiographic aspects of CAD in some of the women, and in view of the fact that eight of the 24 women were on oral contraceptives for a longer period of time, this problem was further analysed. The eight women on oral contraceptives were significantly younger (36 versus 40 years) than the rest of this group. Most interestingly: they also demonstrated a significantly smaller extent of the disease, only 0.62 vessels per patient being involved against 1.625 in the non-oestrogen-group ($p < 0.025$), four of the women on oral contraceptives (50 percent) still exhibiting normal coronary arteries, three single vessel disease at the time of angiography versus only one (6 percent) with normal arteries in the non-oestrogen-group. In contrast, all women on oral contraceptives showed an abnormal left ventricle, six of eight (75 percent) having large akinetic areas.

Table 8.4 Angiographic aspects of CAD in women below age 45 with or without oral contraceptives (HMU, 1/74 - 6/77)

	Oral contraceptives		
	Yes	No	
Age (Years)	36.2	40.1	
Coronary Arteries			
Normal	4	1	
Single vessel disease	3 ⎤	7 ⎤	⎡ Chi-Square ⎤
Double vessel disease	1 ⎬ 4	5 ⎬ 15	6.189
Triple vessel disease	0 ⎦	3 ⎦	p <0.025 ⎦
No, vessels/pat.	0.625	1.625	
LAD	3	14	
LCX	1	5	
RCA	1	7	
LV wall motion			
Normal	0	2	
Hypokinetic	2	6	
Akinetic	6 (75%)	8 (50%)	

It is interesting to note that regional myocardial blood flow, when recorded by the praecordial Xenon residue detection technique using a gamma camera connected to a CDC 1700 computer system (Engel, 1977), in three of the women on oral contraceptives, was found to be reduced by approximately 38 percent — in spite of normal coronary arteries.

Thus, from the angiographic standpoint, it seems that there is a clear distinction between young women with CAD on oral contraceptives as compared to patients without: their coronary arteries are less severely affected by the disease — at least at the time of angiography — than in women not on contraceptives; however, their left ventricles are damaged to a greater extent.

Discussion

As this and other studies have shown (Engel, 1974, 1976), CAD in young women is not only a rare phenomenon (0.65 percent in Engel's series of patients below the age of 40; 0.86 percent in the present study of patients younger than 45 years, considering all coronary angiograms), it is also associated with a smaller extent of the disease (0.81 vessel per patient in Engel's series and 1.29 in our own series, the difference probably being due to the inclusion of patients up to 45 years of age in our series), and a high incidence of severe left ventricular wall damage. When compared with the angiographic appearance of CAD in young patients below 40 years of age in general, the differences are, however, not so striking. In a series of 76 patients below 40 years of age (including only four women), analysed by Bretholz and Lichtlen (1974), single vessel disease was present in 49 percent and triple vessel disease only in 12.5 percent, thus, a distribution similar to the one reported in this study was found. This, of course, contrasts with patients above 55 years of age where the same investigation yielded an incidence of single vessel disease of only 25 percent versus 49 percent of triple vessel disease; in a more recent study, triple vessel involvement amounted even to 76 percent (Lichtlen, 1976). Similarly, the investigation of Bretholz reported an involvement of the LAD in 40 percent of the young patients, 66 percent demonstrating also large akinetic areas. From this point of view, therefore, it seems that in general CAD in young women follows the same trend as in young men, with a predominance for single vessel disease and large akinetic areas due to early manifestation of myocardial infarctions.

The group of women on oral contraceptives, however, seems to represent a special form of the disease in so far as coronary lesions are significantly milder or often absent, left ventricular lesions, however, being frequently extensive and severe. Nevertheless, from the present small series, it is not possible to answer adequately whether one is faced with an early manifestation of typical CAD, or possibly with a separate disease of another pathophysiologic origin, although the latter seems very likely in view of the striking angiographic differences outlined earlier.

References

Bretholz, A., Moccetti, T. & Lichtlen, P. (1974) Koronarsklerose im jungen Erwachsenenalter. *Schweizerische Medizinische Wochenschrift,* **104,** 1600-1601.

Engel, H.-J., Page, H.L. & Campbell, W.B. (1974) Coronary artery disease in young women. *Journal of the American Medical Association,* **230,** 1531-1534.

Engel, H.-J. & Lichtlen, P. (1976) Angina pectoris und Myokardinfarkt ohne Koronarsklerose. *Therapeutische Umschau,* **33,** 75-86.

Engel, H.-J., Hundeshagen, H. & Lichtlen, P. (1977) Transmural myocardial infarction in young women taking oral contraceptives. Evidence of reduced regional coronary flow in spite of normal coronary arteries. *British Heart Journal,* **39,** 477-484.

Lichtlen, P., Engel, H.-J. & Hundeshagen, H. (1976) Regional myocardial blood flow in patients without coronary artery disease, yet proven myocardial infarctions. *American Journal of Cardiology,* **37,** 151.

Lichtlen, P., Rafflenbeul, W., Freudenberg, H. & Bogenstatter, P. (1976) Angiographic findings in angina pectoris. *7th European Congress of Cardiology,* Abstract Book I, 396, Amsterdam.

Maleki, M. & Lange, R.L. (1973) Coronary thrombosis in young women on oral contraceptives. Report of two cases and review of the literature. *American Heart Journal,* **85,** 749-754.

9. Angina in young women with normal coronary angiogram

S. P. SINGH AND J. D. EDDY

It is well recognised that ischaemic heart disease is rare in young women. In most reported cases there have been contributory factors, such as hypertension, significant hyperlipidaemia, diabetes mellitus, excessive chronic smoking or sustained use of the oral contraceptive pill (Malmcrona, 1961, Todd, 1972, Kubik, 1973, Oliver, 1974).

We have studied 23 young women for two to eight years, who had anginal type of chest pain. The youngest was 22 and the oldest 43 years old, three subsequently developed acute myocardial infarction. There were no significant risk factors. Patients with abnormal glucose tolerance test, significant hyperlipidaemia and high blood pressure were excluded. Similarly women who were on the pill for prolonged periods, or who had smoked heavily were not included in this study. None had a significant family history of vascular disease.

The pain was exertional in all but one, in seven it also occurred at rest or was provoked by emotion. The duration of the pain varied from a few minutes up to half an hour and in some an 'aching feeling' continued even up to an hour. The relief was delayed in 4 women to more than five minutes after sublingual administration of nitroglycerine or iso-sorbide dinitrate.

ECG was performed at rest and was normal in 16 and in 7 there were either definite 'T' wave changes or minor repolarisation changes. Exercise ECG (bicycle ergometer) were obtained in 18 and were positive in 15 cases. There was either horizontal ST depression of 2 mm. or more or, actual 'T' wave inversion (3 patients) and in 4 there were multiple ventricular extrasystoles.

There were 7 patients who were hospitalised, had pain and ECG was performed and was abnormal in 6 (ST depression or 'T' wave inversion).

Echocardiogram was performed in 20 (by Dr. R. Behnam) and this showed normal left ventricular function without prolapsed mitral valve or evidence of primary myocardial disease, such as, hypertrophic obstructive cardiomyopathy. The resting left ventricular end diastolic pressure was measured in all the patients and it was more than 12 mmHg. (12 being our arbitrary figure of normality). After exercise it was noted to be elevated in 5 of the 11 cases where it was performed. Lactate estimations were done from the aortic root and from the coronary sinus and they were abnormal in 5 of the 6 cases. Cold vaso-pressor test was performed in 10 patients and was negative in all, the ECG was recorded during the test and showed no change. Left ventricular angiogram was performed in all the patients and it was normal.

I will show you very quickly the coronary angiographic pictures of 2 typical patients

(Figs. 9.1 and 9.2). They both show small spastic-looking coronary arteries. The main branches are unobstructed, but the peripheral branches look thin, sparse or tortuous.

The cause of this syndrome is unknown, in the absence of risk factors. Spasm of the coronary arteries, abnormal left ventricular function and the small vessel disease have to be considered. We were unable to produce angina or ECG changes with cold vaso-pressor test which would be to some extent against the theory of the spasm of coronary arteries giving rise to angina. As far as the abnormal left ventricular function is concerned, echocardiography and haemodynamic studies show satisfactory function in the majority of these women. Small vessel disease in this situation has been excluded by Dr. Richardson and his colleagues from King's College Hospital, London. They performed myocardial biopsies in this group of patients and found them to show no disease of the small vessels.

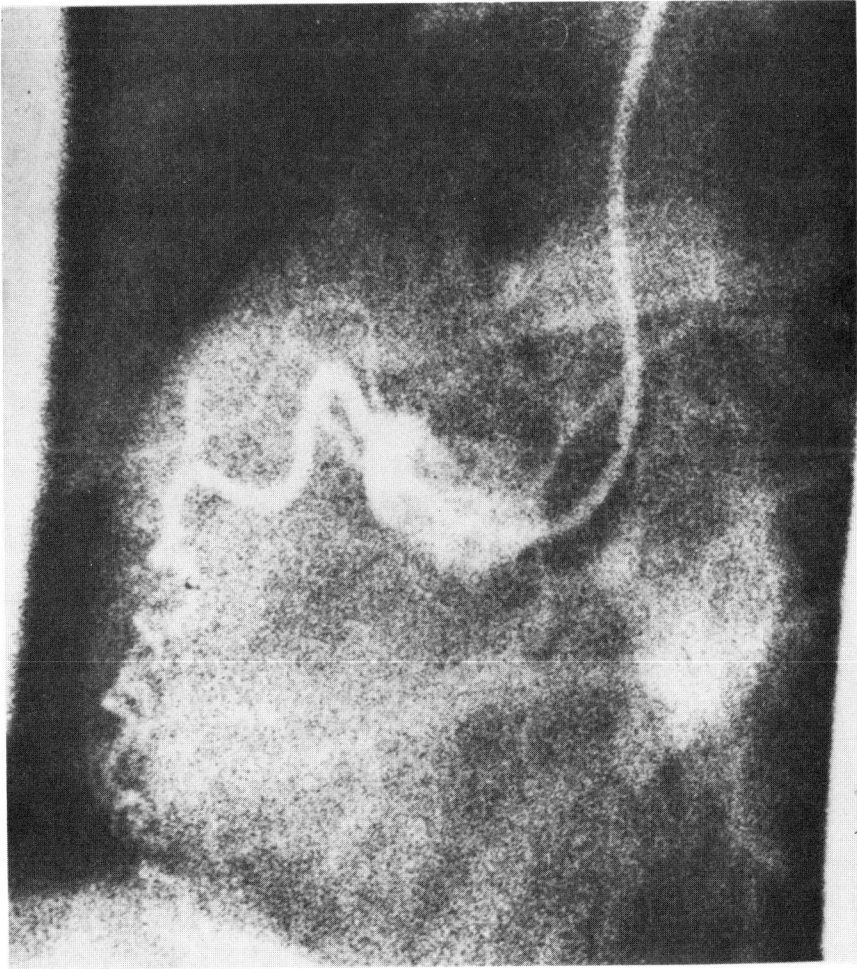

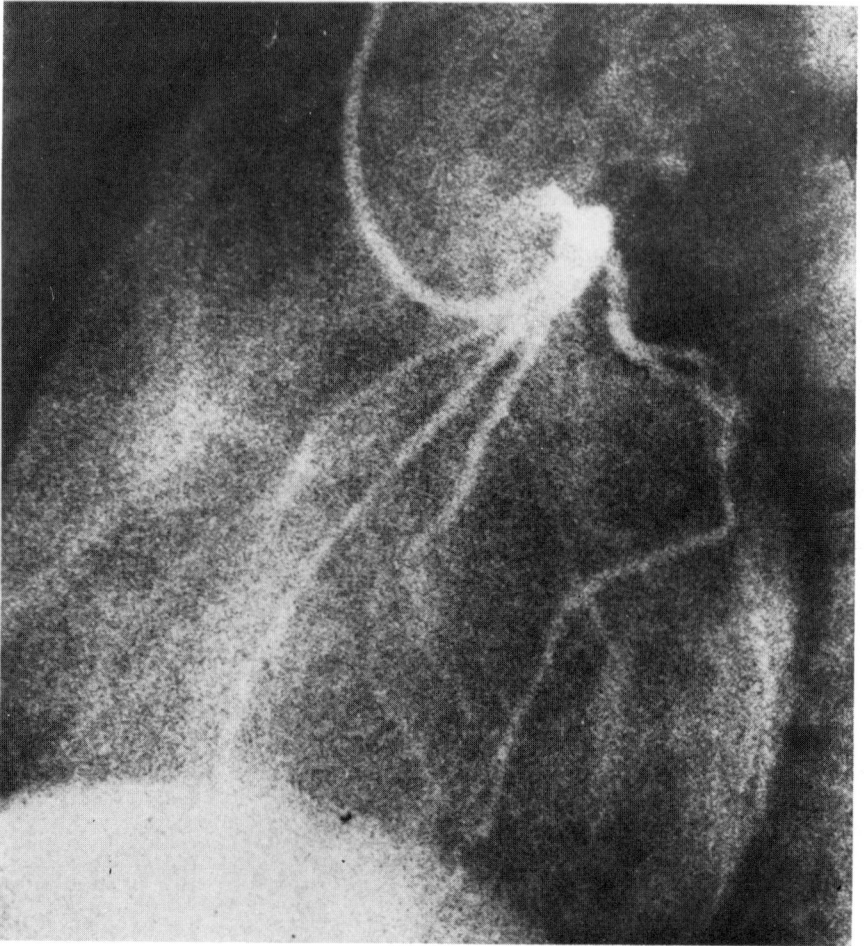

Fig. 9.2 (Left anterior oblique view) Coronary angiogram showing sparse thin branches of the left coronary artery.

We felt that it is possible that some of these cases might have congenitally small coronary arteries with poor collateral circulation and with increasing myocardial oxygen demand in young and middle age, these vessels are unable to supply enough oxygen and thus trigger off angina.

References

Kubik, M.M. & Bhowmick, B.K. (1973) Myocardial infarction and oral contraceptive. *British Medical Journal*, 35, 1271.

Malmcrona, R., Bjorntorp, P., Soderholm, B., Thulesius, O. and Hlyman, F. (1961) Myocardial infarction in the young age group. Clinical review of cases up to the age of 55. *Acta Medica Scan.*, 170, 301.

Oliver, M.F. (1974) Ischaemic heart disease in young women. *British Medical Journal*, **4**, 253.

Todd, G.F. (1972) *Statistics of smoking in the United Kingdom.* London Tobacco Research Council.

Discussion 2B

Oliver (Edinburgh)   Was there any difference in the prevalence of other risk factors, additional to the oral contraceptive, in those patients with two and three vessels disease compared with none and one?

Lichtlen   Of the three women with three vessels disease, two had hypertension and the third had manifest diabetes requiring insulin. So many of those not on oral contraceptives but with abnormal coronary angiograms had additional risk factors, i.e. hypertension, diabetes in two cases, and heavy cigarette smoking.

Oliver (Edinburgh)   It appears as if there are two groups. Women with multiple risk factors and 2 or 3 vessel disease, and women using oral contraception with no other risk factors and little or no evident coronary disease.

Lichtlen   Angiographically they look different.

Mitchell (Nottingham)   Those on the oral contraceptive were on average 5 years younger, how do you know this is not an effect of age?

Lichtlen   There was no male case with normal coronary arteries and infarction. This only occurred in these women. The men were also below the age of 40 and the average was around 36 or 37. The women were under 45 years and the average age of those on the oral contraceptive was 36.

Baird (Edinburgh)   Had all these women had myocardial infarction?

Lichtlen   No, they had either myocardial infarction or angina. Those with akinetic wall motion had myocardial infarction.

Mitchell (Nottingham)   Were they all symptomatic patients?

Lichtlen   All had been symptomatic at one time. Most were studied because they had clear-cut myocardial infarcts; those who had triple vessel disease had angina pectoris; the 5 women with normal coronary arteries who had previously had an infarct were studied because they were young and were asymptomatic at the time of angiography.

Mitchell (Nottingham)   There have recently been a number of reports suggesting that taking oestrogens is sufficient to cause abnormalities in the electrocardiogram in women. I have a group of 150 women with mild hypertension (blood pressure at about 150/90-160/100): 20 percent of them had ECG diagnosed by competent cardiologists as myocardial ischaemia. After taking these women off the contraceptive pill, their electrocardiograms three months later had mostly become normal. I mention this in this audience because I think there is a trap building up here for cardiologists and people working in this epidemiological field. There is an electrocardiographic abnormality which is found in women taking steroidal contraceptives, the significance of which we do not know. Oestrogens may have some effect on the availability of calcium to the myocardium and this may cause changes in electrocardiograms in women on the pill.

Lichtlen The group of women on oral contraceptives, I have reported, all had established Q wave infarcts.

Spain (Brooklyn) The coronary angiographs were taken at varied times after the initial event, in these cases with oral contraceptives. Is there any reduction in size of the obstructive lesions as time goes on with resolution of thrombotic obstruction? There is experimentally, so after 5 months there will be one size of obstruction, a little later there will be less obstructive and a little later even less. Could the absence of any coronary obstruction lesion relate to the duration of time between the initial attack and coronary angiography?

Lichtlen I agree that this is possible. How long does it take for the thrombotic obstruction to resolve? Days, weeks, months or longer?

General discussion

Fulton (Glasgow) In Kenya where the incidence of coronary disease is low in both sexes, there is about 15 percent incidence of diabetes. Women seemed to sustain hypertension in that country very well. I wonder whether enough attention is being paid to give a clue as to why women (and men) are so relatively free of CHD in underdeveloped countries?

Lichtlen (Hannover) How can we relate all these results to the problem of young women with CHD?

Venning (High Wycombe) If we should be looking for something adverse in man rather than something protective in women, how can we reconcile this with the evidence of some protective effect from the ovary? What is it — if not steroidal — from the ovary that appears to provide a protective effect?

Rose (London) I am not entirely convinced that the evidence of a protective effect of oestrogens or of a deleterious effect of ovarian removal can be trusted. The woman who has her ovaries out, or who has an early menopause, is a different kind of person, and I am not convinced that the association is a simple one. The hypothesis that there is an adverse effect related to maleness is not in conflict with a protective female factor. I think both can be true.

Nordin (Leeds) While I accept that women who have had their ovaries out have a higher incidence of coronary heart disease, the evidence that oestrogens and progestogens protect people from the known risk factors associated with CHD is lacking or contrary. We know that there is an association between oestrogen administration in both men and women with CHD, so it seems to me we can't have it both ways.

Gordon (Bethesda) The hormone picture in women is extraordinarily complex and much more so than we have ever entertained in our speculation about the role of oestrogen *per se.* All the epidemiological or clinical evidence shows that oestrogens in women and in men appears to be a cause, rather than a protective, against CHD.

Hazzard (Seattle) It may well be that a woman who has been through an early menopause is prematurely aged. The ageing process may accelerate the atherosclerotic process itself. I think we should ask at what stage in the pattern of atherosclerosis can oestrogens have either a protective or deleterious effect. Oestrogens can promote some and retard other atherogenic mechanisms. Clotting mechanisms, platelets, the arterial endothelium, replication of arterial muscle cells, deposition of lipoproteins, changes in lipoproteins can be effected differently. For instance, we know that oestrogens increase high density lipoproteins and androgens decrease them. This might be associated with protection. On the other hand, we know that oestrogens increase coagulability and decrease fibrinolysis and this would be expected to aggravate the problem of atherosclerosis. The same hormone can accelerate atherosclerosis very radically and also decrease it.

SESSION 3 Endocrine pathophysiology

Chairman: R.V. Short

10. Patterns of sex hormone production in women

D. T. BAIRD

Introduction

Because the menopause is characterised by ovarian failure, the rise in coronary heart disease which occurs in women at this time is usually attributed in part to a relative oestrogen deficiency. However, in addition to oestradiol the ovary secretes a variety of steroid hormones, the production of which changes throughout life (Baird 1971). Moreover, not all 'sex steroids' are secreted exclusively by the ovary. For example androstenedione, the major androgen secreted by the ovary, is also secreted in appreciable amounts by the adrenal glands. It is the purpose of this paper to trace the production and source of 'sex hormones' (oestrogens, androgens and gestogens) in women from infancy to old age.

Synthesis and site of production of sex hormones

Although the ovary and adrenal both have the biosynthetic capacity to synthetise a variety of sex hormones, each gland secretes its own characteristic pattern. Thus in general, although androgens (androstenedione, testosterone and dehydroepiandrosterone) are secreted appreciably by both type of glands, the adrenal secretion of oestrogens and gestogens is minimal. The synthesis of sex steroids from acetate proceeds through the classical route through cholesterol to pregnenolone. This rate limiting step involving the hydroxylation and subsequent removal of the side chain at C_{20}, is stimulated by ACTH and LH in the adrenal and ovary respectively.

Some steroids which circulate in the blood stream are not secreted as such by the endocrine glands but are produced elsewhere in the body by conversion of other steroids which are themselves secreted. The sites of this 'extraglandular' production of steroids is not fully known although the liver, fat cells, skin and muscle all have the enzymes necessary for some of these interconversions (Siiteri and MacDonald, 1973).

Infancy and childhood

Very little is known about the secretion of the ovary in fetal life although very high concentrations of oestrogens and progesterone of placental origin are present in umbilical cord blood (Faiman, Winter and Reyes, 1976). During infancy and childhood the ovary is not inactive although the quantities of steroids secreted are tiny compared to adult life (Fig. 10.1). The concentration of both oestrone and oestradiol rise progressively throughout childhood although it is not until late puberty that the

95

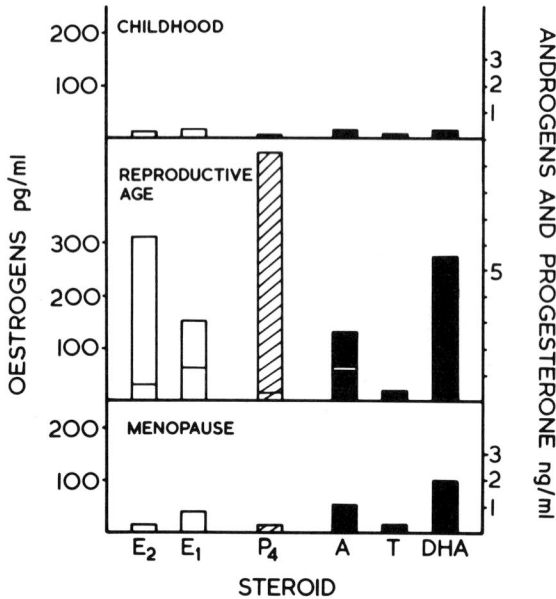

Fig. 10.1 Concentration of sex steroids in peripheral plasma at different stages of reproductive life. In childhood and post-menopause the total height of the bars represent the mean values; during reproductive age the total height of the bar and the horizontal line represent the maximum and minimum value respectively at different stages of the menstrual cycle.

E_2 = Oestradiol E_1 = Oestrone P_4 = Progesterone

A = Androstenedione   T = Testosterone   DHA = Dehydroepiandrosterone

concentration of oestradiol exceeds that of oestrone. This change in the ratio of oestrogen reflects the greatly increased secretion of oestradiol from the maturing Graafian follicles.

There is also a marked increase in the production of androgens in late childhood. The increase in the secretion of androgens from the adrenal mainly in the form dehydroepiandrosterone sulphate (adrenarche) precedes the menarche by one or two years (Ducharme, Forest, de Peretti, Sempé, Collu and Bertrand, 1976). The concentrations of androstenedione and progesterone do not reach adult levels until ovulatory ovarian cycles have become established late in puberty.

Reproductive years

Although the first few menstrual cycles are frequently anovulatory, the reproductive years between the menarche and menopause are characterised by series of ovulatory cycles recurring at approximately 28 day intervals. Except when interrupted by pregnancy and lactation, these cycles persist in most women until ovarian function fails some time between 45 and 55 years. The changes in concentration ovarian hormones are well described and will not be described in detail. There is no evidence that there are differences in the clearance rate of steroids at different stages of the cycle so that changes in concentration probably reflect real changes in secretion.

The two peaks of oestradiol concentration are due to the secretion of preovulatory follicle and corpus luteum respectively while the corpus luteum is responsible for the luteal rise in the concentration of progesterone. While those two steroids are derived virtually exclusively from ovarian secretion, the origin of the other sex steroids is more complicated. The ovary secretes only small quantities of oestrone (30 - 150 µg per day), while the remainder of the blood production rate is either secreted by the adrenal gland directly or derived by extraglandular conversion of oestradiol and androstenedione (Baird, Horton, Longcope and Tait, 1969). The amount of oestrogen produced in this way (40 - 120 µg per day) is probably insufficient in the premenopausal woman to have any significant biological effect when compared to the secretion of the much more potent oestradiol (40 - 400 µg per day). In anovulatory states, however, e.g. polycystic ovarian disease or after the menopause, extraglandular production of oestrone from androstenedione is the major source of oestrogen (Siiteri and MacDonald, 1973).

Androstenedione is secreted by both the ovary and adrenal in approximately equal quantities. As both the Graafian follicle and the corpus luteum secrete androstenedione as well as the ovarian stroma, it is not surprising that its production rate varies throughout the cycle. In addition to being a prehormone for oestrone, androstenedione is the major source of the biologically potent androgens, testosterone and dihydrotestosterone. Extraglandular conversion of androstenedione accounts for over 50 percent of the blood production rate of testosterone, the remainder of which is secreted directly by the adrenals and ovaries. Dehydroepiandrosterone sulphate is secreted exclusively by the adrenal glands, although small quantities of the free steroid originate from the ovaries. The biological action of these androgens in women is unknown although they may be concerned with the growth of sexual hair, muscle and the maintenance of sexual libido as in the rhesus monkey.

Although the extent of extraglandular conversion is small (1 - 2 percent), the production rate of androstenedione (2 - 3 mgm/day) is so much greater than that of oestrone or testosterone (50 - 250 µg/day) that a significant proportion of the production of these latter hormones originates from this source. The percentage conversion of androstenedione to oestrone (1.4 percent) is similar to intact, castrate and adrenalectomised women although it is directly related to both age and body weight (see later).

Pre-menopause

In the few years before the onset of the menopause there is a striking increase in the variation of the length of the menstrual cycle (Treolar, Boynton, Behn and Brown, 1967). A variety of abnormalities in the endocrine control of the ovarian cycle have been described in such women including short luteal phase, anovulatory cycles, long and short follicular phases (Van Look 1976). As the population of oocytes in the ovary becomes depleted there may be a progressive rise in the concentration of both FSH and LH due to the reduced negative feedback effect of oestradiol. Repeated anovulatory cycles result in persistent stimulation of the uterus with oestrogen and consequent cystic hyperplasia of the endometrium. The hormonal characteristics of this period of life, therefore, are highly variable.

Post-menopause

The menopause, which is defined as the last menstrual period, is due to depletion of healthy oocytes from the ovary and consequent failure of follicle growth. Although the post-menopausal ovary secretes virtually no oestradiol or oestrone, small amounts of testosterone and androstenedione continue to be produced (Judd, Judd, Lucas and Yen, 1974). Because the bulk of sex steroids are adrenal in origin, there is a diurnal variation in their concentration with a peak occurring in the early morning (Vermeulen 1976).

In the absence of ovarian secretion the concentration of oestradiol falls to very low levels and the concentration of FSH and LH rise into the castrate range. Although the production of androstenedione also falls, the change in concentration of testosterone and oestrone is much less marked. As noted above, the stroma of post-menopausal ovary continues to secrete testosterone, probably stimulated by the high levels of LH. Small amounts of oestrone are secreted by the adrenal and the percentage conversion of androstenedione to oestrone actually increases. Thus, although there is a reduction in amount of precursor, the quantity of oestrone produced by extraglandular aromatization is the same or greater than the pre-menopausal woman. As mentioned above, the extent of this conversion is related not only to age but to body weight. In some obese women the amount of oestrone produced in this way may be sufficient to stimulate the endometrium and post-menopausal bleeding may result.

In addition to the marked reduction in the secretion of ovarian oestradiol, the secretion of androgens from the adrenal also declines after the menopause. The concentration of androstenedione and dehydroepiandrosterone decline with age in both sexes. The importance of the adrenal glands as a source of sex steroids in the post-menopausal woman is seen by the marked suppression of oestrone, oestradiol, androstenedione, testosterone, dihydrotestosterone and progesterone following administration of dexamethasone (Vermeulen 1976).

In summary, therefore, although the post-menopausal ovary continues to secrete small quantities of testosterone and androstenedione, the adrenal is the predominant source of sex hormone production. Although ACTH is known to stimulate adrenal steroid production, the precise factors regulating the proportion of androgens and oestrogens secreted is unknown. In most post-menopausal women the major circulating oestrogen is oestrone which arises by extraglandular conversion of androstenedione. Very little is known about the biological activity of androstenedione and oestrone, although in experimental animals it has been demonstrated that they influence the feedback control of gonadotrophins. Because of extensive metabolism in the gut and liver, orally administered oestrogens, e.g. oestradiol valerianate, enter the systemic circulation as oestrone and its conjugates. Thus, so called 'hormone replacement therapy' (HRT) does not restore the endocrine environment to the pre-menopausal situation. More research into the biological effect of oestrone and other oestrogen metabolites are required in order to assess the possible role of oestrogens in the development of ischaemic heart disease.

References

Baird, D.T. (1971) Steroids in blood reflecting ovarian function. In: *Control of Gonadal Steroid Secretion.* D.T. Baird and J.A. Strong, Eds. Edinburgh University Press, p.176-187.

Baird, D.T., Horton, R., Longcope, C. & Tait, J.F. (1969) Steroid dynamics under steady state conditions. *Recent Progress in Hormone Research,* **25**, 611-664.

Ducharme, J.R., Forest, M.G., De Peretti, E., Sempé, M., Collu, R. and Bertrand, J. (1976) Plasma, adrenal and gonadal sex steroids in human pubertal development. *Journal of Clinical Endocrinology and Metabolism,* **42**, 468-476.

Faiman, C., Winter, J.S. & Reyes, F.I. (1976) Patterns of gonadotrophins and gonadal steroids throughout life. *Clinics in Obstetrics and Gynaecology,* **3**, 467-483.

Judd, H.L., Judd, G.E., Lucas, W.E. and Yen, S.S.C. (1974) Endocrine function of the post-menopausal ovary: concentration of androgens and oestrogens in ovarian and peripheral vein blood. *Journal of Clinical Endocrinology and Metabolism,* **39**, 1020-1024.

Siiteri, P.K. and MacDonald, P.C. (1973) Role of extraglandular oestrogen in human endocrinology. In: Handbook of Physiology, Section 7 Endocrinology, Vol. 11, Part I. R.O. Greep and E.B. Astwood (Eds). *American Physiological Society,* p.615-629.

Treolar, A.E., Boynton, R.E., Behn, B.G. and Brown, B.W. (1967) Variation of the human menstrual cycle through reproductive life. *International Journal of Fertility,* **12**, 77-126.

Van Look, P.F.A. (1976) Failure of positive feedback. *Clinics in Obstetrics and Gynaecology,* **3**, 555-578.

Vermeulen, A. (1976) The hormonal activity of the post-menopausal ovary. *Journal of Clinical Endocrinology and Metabolism,* **42**, 247-253.

Discussion 3A

Short (Edinburgh) We tend to use oestrogen as a block term, and should distinguish between natural and synthetic oestrogens more carefully. Natural oestrogens might be 'good', but Premarin is not natural to the human because it never occurs in the human. Synthetic oestrogens might be less 'good' and they become absorbed into the circulation as oestrone and not as oestradiol.

Bonnar (Dublin) What is the precise ovarian production of oestrogens in a woman on the pill? Do preparations containing mestranol and oestradiol have the same effect? Does a woman produce any of her own oestrogens when she is taking the contraceptive pill?

Baird I can only give you anecdotal data by saying that we have measured the concentration of oestradiol in a number of women on the pill but cannot comment about the effects of specific pills. The concentrations of oestradiol-17-β are below those of the early follicular phase while on the pill. They rise during the week off the pill.

Venning (High Wycombe) There was good data from Shearman about 10 years ago on people receiving a pill which had a high concentration of ethinyl oestradiol. 109 out of 110 women had total suppression of oestrogen excretion through the menstrual cycle. I have not seen similar data for pills with a lower oestrogen content but I think that the suppression of natural oestrogen production will be less complete.

Rose (London) In the extraglandular conversion of androstenedione, you mention fat as one site. Does the amount of body fat show any association with plasma oestrone levels? Is it a rate-limiting site?

Baird   MacDonald and his group have shown a positive correlation between the percentage conversion of androstenedione to oestrone with body weight. They have also claimed association between percent conversion and age.

Horton (Edinburgh) What are the principal hormonal changes during pregnancy?

Baird   The concentrations of oestradiol and oestrone rise one hundred fold, that of oestriol rises one thousand fold; progesterone rises two hundred fold and the androgens, dehydroepiandrosterone, and androstenedione rise by a factor of about two or three.

11. Patterns of sex hormone production in men

A. VERMEULEN

Biologically the most important circulating sex hormone in the human male is testosterone (T). It is almost exclusively secreted by the testes and circulates in plasma largely bound to two plasma proteins: albumin, with a low affinity but a large binding capacity, and the specific testosterone-estradiol binding globulin (TeBG) or sex hormone binding globulin (SHBG) with a high affinity but a low binding capacity ($\pm 5.10^{-8}$M). Only a small fraction (1 to 2 percent) of T is free, and there is good evidence that only the free (or at least the non specifically bound) fraction is biologically active (Vermeulen et al, 1969; Lasnitzki & Franklin, 1972; Rosenfield, 1975).

Another biologically active plasma androgen is 5αdihydrotestosterone (DHT), which is partially secreted as such by the testes (20 percent), the major fraction (80 percent) originating however from peripheral conversion of T and androstenedione (A) (Mahoudeau et al, 1971). Its concentration in plasma is roughly 1/10th of that of T; it is even more firmly bound to TeBG than T. At least in some tissues, biological activity of T requires its prior reduction to DHT; however some androgenic effects appear to be produced by T itself. It is unlikely however that in males circulating DHT is responsible for any significant androgenic effect. The same applies to 5αandrostanediol, a potent androgen which is present in plasma in minute concentrations (10 ng/dl) (Kinouchi & Horton, 1974). Other androgens circulating in plasma are dehydroepiandrosterone (DHEA) (and its sulphate) and androstenedione (A). These are weakly androgenic steroids and their biological activity requires probably their prior transformation to T or DHT.

Besides androgens, oestrogens are also found in the plasma of men. The concentration of oestradiol (E2) in adult males is of the order of 1-3 ng/100 ml); it is bound to TeBG with an affinity which is somewhat lower than for T: as a consequence, the free estradiol fraction is lower than the free T fraction at low TeBG capacity, and higher at high TeBG capacity (Rubens et al, 1974; Vermeulen, 1977). There are indications that the ratio of free testosterone over free estradiol determines whether either the androgenic or the estrogenic effects will predominate when both steroids are present. Finally, the concentration of oestrone (E1) in male plasma is similar to the concentration found in the female during the early follicular phase. Oestrone and estradiol originate essentially from peripheral conversion of A and T respectively.

The human testes start to secrete T at the 6-8th week of fetal life; this secretion reaches a maximum ($\pm$ 200 ng/dl) between the 11th and 18th week of fetal life, followed by a progressive decline. This early secretion is under the influence of HCG, as in acephalic and apituitary infants genitals differentiate normally. Later in pregnancy, LH is the stimulus and in its absence penis and scrotum are often hypoplastic.

In male newborns plasma T levels are about 300 ng/dl; during the first week of life they decrease to about 30 ng, followed by an increase to $\pm$ 300 ng/dl lasting for about 2 months, followed again by a gradual decrease until the 7th month of life when levels of 7-10 ng/100 ml are reached, which will persist until puberty. Whereas at birth TeBG capacity is extremely low (1.5×10^{-8}M), with as a consequence a high free fraction ($\pm$3 percent) and high free T concentration ($\pm$ 10 ng/dl), by the second week of life TeBG capacity has reached the high level of 1.5×10^{-7}M and consequently the free T fraction has become small (0.7 percent) and remains so until puberty. Hence the apparent free testosterone concentration (AFTC) from the sixth month of life until puberty is extremely low (0.1 ng/dl) (Forest 1975).

Other sex hormone levels are similarly extremely low until prepuberty. Except for the immediate postnatal period, sex hormone levels in boys and girls are rather similar from infanthood until prepuberty. In prepuberty, in both sexes, there appears to occur an activation of the adrenal cortex a few years before activation of the gonadal secretion occurs. This 'adrenarche' is characterised by a rapid increase in DHEA and A levels (Sizonenko & Pannier, 1975). This is followed by initiation of puberty, a consequence of the maturation of the hypothalamic gonadostat, which becomes less sensitive to the feed back by the sex hormones and within a period of 3-4 years adult sex hormone levels are reached. From puberty on until old age important differences in sex hormone levels between males and females are found. In adult males T levels vary between 280 and 1000 ng/dl; parallel with the pubertal increase in T levels in males, TeBG concentration decreases; hence the free T fraction increases from 0.7 percent to about 2 percent and the AFTC increases to a mean value of $\pm$ 10 ng/dl. The increase in DHT levels parallels more or less the T levels, although the increase is not so pronounced; also estradiol levels increase. The mean ratio of free estradiol over free testosterone in adult males is $\pm$0.003; this is to be compared to a mean ratio of $\pm$0.1 during reproductive life in women.

In adulthood, plasma levels remain at a constant level until the sixth decade of life; they then decrease progressively with wide individual variations. As the TeBG concentration increases with aging, the decrease in the AFTC is more important than the decrease in total T. Whereas at 30 years, mean AFTC is $\pm$10 ng/dl, it is only 4 ng/dl in the 8th decade and only 2-3 ng/dl in the ninth decade. This decrease in the free fraction is reflected in a decrease of the metabolic clearance rate in elderly men (Vermeulen et al, 1969).

Not only T as well as DHT concentrations decrease in elderly males, but also DHEA (S) levels show a remarkable decrease from a mean value of $\pm$400 ng/dl (DHEA) and 150 ug/dl (DHEA-S) respectively, to a mean value of 175 ng/dl and 80 ug/dl respectively (Vermeulen & Verdonck, 1976). As the secretion of cortisol does not decrease in old age, this suggests that there occurs a change in the enzymatic activity in the adrenal cortex (adrenopauze). The mechanism of this decrease in adrenocortical activity is unknown. However, when prolactin levels are chronically increased as during sulpiride treatment or in prolactinoma, DHEA (S) levels in elderly males (and females) remain high (Vermeulen *et al*, 1977). As however in elderly males prolactin levels are not decreased when compared to values in younger males, the significance of this observation remains unclear.

Whereas androgen levels decrease in aging males, oestradiol levels show a slight increase. As moreover due to the increase in TeBG concentration the free fraction of E2 becomes relatively more important than the free T fraction, the ratio of free estradiol over free testosterone increases by a factor 3 in elderly males (mean : 0.8×10^{-2}) (Rubens *et al,* 1974). In fact in elderly males, estradiol and free estradiol levels are higher than in postmenopausal women; the ratio of free E2 over free T remains however generally higher in women than in men, as in postmenopausal the mean ratio is 2×10^{-2}. However some overlapping between elderly males and postmenopausal women does occur.

References

Forest, M.G. (1975) Differentiation and development of the male. *Clinics in Endocrinology,* **4**, 569-596.

Kinouchi, T. & Horton, R. (1974) 3α-Androstanediol in human peripheral plasma. *Journal of Clinical Endocrinology & Metabolism,* **38**, 262-277.

Lasnitzki, I. & Franklin, H.R. (1972) The influence of serum on uptake, conversion and action of testosterone in rat prostate glands in organ culture. *Journal of Endocrinology,* **54**, 333-342.

Mahoudeau, J.A., Bardin, C.W. & Lipsett, M.B. (1971) The metabolic clearance rate and origin of plasma dihydrotestosterone in man and its conversion to the 5α-androstanediol. *Journal of Clinical Investigation,* **50**, 1338-1344.

Rosenfield, R.L. (1975) Studies of the relation of plasma androgen levels to androgen action in women. *Journal of Steroid Biochemistry,* **6**, 695-702.

Rubens, R., Dhont, M. & Vermeulen, A. (1974) Further studies on Leydig cell function in old age. *Journal of Clinical Endocrinology & Metabolism,* **39**, 40-45.

Sizonenko, P.C. & Paunier, L. (1975) Hormonal changes in puberty III: Correlation of plasma dehydroepiandrosterone, Testosterone, FSH and LH with stages of puberty and bone age in normal boys and girls and in patients with Addison's disease or hypogonadism or with premature or late adrenarche. *Journal of Clinical Endocrinology & Metabolism,* **41**, 894-904.

Vermeulen, A., Verdonck, L., Van Der Straeten, M. & Orie, M. (1969) Capacity of the testosterone binding globulin in human plasma and influence of specific binding of testosterone and its metabolic clearance rate. *Journal of Clinical Endocrinology & Metabolism,* **29**, 1470-1480.

Vermeulen, A. (1969) Transport of Steroid hormones, in: *Plasma protein turnover* Ed. Bianchi, R., Mariani, J. & McFarlane, A.S. MacMillan Press, London, p.309.

Vermeulen, A. & Verdonck, L. (1976) Radioimmunoassay of 17β-hydroxy-5 -α androstan-3-one, 4-androstene-3, 17-dione, dehydroepiandrosterone, 17 hydroxyprogesterone and progesterone and its application to human male plasma. *Journal of Steroid Biochemistry,* **7**, 1-10.

Vermeulen, A. (1977) Physiological and clinical aspects of androgens. Proceedings of the Vth International Congress on Endocrinology — Hamburg, Ed. James, V.H.T., *Excerpta Medica ICS,* **402**, 41-50.

Vermeulen, A., Suy, E. & Verdonck. (1977) Effect of prolactin on plasma DHEA(S) levels. *Journal of Clinical Endocrinology & Metabolism,* in the press.

Discussion 3B

Rose (London) We considered earlier in this symposium, CHD mortality in the two sexes against age. The mortality, on a logarithmic scale, produces something pretty near a straight line for females. The male line approaches that of the females with advancing age but it can be fairly readily separated into two straight lines with a lower line in parallel with the female line up to age 45, when a change in direction occurs, and thereafter the male mortality line rises less steeply and approaches the female line. It looks as though something happens in man in the fifth decade as a result of which they fail to maintain the force of mortality from coronary disease. We proposed the hypothesis recently that the difference in coronary incidence between the sexes may be not due to a protective factor in the female but to an adverse effect of testosterone in the male, which is withdrawn in the fifth decade. Do you think this is a tenable or testable hypothesis?

Vermeulen I do not know of evidence that testosterone is an unfavourable factor in the pathogenesis of coronary disease. There are minor recorded changes in coagulation and plasma lipids but whether the total effects of testosterone favour development of coronary artery disease is not known.

Nordin (Sheffield) The simultaneous fall in testosterone and rise in oestradiol in elderly men must imply a remarkable rise in the conversion rate, unless there is a change in metabolic substrates. I presume this is a hepatic conversion. Do you know of any direct data showing this tremendous increase in conversion rates with age in men?

Vermeulen We have some data on increased conversion rate. It is not a tremendous increase but at least a doubling of values occurs. The increased oestradiol and the decreased testosterone levels have been observed by several other authors.

Douglas (Aberdeen) I think it is usually accepted that there is a seasonal swing in mortality rates from myocardial infarction — lowest in the summer and highest in the winter. Does that correlate with the seasonal testosterone swing?

Vermeulen There are not many studies on the season fluctuation in plasma testosterone. Our observations and those of a group in Paris suggest that the highest levels of plasma testosterone occur in the autumn — in September/October/November. These were studies in young men and the lowest level was in the spring.

Wynn (London) Did you measure free oestrogen and free androgen or were these values derived from affinity coefficients? What data exists concerning variation in protein binding? The plasma levels quoted may not be of relevant biological significance.

Vermeulen   The free oestradiol and free testosterone concentrations are derived values. They are obtained by dialysis of plasma diluted at 1 in 5 and are calculated taking into account an association constant and the concentration of albumin. We have compared the values for these free fractions obtained by our method with other methods and the correlations are close. During reproductive life, the sex hormone binding levels to globulin are fairly constant except for pregnancy and disease states such as hyperthyroidism. So that the ratio of total oestradiol concentration to free concentration remains fairly constant.

12. Effects of physiological changes in sex hormones on potential coronary risk factors

J. BONNAR

In general, the incidence of death from coronary heart disease increases with age in all populations. In countries with a high incidence of heart disease the death rate in the age group 25 to 55 years is considerably higher in men than in women. For example, in this age group the ratio of male to female deaths was reported to be 5:1 in the United States and in Edinburgh, Scotland, in the age group 30 to 44 years the ratio for sudden cardiac death was 5.5:1 (Oliver, 1974). This sex advantage for women declines with age and finally disappears after the menopause. However, in countries such as Japan, where the population is at low risk, the sex difference is absent in the reproductive age group.

My task is to review physiological events in the female reproductive years, with a view to discussing how these might influence certain high-risk factors for vascular disease. This is a vast and complex field where many gaps in knowledge exist. I have selected the phenomena of:
1. The menstrual cycle and ovulation,
2. Pregnancy and lactation,
3. Age of the menopause.
Risk factors for atherosclerosis and death from coronary artery disease have been identified in relation to carbohydrate and lipid metabolism, blood pressure and the blood clotting mechanism. This is not to suggest that we are dealing with aberrations of isolated aspects of physiology. These processes in vivo are closely intermeshed and biochemically related.

The menstrual cycle and ovulation

The female reproductive years are characterised by the presence of the menstrual cycle reflecting the cyclical changes in the ovary which are interdependent of pituitary and hypothalamic function. The phases of the menstrual cycle are characterised by formation of specific steroid hormones in different parts of the ovary — follicle, stroma and corpus luteum — in response to gonadotrophin stimulation and ultimately related to the age and endocrine state of the ovary. The metabolic pathways for the biosynthesis of ovarian steroid hormones are complex. Cholesterol provides the basis for the formation of the steroid nucleus which is common to all steroid hormones. Acetate conversion to cholesterol initially described in the liver and adrenal also occurs in the ovary. Side-chain cleavage of cholesterol in progesterone and aromatisation of androgens to oestrogens occurs in both the ovary and the placenta.

Lipid and carbohydrate metabolism during the menstrual cycle

In a group of healthy young women, Oliver and Boyd (1953) found definite cyclical changes in the plasma lipids during the menstrual cycle. At mid-cycle a sharp decrease of plasma total-cholesterol occurred and a less marked fall in plasma phospholipids with a resultant fall in the total-cholesterol: phospholipid ratio.

In the follicular and luteal phase of the cycle a greater increase in plasma cholesterol than in phospholipids occurred and therefore a relative increase in the total-cholesterol: phospholipid ratio. Such findings suggest that during the reproductive years the plasma total cholesterol and plasma total-cholesterol: phospholipid ratio are regularly depressed during the menstrual cycle, possibly influenced directly or indirectly by the ovarian hormones. During the menstrual cycle minimal changes of glucose tolerance and insulin secretion have been reported, but on the whole the changes remain within the normal limits of the test systems used.

Ryan (1976) recently reviewed the role of oestrogen and atherosclerosis and the effect of steroids on lipoprotein factors (Table 12.1). Oestrogens tend to increase the cholesterol in high-density lipoproteins and decrease cholesterol in low-density lipoproteins, with often no change in total serum cholesterol.

Table 12.1 Effect of oestrogens on lipid metabolism. From: Ryan, K.J. (1976) Estrogen and atherosclerosis. *Clinical Obstetrics and Gynecology*, **Vol. 19**, No. 4, pp. 805-815.

	Protein: Lipid ratio	Cholesterol: phospholipid ratio	% Triglycerides	Oestrogen effect on lipoprotein concentration
High-density Lipoproteins (HDL)	1	0.8	5	↑
Low-density Lipoproteins (LDL)	0.25	2	‾5	↓
Very low density Lipoproteins (VLDL)	<0.2	1-1.8	15-70	↑

In addition, oestrogens increase very low-density lipoproteins. There appears to be an elaborate feed mechanism whereby dietary and blood borne lipoprotein-bound cholesterol can regulate endogenous cellular cholesterol production.

Blood clotting and platelet function during the menstrual cycle

Coagulation factors and inhibitors do not appear to show any significant variation during the normal menstrual cycle. Likewise, fibrinolytic activity of the circulating blood has been found to be constant throughout. Several authors have reported a decrease in the platelet count at the onset of menstruation. Minimal variations of platelet adhesiveness and aggregation have been reported during the cycle. A significant difference in platelet sensitivity to aggregating stimuli was found between men and women, male sensitivity increasing at a greater rate than female sensitivity (Johnson *et al*, 1975). High-risk age groups showed enhanced platelet responses when compared with low-risk groups. These changes were considered to reflect possibly the effects of androgens in the male rather than oestrogen in females, as no difference between pre- and post-menopausal women was found.

Blood pressure   Arterial blood pressure shows a steady slight rise after the age of 35 years, but no significant variation occurs within the menstrual cycle.

Pregnancy and lactation

In pregnancy, homeostasis undergoes continuous and extensive modifications and manifestly healthy women have many biochemical and physiological measurements which differ considerably from those found in non-pregnant women and men. The total dependence of the fetus on the mother for nutritional support necessitates an extensive adjustment of metabolism in the mother during pregnancy.

Lipid metabolism

An increase in the serum concentrations of the major lipid classes occurs during pregnancy and is most marked at term. Post-heparin esterase activity and lipoprotein lipase determinations indicate inhibition of these activities in late pregnancy, with a rapid return to normal following delivery. The elevation of serum triglyceride is usually the most marked; cholesterol can also rise to around double the normal limit for non-pregnant females of the same age (Fallon, 1975). The changes in serum lipid constituents are a consequence of corresponding increases in low-density lipoproteins.

During pregnancy, the feto-placental unit increases the production of oestrogens approximately one-thousand-fold. Cholesterol cannot be synthesised by the placenta. The placenta is rich in the enzyme (C_{20} - C_{22} - desmolase) which converts cholesterol to pregnenolone — the precursor of progesterone and other steroid hormones. The cholesterol for this process must come either from the mother or the fetus. *Fetal cholesterol* appears to be utilised in oestrogen production in the feto-placental unit and *maternal cholesterol* for progesterone production in the placenta. The roles of these hormones in the physiological and biochemical changes of liver function in normal pregnancy are not yet clear.

Carbohydrate metabolism

The energy requirements of the developing fetus are believed to be met entirely by consumption of glucose (Dawes and Shelley, 1968). It is not surprising, therefore, that pregnancy is accompanied by profound changes in carbohydrate metabolism. In normal pregnancy the circulating levels of glucose and amino acids are reduced, free fatty acids and ketones are increased, while the secretion of insulin in response to glucose is augmented. Pregnancy constitutes a major diabetogenic stress and in genetically predisposed women gestational diabetes develops which reverts completely to normal following delivery. This strongly suggests that the feto-placental unit is responsible for the diabetogenic stress. Enhanced utilisation of fat is also a feature of pregnancy, possibly mediated by human placental lactogen which is immunochemically and biologically similar to growth hormone.

Blood pressure in pregnancy and cardiovascular function

Blood pressure during pregnancy has been the subject of numerous studies. Hytten and Leitch (1971) concluded that systolic arterial pressure was slightly below the non-pregnant level, rising in late pregnancy, and the diastolic pressure was considerably below non-pregnant levels from early in pregnancy until the third trimester.

In a study of 2,000 women with chronic hypertension, approximately one-third were found to remain essentially unchanged, in one-third the blood pressure decreased, and in the remaining one-third the blood pressure increased with evidence of superimposed pregnancy-induced hypertension (Finnerty, 1975). In the hypertensive group whose blood pressure fell, the decrease occurred in the first trimester and the blood pressure remained low throughout pregnancy. After delivery the blood pressure rose to above the non-pregnant level and over several weeks returned to its usual hypertensive range.

In a cohort of 6662 white pregnant women, age and parity were found to have significant effects on blood pressure during pregnancy. For a given age, primigravidas were observed to have higher mean blood pressures than parous women, irrespective of the inclusion or exclusion of women diagnosed as having hypertensive disorders (Christianson, 1976). Within each parity level, the mean systolic blood pressures were similar for pregnant women under 25 years to those 25 to 34 years; after age 35 years the blood pressures showed a slight increase. MacGillivray (1961) found that diastolic pressure rose after the age of 30 years.

Pregnancy is accompanied by circulatory changes which are evident from the first trimester. Increments in cardiac output approach 30 to 40 per cent. by 20 to 24 weeks, heart rate increases by around 15 beats per minute and blood volume by 20 to 100 per cent. above non-pregnant values. These changes in cardiovascular function during pregnancy are probably major factors which counter-balance any potential hazards arising from the metabolic and coagulation system changes which accompany normal pregnancy.

Blood coagulation and fibrinolysis in pregnancy

The adaptations of the utero-placental blood supply to meet the needs of the growing fetus involve fibrin deposition in the expanded spiral arteries. In these vessels mural thrombi are found in apparently normal pregnancy in healthy young women. The increased production of fibrinogen and coagulation factors during pregnancy appear to be partly a compensatory response to utilisation in the utero-placental circulation. Fibrinolytic activity is markedly depressed during pregnancy and returns to normal within one hour of placental delivery. In pregnancies complicated by severe fetal growth retardation, placental infarction is almost invariably present. In these pregnancies, extensive atheromatous-type lesions are found in the utero-placental arteries (Fig. 12.1). Partial or complete occlusion of the spiral arteries occurs which is associated with ischaemic areas or infarcts in the placenta (Sheppard and Bonnar, 1976). This type of vascular pathology is most often found in pregnancies complicated by hypertension, but similar lesions can occur in the absence of hypertension and

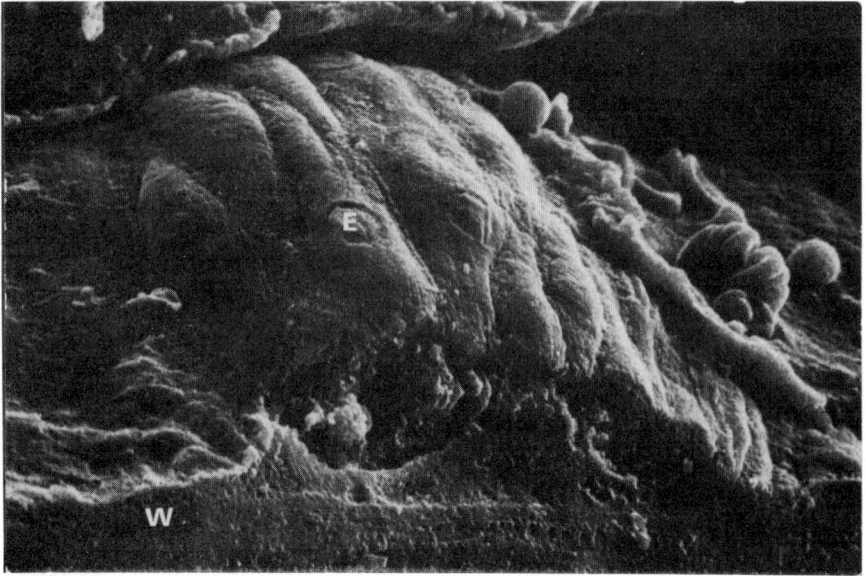

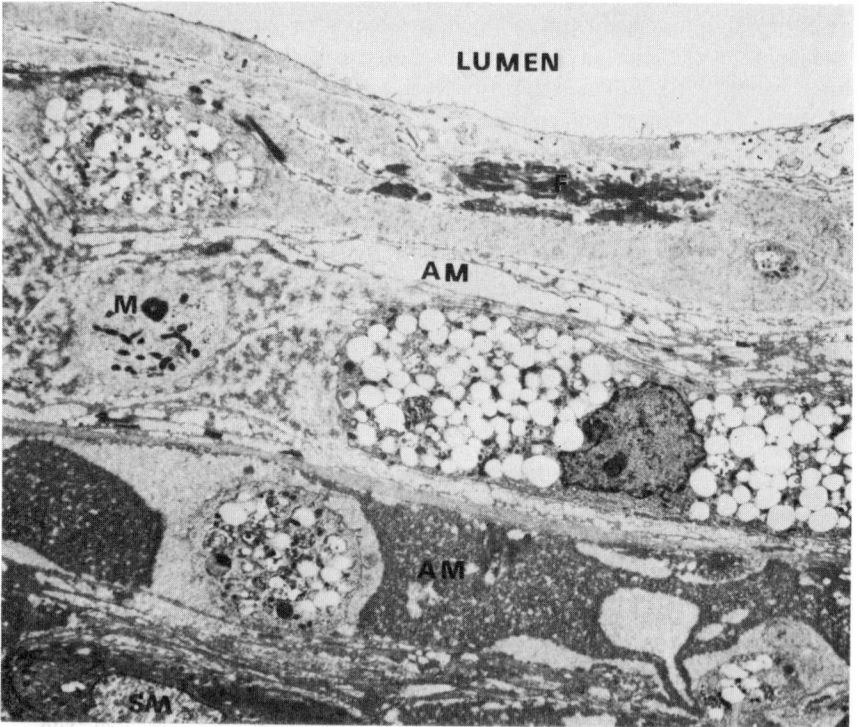

Fig.l2.1 (a) Scanning electron micrograph of a longitudinal section through a utero-placental spiral artery in a pregnancy complicated by severe fetal growth retardation. The atheromatous lesion in the vessel wall (W) is lined by endothelium (E) (x 1500)

(b) Transmission electron micrograph through part of the lesion shown above. Mononuclear cells (M), some of which contain lipid (L), smooth muscle cells (SM), fibrin (F) and amorphous material (AM) of varying electron density are seen within the lesion beneath the endothelial lining (E) (x 5000).

From: Sheppard, B.L. and Bonnar, J. The ultrastructure of the arterial supply of the human placenta in pregnancy complicated by fetal growth retardation. *British Journal of Obstetrics and Gynaecology*, 83, No. 12, 948-959, 1976.

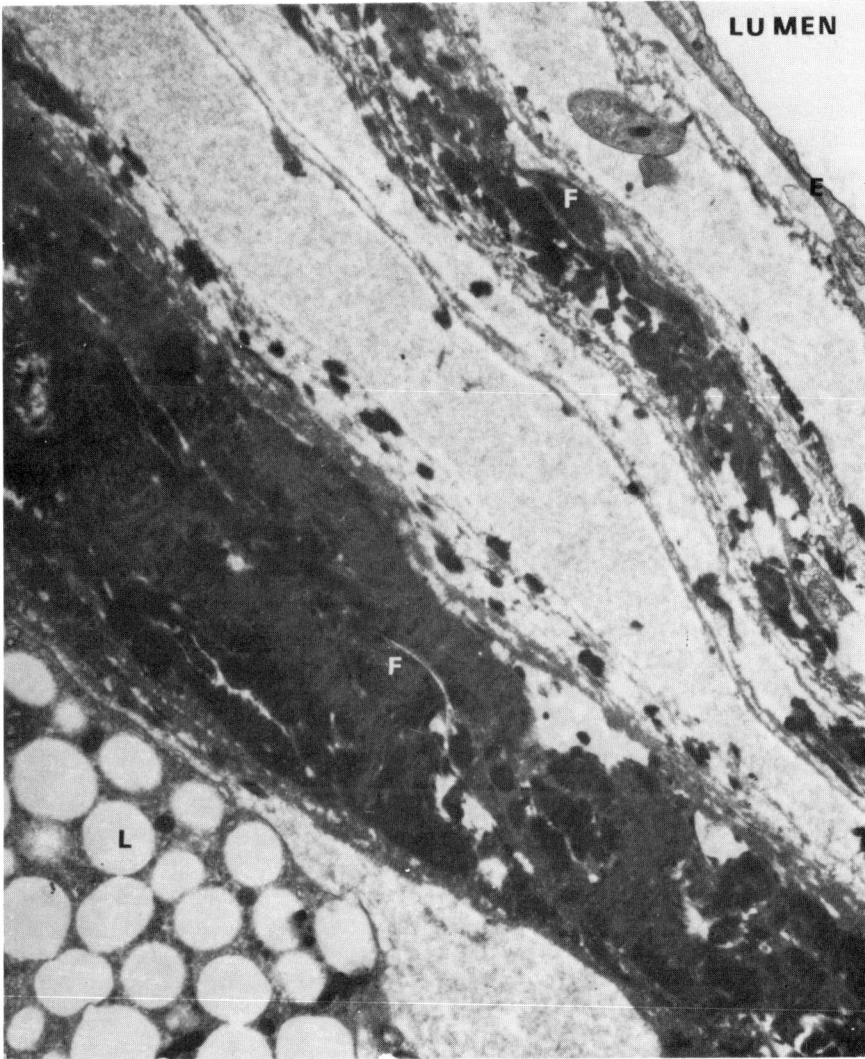

Fig. 12.2 Part of an atheromatous-type lesion in a spiral artery of a pregnancy complicated by severe fetal growth retardation. Part of a lipid-laden cell (L) is shown below the endothelium (E) but layers of fibrin (F) are the main feature of the lesion. (x 10,000). From: Sheppard, B.L. and Bonnar, J. The ultrastructure of the arterial supply of the human placenta in pregnancy complicated by fetal growth retardation. *British Journal of Obstetrics and Gynaecology*, 83, No. 12, 948-959, 1976.

also in association with heavy smoking. The atheromatous lesions in the spiral arteries show a considerable amount of fibrin deposition (Fig. 12.2). These pathological changes in the spiral arteries appear to develop rapidly, probably within three months. Given that the life span of the utero-placental circulation is limited to nine months, such a rapid atherogenesis is not surprising.

Myocardial infarction and pregnancy   Acute myocardial infarction is very rare during pregnancy and the incidence is estimated at less than 1 in 10,000 deliveries. Ginz (1970) found the frequency of myocardial infarction was highest during the third trimester, but the mortality rate was highest (50 per cent.) in the puerperium. Parity does not appear to be a factor contributing to ischaemic heart disease occurring in the pregnant or the non-pregnant state. Maternal death studies over the last 25 years show no evidence of any increase in deaths due to coronary heart disease, despite the marked rise of cigarette smoking in young women during this period.

Lactation

In recent years, in developed countries, the practice of breast feeding has largely been dispensed with. In women who do breast feed, lactation is usually only for a brief period. During pregnancy, an important physiological change is the deposition of fat. The amount varies from woman to woman, but the average is calculated to be around 4 kg. Women who breast feed seem to lose most of their recently acquired fat, but in the mother who does not breast feed this additional fat will remain unless she restricts her food intake. The decline in breast feeding in Western societies may therefore be a contributory factor to the serious problem of obesity. Many women certainly seem to date the start of their obesity problem to pregnancy.

The menopause and age

The sex differences in cardiovascular disease decrease with advancing age and for many years the age of the menopause has appeared to be a relevant factor.

Cholesterol and triglyceride levels are known to increase after the menopause. Several reports strongly suggest that a premature menopause appears to be a contributory factor to coronary heart disease. In a study of 150 women with ischaemic heart disease, Oliver (1974) found a premature menopause had occurred in 20 per cent., and most of these women had hyperlipidaemia. No relationship was found between ischaemic heart disease and age of the menarche, parity or number of abortions.

In a study of 21 women with advanced coronary atherosclerosis, aged 40 years or younger, Engel and colleagues (1974) found that common predisposing factors were family history, hypertension, glucose intolerance and cigarette smoking (Table 12.2). Oophorectomy had been performed in 4 out of the 21 patients and each had received supplementary oestrogen therapy (Table 12.3).

The relation of the age of the menopause to the incidence of cardiovascular disease was investigated in the Framingham Study (Kannel *et al*, 1976). In the 20 years of follow-up, 20 cardiovascular events occurred among pre-menopausal women aged 40 to 54 years and 70 events among post-menopausal women of the same age. Although

Table 12.2 Risk factors for coronary artery disease in 21 young women aged 40 years or younger. Adapted from: Engel *et al*, (1974) Coronary heart disease in young women. *Journal of American Medical Association*, **230**, No.11, 1531-1534.

Family history of myocardial infarction		17/21	(81%)
	hypertension	4/21	
	diabetes	6/21	
		20/21	(95%)
Smoking		16/21	(76%)
Obesity		10/21	(48%)
Hypertension		11/21	(52%)

Table 12.3 Gynaecological data from 21 young women aged 40 years or younger with coronary artery disease. Adapted from: Engel *et al*, (1974) Coronary heart disease in young women. *Journal of American Medical Association*, **230**, No. 11, 1531-1534.

Normal menstruation	8/21	(38%)
Definitely premenopausal	9/21	(43%)
Probably premenopausal	8/21	(38%)
Hysterectomy	6/21	(29%)
Bilateral oophorectomy and oestrogen replacement	4/21	(19%)
Oral contraception	4/21	(19%)
All parous (Mean 2.9)		

the numbers are small, comparison of the incidence of cardiovascular disease at specified ages showed up to age 55 a two-fold incidence among post-menopausal versus pre-menopausal women; this was highly significant.

The study also suggested that the menopause had a greater impact at younger ages than older. The data of the Framingham Study would certainly suggest that women tend to lose their relative immunity to cardiovascular disease on going through the menopause.

In a report (Parrish *et al*, 1967) based on autopsy material, women who had undergone castration up to 15 years previously were compared with non-castrated controls of the same age and race; excessive coronary atherosclerosis was not seen unless the castration was performed before the age of 40 years and the individual survived 14 years beyond the operation.

Conclusion

During pregnancy, the female has an extensive modification of her metabolism to meet the needs of the fetus. These involve changes of lipid and carbohydrate metabolism and the haemostatic system, and are accompanied by altered cardiovascular dynamics. This would suggest that the female of the species, through the evolutionary process, has developed a greater ability than the male to cope with such stresses, at least during her reproductive years.

The sex advantage of women over men is found only in high-risk relatively affluent

E

populations. The presence of predisposing factors, such as diabetes and severe hypertension, virtually eliminates the female advantage in ischaemic heart disease. The weight of evidence indicates that normal ovarian function is important in women in the reproductive stage of their life, as this offers protection from atherosclerotic heart disease; women who suffer a premature menopause below 40 years are at increased risk. The precise mechanism whereby protection against atherosclerosis is lost during and after the menopause is still unknown.

As yet there is no evidence that oestrogen therapy after the menopause will reduce or increase this hazard. The oestrogen preparations at present being used, however, are known to alter components of the coagulation system.

Oestrogen therapy prior to the menopause, which suppresses normal ovarian function, increases the hazard of vascular complications, particularly in women who are already at risk due to other risk factors.

References

Christianson, R.E. (1973) Studies on blood pressure during pregnancy. *American Journal of Obstetrics and Gynecology,* **125**, No. 4, 509-513.

Dawes, G.S. and Shelley, H.J. (1968) Physiological aspects of carbohydrate metabolism in the fetus and newborn. In: *Carbohydrate Metabolism and its Disorders,* Vol. 2, Eds. Dickens, F., Randle, R.J. and Whelan, W.J. Academic Press, New York.

Engel, H.J., Page, H.L. and Campbell, W.B. (1974) Coronary heart disease in young women. *Journal of American Medical Association,* **230**, No. 11, 1531-1534.

Fallon, (1975) In: *Medical Complications of Pregnancy.* Eds. Burrow, G.N. and Ferris, T.F. W.B. Saunders, Philadelphia and London. 351-356.

Finnerty, F.A. (1975) Hypertension in pregnancy. *Clinical Obstetrics and Gynecology,* **18**, No. 3, 145-154.

Ginz, B. (1970) Myocardial infarction in pregnancy. *Journal of Obstetrics and Gynaecology of the British Commonwealth,* **77**, 610.

Hytten, F.E. and Leitch, I. (1971) *The physiology of human pregnancy,* Ed. 2, Blackwell Scientific Publications, Oxford, p.83.

Johnson, M., Ramsey, E. & Ramwell, P.W. (1975) Sex and age differences in human platelet aggregation. *Nature,* **253**, 355-357.

Kannel, W.B., Hjortland, M.C. and McNamara, P.M. (1976) Menopause and risk of cardiovascular disease The Framingham Study. *Annals of Internal Medicine,* **85**, 447-452.

MacGillivray, I. (1961) Hypertension in pregnancy and its consequences. *Journal of Obstetrics and Gynaecology of the British Commonwealth,* **68**, 557.

Oliver, M.F. (1974) Ischaemic heart disease in young women. *British Medical Journal,* **4**, 253-259.

Oliver, M.F. and Boyd, G.S. (1953) Changes in the plasma lipids during the menstrual cycle. *Journal of Clin. Sci.,* 217.

Parrish, H.M., Carr, H.A., Hall, D.G. and King, J.M. (1967) Time interval after castration in premenopausal women to development of excessive coronary atherosclerosis. *American Journal of Obstetrics and Gynecology,* **99**, 155.

Ryan, K.J. (1976) Estrogen and atherosclerosis. *Clinical Obstetrics and Gynecology,* **Vol. 19,** No. 4, 805-815.
Sheppard, B.L. and Bonnar, J. (1976) The ultrastructure of the arterial supply of the human placenta in pregnancy complicated by fetal growth retardation. *British Journal of Obstetrics and Gynaecology,* **83,** No.12, 948-959.

Discussion 3C

Marquis (Edinburgh)   I was interested in your remark that multiparity was not associated with an increased instance of myocardial infarction in women. I had understood otherwise.

Bonnar   The problem is complicated by age insofar as the greater the parity, the more likely it is that women will be in the age group 35/45, but the evidence that we have does not point to any greatly increased risk. They are often also very obese and perhaps more hypertensive but on its own parity does not increase risk of coronary heart disease.

Oliver (Edinburgh)   We made a study of this some years ago and found that significantly more female coronary patients had 4 or more pregnancies than aged-matched controls. Also, in the 'normal' population selected at random those with 4 or more pregnancies had significantly more coronary disease. But the same was true for fathers!

Gordon (Bethesda)   In the Framingham study we found no association between parity and coronary heart disease in women.

Bengtsson (Goteborg)   In Goteborg we found that women who have borne many children, there was a statistically significant increased number of women with myocardial infarction, although the difference was not great.

Wynn (London)   I understand that there is no difference in CHD incidence between young and middle aged black men and women in America.

Morris (Birmingham, Ala.)   No, there is still a slight male predominance.

Doll (Oxford)   The only coloured population I know with equally high incidence in women as in men is the Maori population in New Zealand with the same myocardial infarction mortality rate.

Spain (Brooklyn)   The sudden death rate in white men exceeds that of women by a 10/1 ratio, but in the black population the number of sudden deaths from coronary heart disease in women is somewhat more than the male.

Bonnar   This all refers to high risk populations. In the Japanese population, there is no difference during the reproductive years. When other factors come in, the male appears to cope less adequately with them than perhaps the female. This is my conclusion on the available data.

Spain (Brooklyn) Certainly, an explanation for sudden death is that there was a much higher proportion of hypertension in the black female.

Hazzard (Seattle) It is my impression that the only risk factor which clearly obliterates the sex differential is diabetes mellitus. All other risk factors give an increase in risk relevant to women without the same risk factor, but to men they still are of little importance and CHD occurs about 10 years later or so.

Wynn (London) In the low risk groups, such as the Japanese, diabetes is not a risk factor in women.

Bonnar   I think severe hypertension in a woman would also eliminate any sex advantage.

General discussion

Nordin To amplify what Professors Baird and Vermeulen have said, a close relationship exists between plasma androstenedione and oestrone levels in post-menopausal women (Fig. GD3.1). The solid circles represent untreated normal

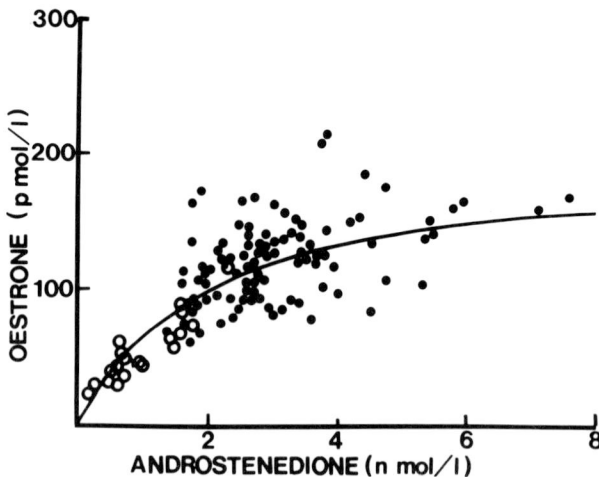

Fig. GD3.1   The relationship between plasma androstenedione and plasma oestrone is untreated ( ) and steroid-treated (o) post-menopausal women.

and oophorectomised post-menopausal women and the open circles corticosteroid treated cases. The data form a continuous series which goes through the origin and make it clear that what matters to the post-menopausal women in terms of her oestrogen status is her plasma androstenedione level. About 66 percent of the variance on plasma oestrone is accounted for by the androstenedione level, so the actual conversion rate in any individual patient is less important than the plasma androstenedione concentration. The latter is of course mainly adrenal in origin but there is also a significant contribution from the post-menopausal ovarian stroma which explains why oophorectomised women tend to have lower androstenedione and therefore oestrone levels than women with intact ovaries. Osteoporotic women have lower androstenedione and oestrone levels than age-matched normal women and resemble oophorectomised women in this respect — even if they have not been oophorectomised. Corticosteroid treatment suppresses the pituitary and produces low androstenedione levels and, therefore, low oestrone and (incidentally) low testosterone levels. Again, what matters to the woman is what her androstenedione level is, not what the rate of conversion happens to be. The low oestrone levels in steroid-treated post-menopausal women probably explain their high risk of osteoporosis and constitutes an indication for oestrogen therapy in this group, who also have very low oestradiol and testosterone levels.

Professor Vermeulen shows data of the oestradiol/testosterone ratio but I question the validity of the ratio which must, by virtue of these data, be varying according to what the androstenedione level or the testosterone level is.

Vermeulen   In man, the origin of oestradiol is mostly from testosterone and not from androstenedione.

Nordin (Sheffield)   Our corresponding data on men suggest that plasma oestrone depends on plasma androstenedione, but plasma oestradiol depends on plasma testosterone. I was rather surprised by your data inferring that oestradiol goes up with age in men while testosterone is going down because that would suggest a large change in conversion rate.

Short (Edinburgh)   But do we know about the testicular secretion rate for oestradiol in elderly men? Perhaps that goes up as the testosterone level comes down?

Nordin (Sheffield)   Of course, as the testosterone level declines, the level of sex hormone-binding globulin is going up and, as oestradiol has a high affinity of sex hormone globulin, it will increase.

Vermeulen   Metabolism is a direct function of the free fraction of oestradiol. This free fraction changes relative to the free fraction of testosterone, so I think the situation is rather complex. While oestrone levels may be a direct function of androstenedione in elderly men the androstenedione level is constant.

SESSION 4 What are the coronary risk factors in young women?

Chairman: J.R.A. Mitchell

13. Hormones and lipoprotein metabolism

B. LEWIS

Lipoproteins: Composition and functional roles

The plasma lipoproteins have evolved to permit transport of the sparingly soluble lipids between the liver and small intestine (the sites of lipoprotein synthesis) and adipose tissue, muscle and most other peripheral tissues. The lipoproteins are partly metabolised within the plasma, and exchange certain lipid and protein components between them. Current concepts suggest that there are two systems of plasma lipoproteins, one concerned with the outward transport of lipids to peripheral tissues, the other with centripetal transport. The first system includes chylomicrons, very low density lipoproteins (VLDL) and low density lipoprotein (LDL), the second is the high density lipoproteins (HDL). Normal and abnormal lipoprotein metabolism has recently been reviewed (Lewis, 1976) and will not be discussed at length in this chapter.

Chylomicrons carry dietary triglyceride from the small intestine during alimentary lipaemia, and have this lipid as their main component. VLDL is the major form in which triglyceride of endogenous origin is transported. These particles also bear absorbed cholesterol and cholesterol synthesised in the liver and small intestine. Both particles are metabolised at the vascular endothelial surface, particularly in the capillary beds of muscle and adipose tissue. The essential and rate-limiting enzyme lipoprotein lipase, sited in endothelial cells hydrolyses much of this triglyceride and some phospholipid of these lipoproteins. The fatty acids enter the parenchymal cells, while smaller lipoprotein products remain in plasma. These products known as remnant particles, still contain their structural protein and cholesteryl ester moieties. They are further metabolised in the liver, where they may be converted largely or almost quantitatively to low density lipoprotein. This is true of normal man and is the source of LDL. However these relationships differ in certain hyperlipidaemic states, and in other species.

LDL, carrying some 60-70 per cent of the plasma cholesterol, appears to be metabolised intracellularly in peripheral tissues, fibroblasts, smooth muscle cells, adipocytes and monocytes being amongst the cell types known to have this property. The cholesterol is stored or utilised, and the protein is hydrolysed. Thus tissue accumulation of cholesterol is in part determined by LDL turnover.

HDL is also secreted by the liver and contains cholesterol and other lipids. There is strong evidence that it acquires further cholesterol from peripheral tissues. Its site of catabolism appears to be the liver. Hence HDL may constitute an important vehicle for cholesterol mobilisation from such tissues; the lipid is ultimately excreted or catabolised by the liver.

F*

Accumulation of cholesterol in the arterial intima may therefore be influenced by the balance between LDL and HDL metabolism (Fig. 13.1). Epidemiological data is compatible with this. The flux of cholesterol into the intima correlates closely with plasma LDL concentration (Niehaus *et al*, 1977). Conversely the size of the exchangeable pools of cholesterol in the tissues is inversely related to plasma HDL levels (Miller *et al*, 1976).

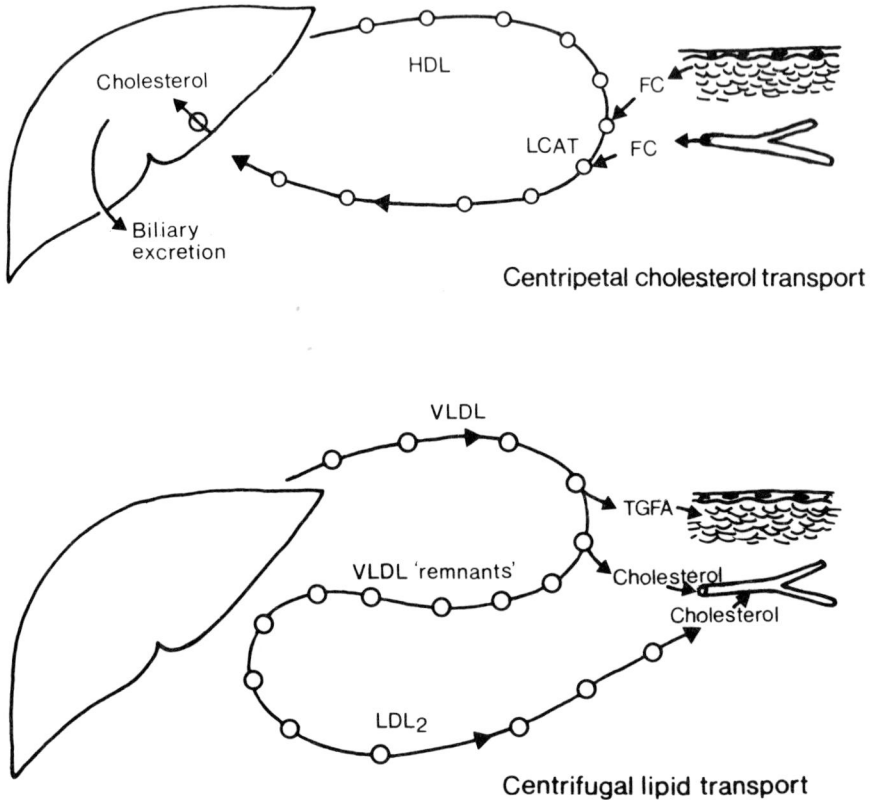

Centripetal cholesterol transport

Centrifugal lipid transport

Fig. 13.1

Hormonal influences on plasma lipoproteins

Some of these effects are summarised in Table 13.1. Insulin has at least two sites of action on plasma lipoprotein metabolism. By decreasing free fatty acid release from adipose tissue it limits the supply to the liver of a major substrate for VLDL triglyceride synthesis. A second effect also tending to increase VLDL levels is induction of lipoprotein lipase activity in adipose tissue.

It has further been suggested that insulin has an opposite, direct effect on the liver, increasing triglyceride synthesis and VLDL production; if true this might be the mechanism at least of a subgroup of endogenous hypertriglyceridaemias. Though such patients are often hyperinsulinaemic there is little experimental evidence that this association is one of cause and effect. In a study on a single hyperinsulinaemic patient, Chait, Janus and Lewis (unpublished data) have shown that suppression of insulin production by diazoxide-reduced VLDL production by 50 per cent led to a marked fall in initially raised serum triglyceride levels.

A hypolipidaemic effect of glucagon has been demonstrated but it is not certain that this response is specific as the dosages used were probably unphysiological.

In thyroid insufficiency, elevated LDL levels are attributable to subnormal excretion and catabolism of cholesterol; hypertriglyceridaemia is also probably due to impaired clearance from plasma.

Table 13.1 Some hormonal effects on plasma lipid and lipoprotein concentrations.

Insulin	In diabetes:	triglyceride ↓ cholesterol ↓
		free fatty acids ↓
		VLDL ↓ HDL ↑
	In primary hypertriglyceridaemia:	VLDL ↑ ?
Glucagon	cholesterol ↓ triglyceride ↓	
Thyroxine	cholesterol ↓ triglyceride ↓	
	free fatty acids ↑	
	VLDL ↓ LDL ↓	
Catecholamines	β-receptor:	triglyceride ↑ cholesterol ↑
	free fatty acid ↑	
	VLDL ↑	
	β-receptor:	free fatty acids ↓
Corticosteroids	cholesterol ↓ ↑ triglyceride ↓ ↑	
	free fatty acids ↑	

Catecholamines have a powerful effect (mediated by β-adrenergic receptors) in increasing release of free fatty acids from adipose tissue. The consequent increased fatty acid flux into the liver leads to enhanced VLDL production. Corticosteroids lead to biphasic changes in serum lipid levels — in susceptible individuals the second hyperlipidaemic stage may be pronounced.

Sex differences in serum lipoprotein concentrations

Throughout adult life, serum triglyceride levels are lower in women than in men, reflecting differences in VLDL concentration (Lewis, 1976). The isolated perfused liver from male rats shows a greater rate of VLDL production than that by female livers; and the clearance of circulating triglycerides appears to be more rapid in women than men, as assessed by the fractional catabolic rate of injected triglyceride emulsion. VLDL cholesterol as well as triglyceride levels are higher in men than in women.

In young women, serum LDL concentrations and total cholesterol levels are somewhat lower than in men of similar age; the increase in LDL levels during middle age is steeper in women than in men, and above age 45 mean LDL concentrations are higher in women.

High density lipoprotein levels in women exceed those of men at all ages; our own data do not show any significant age-related trends. This sex difference is largely due to higher concentrations of the less-dense subfraction HDL_2.

Sex hormone effects on lipoprotein metabolism

Oestrogens increase VLDL and HDL concentrations and decrease LDL concentration. The rise in VLDL levels is accompanied by compositional changes, particularly a decrease in the proportion of one of the several apoproteins, apo CII. This protein is of functional importance, for it is a specific activator of lipoprotein lipase. Yet oestrogens have not been shown to alter the fractional catabolic rate of endogenous triglyceride. There is good evidence in man and in the rat that their effect on VLDL concentration is due to increased secretion of this lipoprotein. Oestradiol increases the synthesis of VLDL apoprotein by the isolated rat liver. It is possible that certain oestrogens have a greater effect on VLDL levels than others; it has been reported that a so-called 'natural' oestrogen did not increase serum triglyceride, while ethinyl oestradiol did. Such studies are susceptible to the difficulty of choosing oestrogenically-equivalent doses of different hormones.

Although LDL is normally a product of VLDL metabolism its concentration is decreased by oestrogens. The mechanism is unknown: LDL catabolism could be enhanced, or possibly the conversion of VLDL remnant particles to products other than LDL is increased. A decrease in the cholesterol:protein ratio of LDL has been reported.

Though oestrogenic hormones increase total HDL concentration there is an apparent inconsistency as to which HDL subclass is affected. While HDL_2 levels fluctuate during the menstrual cycle and are considerably higher (about two-fold) in premenopausal women than in men, it has recently been claimed that oestradiol administration selectively elevates HDL_3 concentration.

Despite the usual hypertriglyceridaemic effect of oestrogens, one situation has been identified in which a paradoxical response occurs: Hazzard et al (Gagne, 1975) have shown that in women with remnant hyperlipoproteinaemia (Type III; broad β disease), the subnormal clearance of remnant particles is enhanced by oestrogens.

Androgens, generally, have opposite effects to oestrogens on plasma lipoprotein concentrations.

Progestogens have been inadequately studied. There is evidence to suggest that VLDL concentrations are reduced, due to enhanced clearance from plasma.

Sex differences in serum lipoprotein levels are partly attributable to known effects of androgens and oestrogens. In particular differences in LDL and total HDL concentrations may be so explained. The lower VLDL level in women of all ages are not readily accounted for; conceivably this may be proved to be related to a progesterone effect.

Oestrogen – progestogen combinations: the contraceptive pill

In premenopausal women, the effect of earlier, high-oestrogen oral contraceptives in increasing serum triglyceride levels was well documented by Wynn and his colleagues (Wynn, 1966) and by others. Serum cholesterol concentration is increased to a lesser extent. Postmenopausally, a sequential oestrogen-progestogen

preparation studied by Magnani (Magnani and Moore, 1976) also increased triglyceride levels, but serum cholesterol levels were decreased.

Studies on the effect of the contraceptive pill on the plasma lipoprotein classes
appear to be separable into two phases. The high-oestrogen preparations were
found to increase VLDL levels as their major effect. Rossner *et al* (Rossner, 1971)
and Dr. George Miller and I (to be published) have obtained data on newer lower
dose oral contraceptives. Rossner's study was an internally-controlled one. The main
findings were that the triglyceride content increased in all three lipoprotein classes;
the contribution of LDL and HDL triglycerides changes to the rise in total plasma-
triglyceride was substantial. Changes in the cholesterol content of the individual
lipoproteins did not attain statistical significance though total cholesterol levels
rose significantly.

Our own findings are based on a population survey completed in 1974. We too
found that users of oral contraceptive preparations (mostly 'Minovlar') had increased
triglyceride concentrations in all lipoprotein classes; LDL triglyceride levels in women
on the pill (0.38 mmols/1) exceeded even male concentrations (0.29 mmol/1).
VLDL cholesterol was slightly increased; and LDL cholesterol decreased (3.16 mmol/1)
compared with 3.45 mmol/1) in pill-users. When HDL cholesterol levels were directly
compared, similar values were observed in those taking oral contraceptives and those
not on the pill. Using the method of multiple regression analysis, however, it was
found that women on the pill had higher levels of HDL cholesterol than non-users
when data were adjusted for age, alcohol intake and VLDL-triglyceride concentration.
Oral contraceptives have recently been reported to increase HDL apoprotein levels
(Albers and Cheung, 1976).

In Rossner's and our studies, the increase in triglyceride levels was most often
modest in extent. The highest serum triglyceride level in the former study was
2.35 mmol/1, and in the latter only one woman receiving an oral contraceptive was
amongst those with triglyceride levels exceeding the 95th percentile. It is important
to note that individual susceptibility to the hyperlipidaemic effect of oestrogens
and oral contraceptives may be widely variable. In hyper-responders intense lipaemia,
complicated by acute pancreatitis has been reported. Zorilla *et al*, (1968) suggest
that women with primary hypertriglyceridaemic states and diabetics are particularly
susceptible.

Sex hormones and lipoprotein risk factors for coronary heart disease

Only tentative conclusions may be drawn from the data presently available. LDL
cholesterol levels are reduced by oestrogens and, modestly, by oral contraceptive
combinations. VLDL triglyceride and cholesterol levels in our study were increased
only slightly in most women on the pill, but pronounced elevation has been
observed in a minority. HDL levels are increased by oestrogens, and oral contraceptives may have a similar effect when other variables are held constant; this may be
interpretable as a protective effect against coronary heart disease (Miller and Miller,
1975).

The search for lipoprotein changes which might explain, in part, the association
between oestrogen medication and coronary heart disease has at present yielded
somewhat inconclusive results. Clearly other mechanisms may be operative. But

there is an impressive individual variation in the hyperlipidaemic response to exogenous oestrogens, as in oral contraceptives; it suggests the possibility that a small minority of women may be uniquely susceptible to this effect. If so, baseline screening for hyperlipidaemia may be of less value than assessment at 3 months after commencing treatment. Baseline screening for hyperlipidaemia and impaired glucose tolerance should however be considered in all women with characteristics suggestive of high risk: such features include a positive family history of early-onset coronary heart disease or stroke, and, of course, of overt hyperlipidaemia or diabetes. Suggestive physical signs such as tendon thickening, corneal arcus and xanthelasmas should be sought. Widespread use of such screening would tax existing laboratory facilities in the United Kingdom. On current evidence, it is likely that the best indicator of enhanced risk from oral contraceptive medication is coincident cigarette smoking (Ory, 1977).

References

Albers, J.J. and Cheung, M.C. (1976) Quantitation of apolipoprotein A II of human plasma high density lipoprotein. *Circulation,* **53**, II-93 (abstract).

Gagne, C., Kushwala, R., Abbers, J., Brunzell, J. and Hazzard, W. (1975) Type III hyperlipidemia: implications of paradoxical hypolipidemic response to estrogen. *Circulation,* **52**, II-39 (abstract).

Lewis, B., Chait, A., Wootton, I.D.P., Oakley, C.M., Krikler, D.M., Sigurdsson, G., February, A., Maurer, B. and Birkhead, J. (1974) Frequency of risk factors for ischaemic heart disease in a healthy British population. *Lancet,* **i**, 141-146.

Lewis, B. (1976) *The Hyperlipidaemias Clinical and Laboratory Practice.* Oxford. Blackwell.

Magnani, H.N. and Moore, B. (1976) The effect of sequential mestranol — norethisterone on the circulating lipid levels of pre- and post-menopausal women, and its possible significance. *Postgraduate Medical Journal,* **52** (suppl.6), 55-58.

Miller, G.J. and Miller, N.E. (1975) Plasma — high — density — lipoprotein concentration and development of ischaemic heart-disease. *Lancet,* **i**, 16-19.

Miller, N.F., Nestel, P.J. and Clifton-Bligh, P. (1976) Relationship between plasma lipoprotein cholesterol concentrations and the pool size and metabolism of cholesterol in man. *Atherosclerosis,* **23**, 535-547.

Niehaus, C.E., Nicoll, A., Wootton, R., Williams, B., Lewis, J., Coltart, D.J. and Lewis, B. (1977) *Transfer of plasma lipoprotein into human arterial intima: the influence of lipid levels and age.* Submitted for publication.

Ory, H.W. (1977) Association between oral contraceptives and myocardial infarction. *Journal of the American Medical Association,* **237**, 2619-2622.

Rossner, S., Larsson-Cohn, U., Carlson, L.A. and Boberg, J. (1971) Effects of an oral contraceptive agent on plasma lipids, plasma lipoproteins, the intravenous fat tolerance and the post-heparin lipoprotein lipase activity. *Acta Medica Scandaninavica,* **190**, 301-305.

Wynn, V., Doar, J.W.H. and Mills, G.L. (1966) Some effects of oral contraceptives on serum-lipid and lipoprotein levels. *Lancet,* **ii**, 720-724.

Zorrilla, E., Hulse, M., Hernandez, A. and Gershberg, H. (1968) Severe endogenous hypertriglyceridemia during treatment with estrogen and oral contraceptives. *Journal of Clinical Endocrinology and Metabolism,* **28,** 1793-1796.

Discussion 4A

Jarrett (London)   Is it the apoprotein or the cholesterol levels which vary with oestrogens?

Lewis   I don't think it is possible to answer that. HDL composition does vary widely and I suppose there is a capacity for HDL to acquire more cholesterol but it might be the protein structure which is the limiting factor.

Horton (Edinburgh)   Was the oestrogen you used synthetic? The dose you used could be very critical. Were all these various effects produced by a single dose or were they effectively the same if you vary the dosage?

Lewis   Doses of 20, 50 and 100 µg of oestradiol were compared.
So-called 'natural' oestrogen, which is more the advertisers' name for Premarin than reality, is, by no means natural to human beings. It must be extremely difficult, if not impossible, to obtain comparable doses of natural and synthetic oestrogen. How does one know one is giving exactly the same dose? But, the evidence is that changes in VLDL are smaller with Premarin at a dose of 1.25 mg a day, which should be an adequate replacement dose for an ovariectomised woman, than 50 µg of oestradiol.

Oliver (Edinburgh)   Oestriol and oestrone given to men lower serum cholesterol and alter the ratio of LDL to HDL less than ethinyl oestradiol. Of course, one can't be sure about equivalency in oestrogenic dose. Androgens — methyl testosterone — have a striking effect in the opposite direction. Progesterone had no effect on serum cholesterol or LDL/HDL ratio.

Loudon (Edinburgh)   There is a wide variety in the combination of oestrogen and progestogen in the oral contraceptives. Were you using one specific pill and if so, which one?

Lewis   The population study is the only one which is my own work and in it the majority of pill users were using Minovlar, which is a 50 µg preparation.

Loudon (Edinburgh)   Have you any results using a 30 µ pill?

Lewis   No, this will be very interesting.

Bonnar (Dublin)   What are the differences in the lipoproteins in post-menopausal women compared with younger women put on to a low oestrogen contraceptive pill?

Lewis   The difference between pill users and non-users is smaller than the difference between pre-menopausal women and post-menopausal women in respect of LDL levels and VLDL levels.

Oliver (Edinburgh)   In 1955 we examined healthy men and women in practices in Edinburgh selected on a random basis. The post-menopausal rise in total serum cholesterol is quite marked. This earlier observation has not been amplified adequately with lipoprotein analysis on another population randomly selected.

Somerville (London)   You said it might be advisable to screen women for suscept-ibility before starting an oral contraceptive. Do you mind saying again how you would do this screening and to whom is the screening addressed? Do you mean *all* women, or a particular sub-set of women?

Lewis   It is disappointingly difficult to find any way in which plasma lipoprotein levels mediate between the rather definite relationship of exogenous oestrogens and premature vascular disease. On the other hand, occasional women develop intense lipaemia when exposed to oestrogens. These are people with mild endogenous hypertriglyceridaemia and diabetics. In these two categories at least serum lipid measurements should be made before instituting oestrogens. Perhaps also those individuals who have a strong family history of ischaemic heart disease could justifiably be screened before allowing them to have oestrogen-containing contraceptives.

14. Metabolic effects of oral contraceptives in relation to coronary heart disease in young women

VICTOR WYNN

In 1966 my co-workers and I suggested that there would be cardiovascular hazards for young women taking the currently available oral contraceptives (Wynn and Doar, 1966; Wynn, Doar and Mills, 1969). Our predictions were based upon observations of untoward metabolic effects produced by oral contraceptives which could be considered to be atherogenic in nature. Our main findings were supplemented by later publications (Wynn and Doar, 1969; Wynn, Doar, Mills and Stokes, 1969). We showed that oral contraceptives caused impairment of glucose tolerance, hypo- or hyperinsulinism, elevated blood pyruvate and lactate levels and elevated serum lipids, including cholesterol and triglyceride. We described changes in serum lipoproteins measured by an analytical ultracentrifugal method. Certain fractions of LDL were increased, VLDL was increased and there was a decrease in HDL lipoproteins. Subsequent work has added to this list of metabolic changes. We have shown, for example, that the rise in serum triglyceride is dependent upon the dose of oestrogen but modified by the amount of progestogen (Stokes and Wynn, 1971). For a given oestrogen dose, the cholesterol rise is dependent upon the dose of progestogen when this is a 19-nor testosterone derived drug. This and other points will be elaborated upon later in the present communication. We have also found that the oestrogen is responsible for increasing the rate of triglyceride production in the liver and the progestogen for increasing its rate of removal by the peripheral tissues (Kissebah, Harrigan and Wynn, 1973). Recently we showed that the changes in serum lipids with oestrogen can be explained by an increase in the molar ratio of insulin:glucagon in the portal vein blood (in the rat) together with an oestrogen-induced resistance to glucagon effects in the liver (Mandour, Kissebah and Wynn, 1977). Further metabolic changes which may be induced by oral contraceptives are the production of pyridoxal phosphate (vitamin B_6) deficiency (Adams, Wynn, Folkard and Seed, 1976) causing an impairment in carbohydrate metabolism. The metabolism of methionine and homocystine may be altered due to reduced activity of the pyridoxal phosphate dependent enzyme cystathionine synthetase (McCully, 1975). In this respect vitamin B_6 deficiency could have a pathological effect on the coronary arteries, mimicking the inherited disorder of homocystine metabolism seen in children with homocystinuria in whom accelerated atherosclerosis has been described.

While the reports of adverse metabolic effects of oral contraceptives increased, so did the consumption of these compounds, which were promoted with little regard to the possibility of any adverse pathological effect or risk to health. The situation changed dramatically when venous thrombosis and thromboembolism, and cerebrovascular disease were described as a serious hazard of taking oral contraceptives in a series of classic papers by Inman, Vessey and Doll and co-workers, and finally linked with an increased risk of coronary heart disease by Mann and Inman, (1975) and Mann, Inman and Thorogood (1976).

In addition to thrombotic and thromboembolic disease a new hazard to the cardiovascular system of young women became apparent with numerous descriptions of hypertension induced by the pill or aggravated by it, the latest of these reports being by Fisch and Frank (1977). A recent report has shown that the incidence of hypertension in oral contraceptive users increases progesssively when the progestogen (norethisterone acetate) is increased from 1 mg to 3 mg and 4 mg, the amount of oestrogen (ethinyl oestradiol) remaining constant at 50 µg. At the 1 mg dose the incidence of hypertension was about twice that in the control subjects and at the 4 mg dose it was three and a half times greater (Royal College of General Practitioners' Oral Contraceptive Study, 1977). It has taken 22 years of oral contraceptive usage to reach the point where we now realise that both the oestrogen and progestogen have their own pathological effects and the combination of the two steroids has to be taken clearly into account in deciding what the metabolic effects and their consequence would be in the case of individual women.

The metabolic literature on the effects of oral contraceptives is now very large and much of it is inconclusive and contradictory. In the past insufficient attention has been given to the method of patient selection and studies have been written up in which fewer than 20 subjects have been investigated for as short a period as 14 days of oral contraceptive administration. It is not surprising, therefore, that it is difficult to give an account of the metabolic effects of the pill which will not be challenged by some contradictory study or other. The difficulties are further compounded by the fact that there are at least 80 different formulations of oral contraceptives in use at the present time, that duration of use is an important factor in producing metabolic effects and that there are differences between women of various ethnic origins, economic status, and cultural habits. In the studies reported here only ethnic European women are included. The results of our studies in Black, Indian and Asian women are in preparation.

Fig. 14.1 shows the results of a study of the effects of various oral contraceptives on carbohydrate metabolism which we carried out on a group of 142 women acting as their own controls and taking the contraceptives for a period of about six months. The impairment of oral glucose tolerance, hyperinsulinaemia and the elevated serum pyruvate levels are clearly shown. We have defined these changes as showing the effects of steroid diabetes because they are the metabolic changes found when small doses of glucocorticoids are given to women. Similar changes to these are found in obesity and we have previously described how oral contraceptives cause the glucose and lipid metabolism of women on oral contraceptives to resemble that of obese women and how the metabolism of obese women is impaired even further by their use of oral contraceptives (Doar and Wynn, 1970). We have also shown that in hypertensive women on oral contraceptives the impairment of glucose tolerance and the hyperlipidaemia is greatest in women with the highest blood pressure (Mason, Oakley and Wynn, 1973). It is not surprising, therefore, that untoward thrombotic effects involving the cerebral and coronary arteries should be found in young women on oral contraceptives especially if a number

Before O.C. •– – – •   On O.C. o———o

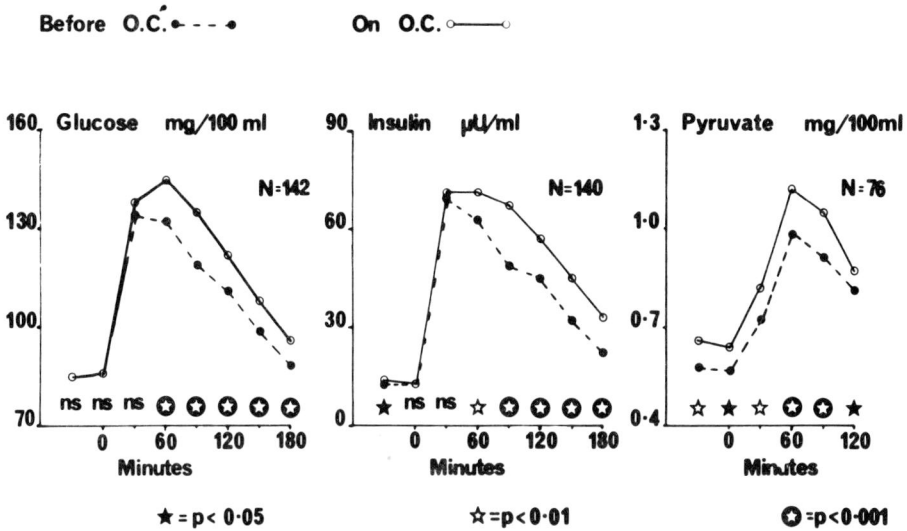

Fig. 14.1 Glucose tolerance, serum insulin and blood pyruvate in 142 women taking various oral contraceptive preparations for a minimum of six months.

of risk factors come together simultaneously, namely hyperglycaemia, hyperinsulinaemia, hyperlipidaemia, and hypertension. If one considers also the well known effects of oral contraceptives on increasing the coagualability of the blood and in altering the behaviour of the blood platelets in an untoward way and the possibility of oral contraceptive-induced pathological changes in the vessel intima, we add yet more factors increasing the risk of thrombotic complications, both arterial and venous, by the use of the oral contraceptive method.

In our more recent metabolic studies on carbohydrate and lipid metabolism, we have been able to separate the effects of the dose of oestrogen and the type of progestogen. In the first place, we have been unable to find any difference in metabolic effect between ethinyl oestradiol and mestranol, the latter being the 3 methyl ether of ethinyl oestradiol. It has long been claimed in the contraceptive literature that mestranol is a weaker oestrogen than ethinyl oestradiol. In fact, mestranol itself is inactive until the 3 methyl group has been removed by enzymatic action in the liver, as the oestrogen receptor will not combine with mestranol. This transformation occurs rapidly and probably completely in women, although progestogens in large doses may inhibit it in animals. We have been able to show quite consistently that when oral contraceptive pills contain 75 µg or more of ethinyl oestradiol or mestranol combined with any progestogen, there is a substantial deterioration in glucose tolerance and a characteristic alteration in the insulin response. The first phase insulin response is suppressed and it is only later in the glucose tolerance test that the insulin levels rise above the control values. This abnormality of suppressed and delayed insulin secretion is similar to that found in pre-clinical or sub-clinical diabetic individuals in whom, as is well known, a high risk of accelerated atherosclerosis exists, especially in women. This abnormality is illustrated in Fig. 14.2. Here, glucose tolerance in 129 apparently healthy women using Ovulen (100 µg mestranol and 1 mg of ethynodiol acetate) for an average period of 20.9 months is compared with an age weighted control group of 583 women who have never used oral contraceptives. In the Ovulen users there is marked deterioration of glucose tolerance and clearly a suppressed insulin response. In 22 per cent of the Ovulen users glucose tolerance was abnormal as judged by classical criteria compared to 1 per cent of abnormal cases in the controls. Eight per cent of the users had frankly diabetic glucose tolerance tests compared to 0.2 per cent of the controls.

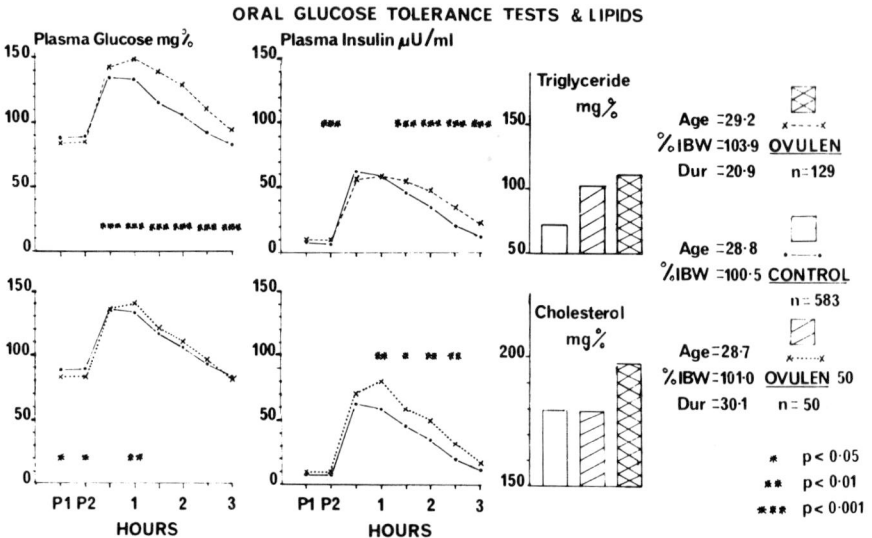

Fig. 14.2 Carbohydrate and lipid results in women taking Ovulen or Ovulen 50 compared with age-weighted control subjects.
N = No. of subjects.   Age is in years.   Dur is in months.

The serum lipid values in these individuals using Ovulen were also grossly abnormal. The mean triglyceride value was 111 mg/100 ml compared with a mean value of 72 mg/100 ml in the controls. The mean serum cholesterol in Ovulen users was 197.4 mg/100 ml compared with 182.0 mg/100 ml for age matched controls. Both the cholesterol and triglyceride values are highly significantly different from the control values ($P < 0.001$). As with carbohydrate intolerance, all the combined oral contraceptive pills with 75 µg or more of oestrogen which we studied showed similar effects. It should be stressed that up until 1969, about 50 per cent of oral contraceptives used throughout the world contained 75 µg or more of oestrogen combined with a progestogen, the metabolic consequences of which would have been those described above. In a lecture given by Dr. Gregory Pincus at the Royal Society of Medicine in London on May 4 1966 (courtesy of the library of Searle Laboratories, High Wycombe, Bucks) he referred to his studies of women using oral contraceptive pills, mainly Ovulen, and described them as possibly an improvement on nature, his exact words being, 'Perhaps in upsetting the endocrine balance we are establishing one which is superior to that which nature provides. This is always possible'. I am afraid that this is an opinion which I did not share at the time, and subsequent events have not justified Dr. Pincus' optimism. It is indeed fortunate that in 1969 the British Committee on the Safety of Medicines strongly urged that oral contraceptives containing more than 50 µg of oestrogen should not be prescribed. This recommendation was based upon the data of Inman, Vessey, Westerholm and Engelund (1970) which showed a correlation between the thrombotic risk and the dose of oestrogens, although it was admitted at the time that the data were incomplete and that there were certain inconsistencies. The metabolic data, reported here in the users of Ovulen (which I must stress we have obtained in other combined pills containing 75 µg or more of oestrogen) leave me in no doubt that the British Committee on the Safety of Medicines made the correct decision and that opposition to it, which was widespread, especially in the U.S.A. was ill-advised.

In the lower half of Fig. 14.2, one can see comparable data for the pill Ovulen 50, which is similar to Ovulen except that the oestrogen dose is 50 µg of ethinyl oestradiol. The difference in metabolic effects is striking. There is a small but still significant deterioration of glucose tolerance and a considerable increase in the amount of insulin secreted in the users during the course of the glucose tolerance test. In other words, the suppressed insulin response seen with Ovulen has been replaced by hyperinsulinism and a much less obvious deterioration of glucose tolerance. We have studied numerous other combinations of oral contraceptives containing 50 µg of ethinyl oestradiol combined with various progestogens derived from the oestrane nucleus (19 nor-testosterone progestogens) and we have found comparable results on glucose tolerance to those reported here. The serum lipid results are also different in the Ovulen 50 users compared to the higher dose oestrogen pill. With Ovulen 50, the mean serum triglyceride levels were 103 mg/100 ml compared to the control group of comparable age whose triglyceride values were 72 mg/100 ml. There was no difference in the mean cholesterol values between Ovulen 50 users and the controls (179 mg/100 ml and 182 mg/100 ml respectively). The difference in cholesterol values between Ovulen and Ovulen 50 users was 18 mg/100 ml, which is a highly significant difference.

Fig. 14.3 shows the effects on carbohydrate and lipid metabolism of two pills containing as their progestogen the gonane derivative norgestrel. Ovran (50 µg of ethinyl oestradiol, 500 mg of dl-norgestrel) produced little deterioration in glucose tolerance but there was a striking insulin response in 44 users who had taken the pill for a mean duration of 18.7 months. We found this pattern of effects consistently in all the pills we have studied so far containing norgestrel, namely that there is little change in glucose tolerance but marked hyperinsulinism, suggesting that this progestogen causes peripheral insulin resistance but does not impair the ability of the pancreas to respond. The serum lipid response in these Ovran users is important. The mean triglyceride value was 76 mg/100 ml compared with 69 mg/100 ml for a group of control women of comparable age. This is only a small difference but is statistically significant. There is no difference in serum cholesterol value which was 170 mg/100 ml for the Ovran users compared with 173 mg/100 ml for the matched control group. I should point out that the progestogen dl-norgestrel is a racemic

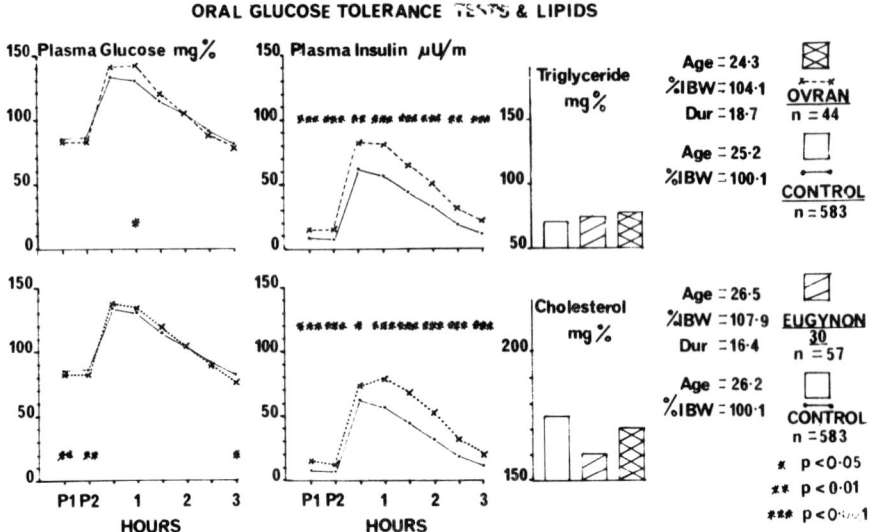

Fig. 14.3 Carbohydrate and lipid results in women taking Ovran or Eugynon 30 compared with age-weighted control subjects.
N = No. of subjects.   Age in in years.   Dur is in months.

mixture of an active d isomer and an inactive l isomer. The lower half of Fig. 14.3 shows the metabolic effect of Eugynon 30 (also marketed as Ovran 30) which contains 30 µg ethinyl oestradiol and 250 mg of d-norgestrel. There is an insignificant effect on glucose tolerance but again the hyperinsulinism found with Ovran is observed. In other words the two norgestrel containing pills show clearly an effect on pancreatic response to glucose administration. In the users of norgestrel pills there is a brisk insulin response which moderates or almost abolishes the expected hyperglycaemia. The serum triglyceride level found in the Eugynon 30 group was 75.1 mg/100 ml, which was a small but significant increase over the control value, 69 mg/100 ml. The serum cholesterol, however, was 160.1 mg/100, which was significantly lower than in the control group (170 mg/100 ml). P<0.01. If we take one metabolic change alone, namely serum cholesterol and compare Ovulen with Eugynon 30, the difference in serum cholesterol is 37.4 mg/100 ml. Here we see clearly the operation of a potential cardiovascular risk factor due to the unnecessarily high dose of oestrogen used initially in the contraceptive pill.

Fig. 14.4 summarises these changes in carbohydrate and lipid metabolism. Before describing these effects, it is necessary to mention two variables, namely the incremental mental glucose area and the insulin area. The incremental glucose area is the area under the glucose tolerance curve which lies above the fasting values. This area gives a composite value for glucose tolerance and is also an index of the rate of glucose dissimilation since the smaller the incremental area, the more rapid is the rate of glucose dissimilation and the larger the area the smaller is the removal rate of glucose and the greater the hyperglycaemia. Similarly the area under the

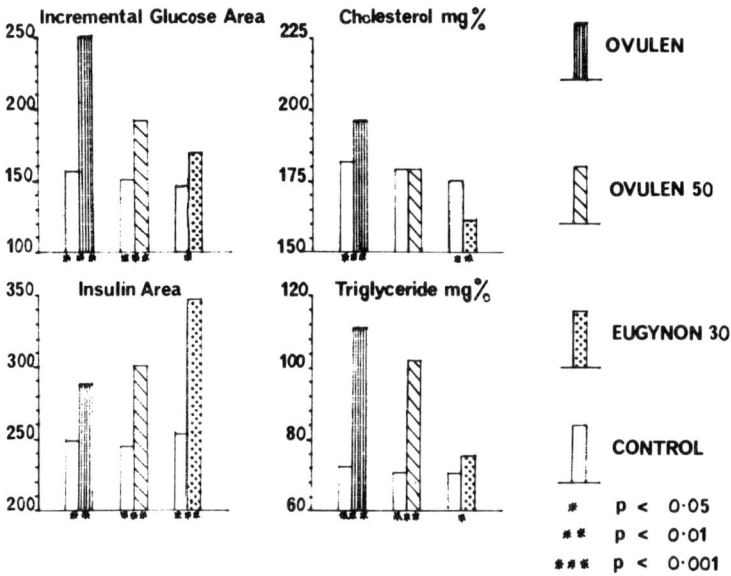

Fig. 14.4 Carbohydrate and lipid parameters measured in women taking Ovulen 50 and Eugynon 30 compared with age-weighted control subjects.

insulin curve during the course of the glucose tolerance test gives a composite value for the amount of insulin secreted during the test. One can measure the whole area, that is to say, the area of the curve above the base-line (insulin area) or one can measure the incremental area by subtracting the fasting values. As the fasting values are usually quite low, it is generally acceptable to measure the whole insulin area rather than the incremental insulin area. It should be pointed out, however, that although the area under the insulin curve gives a good index of total insulin secretion, it does not take into account any influence on the initial first phase insulin response which of course is important for the biological control of glucose homeostasis.

Fig. 14.4 shows that the incremental glucose area is greatly increased in the Ovulen users; there is less effect on this index with Ovulen 50 and least effect with Eugynon 30, but the incremental glucose area is significantly increased above control values with the three pills mentioned. The effect on the insulin area is the converse of that described for incremental glucose area. Ovulen produces the least increase in insulin area, Ovulen 50 has a more marked effect, but the most striking increase in insulin area is found with Eugynon 30.

The serum lipid changes are also clearly summarised in Fig. 14.4. Ovulen produces a large rise in serum cholesterol. With Ovulen 50 there is no change and with Eugynon 30 there is a fall in serum cholesterol. In the case of serum triglyceride, Ovulen produces the largest rise. With Ovulen 50 there is also a very substantial increase in serum triglyceride level but with Eugynon 30 the serum triglyceride levels are only slightly increased above the control values.

It can therefore be seen that combined oestrogen-progestogen oral contraceptive pills may produce changes in metabolic parameters which are in any other context, generally accepted as being risk factors in the accelerated development of atherosclerosis. Confronted with the fact that both prospective and retrospective studies of users of oral contraceptive pills show an increased incidence of thrombotic and thromboembolic phenomena, there is reason to suppose that the metabolic changes described here have direct clinical relevance. While the changes reported in most women may be small, there are obviously predisposed women in whom the changes are pronounced and hardly likely to be without serious clinical significance. As the methods of surveillance which would be required to detect such women are costly and not generally available, it is from a practical point of view, virtually impossible to offer oral contraceptive methodology to all women combined with the appropriate metabolic measurement which could add to the safety of the medication. It is therefore important for doctors to be cautious in the prescription of oral contraceptives and to try to identify on clinical grounds alone those women for whom this sort of medication could be potentially dangerous and at the same time to prescribe contraceptive formulations which produce the minimum of metabolic effect, avoiding especially oral contraceptives containing high doses of oestrogen.

References

Adams, P.W., Wynn, V., Folkard, J. & Seed, M. (1976) Influence of oral contraceptives, pyridoxine (vitamin B_6) and tryptophan on carbohydrate metabolism. *Lancet,* **1,** 759-764.

Doar, J.W.H. & Wynn, V. (1970) Effects of obesity, glucocorticoid, and oral contraceptive therapy on plasma glucose and blood pyruvate levels. *British Medical Journal,* **1,** 149-152.

Fisch, I.R. & Frank, J. (1977) Oral contraceptives and blood pressure. *Journal of the American Medical Association,* **237,** 2499-2503.

Inman, W.H.W., Vessey, M.P., Westerholm, B. & Engelund, A. (1970) Thromboembolic disease and the steroidal content of oral contraceptives: A report to the Committee on Safety of Drugs. *British Medical Journal,* **ii,** 203-209.

Kissebah, A.H., Harrigan, P. & Wynn, V. (1973) Mechanism of hypertriglyceridaemia associated with contraceptive steroids. *Hormone and Metabolic Research,* **5,** 184-190.

McCully, K.S. & Wilson, R.B. (1975) *Homocysteine Theory of Arteriosclerosis Atherosclerosis.* Vol. **22,** 215-227.

Mandour, T., Kissebah, A.H. & Wynn, V. (1977) Mechanism of oestrogen and progesterone effects on lipids and carbohydrate metabolism: glucagon molar ratio and hepatic enzyme activity. *European Journal of Clinical Investigation,* **7,** 181-187.

Mann, J.I., Vessey, M.P., Thorogood, M. & Doll, R. (1975) Myocardial infarction in young women with special reference to oral contraceptive practice. *British Medical Journal,* **2,** 241-245.

Mann, J.I. & Inham, W.H.W. (1975) Oral contraceptives and death from myocardial infarction. *British Medical Journal,* **2,** 245-248.

Mann, J.I., Inman, W.H.W. & Thorogood, M. (1976) Oral contraceptive use in older women and fatal myocardial infarction. *British Medical Journal,* **3,** 445-447.

Mason, B., Oakley, N., Wynn, V. (1973) Studies of Carbohydrate and Lipid Metabolism in Women Developing Hypertension on Oral Contraceptives. *British Medical Journal,* **iii,** 317-320.

Pincus, G. (1966) Unpublished communication to the Royal Society of Medicine, 4 May 1966.

Royal College of General Practitioners Oral Contraceptive Study (1977) Effect of hypertension and benign breast disease of progestogen component in combined oral contraceptives. *Lancet,* **i,** 624.

Stokes, T. & Wynn, V. (1971) Serum – Lipids in Women on Oral Contraceptives. *Lancet,* **ii,** 677-681.

Vessey, M.P. & Doll, R. (1969) Investigation of relation between use of oral contraceptives and thromboembolic disease: A further report. *British Medical Journal,* **ii,** 651-657.

Wynn, V. & Doar, J.W.H. (1966) Some effects of oral contraceptives on carbohydrate metabolism. *Lancet,* **ii,** 715-719.

Wynn, V. & Doar, J.W.H. (1969) Some effects of oral contraceptives on carbohydrate metabolism. *Lancet,* **ii,** 761-766.

Wynn, V., Doar, J.W.H. & Mills, G.L. (1969) Some effects of oral contraceptives on serum lipids and lipoprotein levels. *Lancet,* **ii,** 720-723.

Wynn, V., Doar, J.W.H., Mills, G.L., Stokes, T. (1969) Fasting serum triglyceride, cholesterol, and lipoprotein levels during oral-contraceptive therapy. *Lancet,* **ii,** 756-760.

Discussion 4B

Weir (Glasgow)   The exact definition of hypertension is extremely important. To my knowledge, the readings of blood pressure in the general practice study were taken by a large number of different people under different conditions and we should be cautious in their interpretation. Using standardised techniques in our prospective survey, we looked at different levels of progesterone-containing preparations, each of them containing 50 µg. oestrogen, and found no difference at all in the effect on blood pressure.

Lewis (London)   Is the negative dose response relationship between the oestrogen doses of the different formulations and insulin increment related to their progesterone content?

Wynn   Yes. It is the effect of norgesterol on the insulin receptors in the pancreas. Progesterone alone is insulinogenic and norgesterol is the most insulinogenic progestogen we are now using.

Venning (High Wycombe)   Would you clarify what appears to be conflicting information about whether it is the oestrogen dose or progestogen dose which affects serum cholesterol?

Wynn   The most highly cholesterolaemic drugs are those containing more than 75 micrograms of oestrogen. These effects are found more in women who have been taking a pill for longer than a year.

15. Coronary heart disease in young female diabetics

R. J. JARRETT AND J. H. FULLER

Clinical, epidemiological and pathological investigations (for review see Jarrett and Keen, 1975; Jarrett, 1977) agree that the degree of atherosclerosis and the consequent morbidity and mortality are increased in diabetics. However, there remain problems in analysis and interpretation, partly because of the mode of presentation of data, so that it is not always possible to relate observations to the age and sex of the diabetics, and partly because, in relation to cardiac morbidity and mortality, there are two other factors associated with the diabetic state, particularly in insulin-dependent diabetics, which complicate the attribution of coronary heart disease.

The first of these is the possible existence of a specific diabetic cardiomyopathy. Rubler *et al* (1972), who studied 27 patients with proven diabetic glomerulosclerosis, observed that four had cardiomegaly and congestive heart failure of no known cause. Histological examination at necropsy revealed diffuse fibrotic strands extending between bundles of muscle fibres and myofibrillar hypertrophy. In one case, the small intramural coronary arterioles had thickened walls and luminal narrowing due to deposition of acid mucopolysaccharide material in the sub-epithelial layers. The authors postulated that the myocardial disease was secondary to diabetic microangiopathy, although they could not exclude possible additional or alternative direct effects of an abnormal myocardial metabolism. Hamby *et al* (1974) noted a high frequency of diabetes among their patients with idiopathic cardiomyopathy. Necropsies were performed on three of their diabetic patients and pathological changes were found in the small coronary arteries in each case. By contrast, in only one of 28 non-diabetic patients with cardiomyopathy were there small vessel abnormalities. In the Framingham study (Kannel *et al*, 1974) it was found that the incidence of congestive heart failure was increased in the diabetic population and that the increased risk was apparently independent of hypertension and large coronary artery disease. It was also confined to those treated with insulin. More recently, Seneviratne (1977) has studied left ventricular function in insulin-requiring diabetics with and without clinically significant microangiopathy. Patients with angina, previous myocardial infarction, hypertension and known alcoholism were excluded and all had normal electrocardiograms. The mean systolic time interval was normal in the patients without microangiopathy, but significantly increased in the remainder. In four of these echocardiography was performed and confirmed impaired left ventricular function.

The other complicating factor is diabetic neuropathy. Lloyd-Mostyn and Watkins (1975) demonstrated abnormalities in autonomic control of the heart in diabetics with neuropathy and Page and Watkins (1977) have reported several episodes of cardiorespiratory arrest and of sudden death in young, insulin-dependent diabetics which appear to have been a consequence of autonomic neuropathy. Twelve cardio-resporatory arrests occurred in eight diabetics with severe autonomic neuropathy, all of whom were under the age of 42 years. They were shown to have impaired cardiac innervation by measurement of beat-to-beat variation of heart rate. Five arrests occurred after anaesthesia and it is interesting, in this context, that Partamian and Bradley (1965) commented on the frequency of 'coronary thromboses' occurring after anaesthesia in their series of diabetics. Two of the eight patients of Page and Watkins subsequently died suddenly at home, with no obvious cause discovered, even at necropsy.

Thus, cardiac morbidity and mortality in diabetics may be due to factors other than atherosclerotic coronary artery disease and the statistics derived from death certification must be interpreted with even more than the usual caution.

Data from the United States (Kessler, 1971; Garcia et al, 1974; Bradley and Partamian, 1965) indicate that the incidence of coronary heart disease (CHD) is similar in male and female diabetics, so that the excess over the non-diabetic is greater in the females. This is probably true of the younger females also, though the Framingham data (Garcia et al, 1974) is not clear on this point. The only British study providing a comparison of diabetic mortality with a non-diabetic population is that of Hayward and Lucena (1965) who compared the diabetics of the Birmingham clinic with the population of the West Midlands Conurbation for the period 1945-1959. Table 15.1 gives their data on overall mortality and mortality from 'diseases of the circulatory system' (ICD codes 400-468). Below the age of 40 there was a clear excess of total mortality in the diabetics in each of the quinquennia of diagnosis. However, of the 17 deaths only one was ascribed to a cardiac cause (Table 15.2). Between 1955 and 1959 (Jarrett, 1961) 68 diabetics and 325 non-diabetics were admitted to King's College Hospital with a diagnosis of myocardial

Table 15.1 West Midlands Study (from Hayward and Lucena, 1965)

| | Actual deaths/expected deaths | | | |
| | Females | | Males | |
Treatment	All causes	Codes 400-468	All causes	Codes 400-468
Diet	1.49	1.66	1.23	1.51
Insulin	2.04	2.13	1.57	1.83

Table 15.2 Causes of death in 17 female diabetics below the age of 40 (from Hayward and Lucena, 1965)

Ketosis	8
Uraemia	1
Respiratory	2
Hypoglycaemia	1
Coronary thrombosis	1
Tuberculosis	1
Cirrhosis	1
Unknown	2

infarction. Amongst the diabetics the sex ratio was almost 1 (33 males; 35 females), but none of the women was below the age of 50, whereas in the Joslin Clinic series of hospitalised patients (Partamian and Bradley, 1965) there were 88 men and 117 women and 19 of the women were less than 50 years old. In the Warsaw study (Królewski et al, 1975) of 73 diabetic women hospitalised for cardiac infarction between 1964/74 there were none below the age of 45 and only 8 between the ages of 45 and 54. In the Tecumseh community study (Ostrander et al, 1965) there were only 15 female diabetics below the age of 50 and none had any manifestation of CHD.

The most recent incidence study was also performed in Warsaw (Królewski et al, 1977). In Poland all diabetics are registered, which facilitates epidemiological studies. In Warsaw itself there are four specialist clinics for diabetics. Between January 1, 1963 and June 30, 1973 5261 newly diagnosed diabetics aged 30-68 were diagnosed. Mortality rates were calculated for the period from registration to December 31, 1973 and compared with that of the general population of Warsaw. Table 15.3 shows the data for CHD as well as total mortality. The results differ from the American studies in that, although there is an excess mortality from CHD in the female diabetics, compared with the general population it is almost identical with that of the male diabetics, results which are similar to those of the West Midlands Study. The Warsaw findings, however, agreed with those at Framingham (Garcia et al, 1974) in that the excess mortality from CHD in women was largely confined to the insulin-dependent patients (Table 15.4).

Table 15.3 Diabetic mortality — Warsaw 1963-73*

Age at diagnosis	Sex	CHD deaths			All deaths		
		O	E	O/E	O	E	O/E
30-49	M	18	5.3	3.40	52	24.4	2.13
	F	6	1.8	3.33	21	13.0	1.61
50-68	M	67	38.2	1.75	171	145.1	1.17
	F	31	19.3	1.60	126	102.9	1.22

* Source: Królewski et al, 1977.

Table 15.4 Diabetic mortality — Warsaw 1963-73*

Age standardised mortality rates from CHD according to sex and treatment.

Treatment	Male		Female	
	No. person years	SMR	No. person years	SMR
Insulin	1896	8.5	2273	6.2
Oral agents	7066	9.2	8664	2.5
Diet only	785	5.4	1096	0.8

SMR — age standardised mortality rates on 1000 person years.

* Source: Królewski et al, 1977.

Although it is clear from the various reports referred to that young diabetics — male and female — do have an increased risk of CHD which is relatively greater than that of the older diabetic, the precise degree of risk is not definable. This is partly due to the problem of ascertainment of cause of death, discussed above, and partly due to the heterogeneous nature of any group of diabetics when considered by attained age. Within an age group there will be wide variations in disease duration. This is known to relate closely to the microvascular complications, but its relationship to atherosclerosis and to its clinical manifestations is more complex and less well studied. There may also be differences between populations in the relative risk of female diabetics.

Risk factors for CHD in diabetics

The elucidation of risk factors — or risk indices — for CHD has arisen from studies of populations from which diabetics have been excluded or within which diabetics form a small minority. Within diabetics, the influence of other risk factors and their prevalence has been little studied (see Jarrett, 1977 for discussion). We are currently studying a stratified random sample of diabetics as part of the World Health Organisation Multinational Study of Vascular Disease in Diabetics and have, in addition to the core study, looked at a number of putative risk factors. As controls we have studied a stratified random sample of the employees of the Greater London Council (GLC) and the Inner London Education Authority (ILEA). Controls for the haemostatic parameters are derived from the population under study by Meade and Chakrabarti (Meade, 1973). The data presented is preliminary as the study is still unfinished.

The diabetics attend the clinics at King's College Hospital and Guy's Hospital. They were selected from the age group 35-55 so as to ensure a wide representation of diabetes duration. Table 15.5 gives the age distribution of the diabetic and control females in the age range 35-40. Of the 44 diabetics, 38 were insulin-dependent. Tables 15.6 and 15.7 present mean figures for a number of measured variables which may be factors concerned in the aetiology of arterial disease. As the data is preliminary, we have not calculated levels of significance of the differences. From Table 15.6 it can be seen that the mean levels of systolic blood pressure, total cholesterol, LDL cholesterol and triglycerides are all substantially higher in the diabetics and all are putative risk factors for CHD. It is noteworthy, however, that total HDL cholesterol, currently canvassed as 'protecting' against CHD, is actually higher in the diabetics. Furthermore the prevalence of normal electrocardiograms — assessed according to the Minnesota Code — is also higher amongst the diabetic group. Table 15.7 shows that mean levels of plasma fibrinogen, Factors V, VII and VIII are all higher in the diabetics. Fibrinolytic activity is diminished and platelet adhesiveness slightly increased. Thus a number of factors which have been implicated in the aetiology of vascular disease are present in the diabetic group, but the relevance of these findings must await a prospective study which relates the incidence of vascular disease in diabetics to the prevailing levels of these variables.

Table 15.5   Age distribution of young female diabetics in the W.H.O. Study and in the Controls from the GLC/ILEA.

Age group	Diabetics	Controls
35-39	9	6
40-44	12	6
45-49	23	14
Total	44	26
Mean Age	43.8	43.8

Table 15.6   Comparison of young female diabetics and controls (mean data only).

	Diabetics	Controls
Systolic B.P.	130.3	118.6
Diastolic B.P.	79.4	78.8
Body Mass Index	23.5	23.14
Total cholesterol (mmol/l)	5.82	5.07
LDL cholesterol ''	3.74	3.25
HDL cholesterol ''	1.85	1.70
Total triglyceride ''	0.98	0.69
Normal E.C.G. (%)	89.0	72.0

Table 15.7   Comparison of haemostatic variables: women aged 35-49 years.

	Non-Diabetics (n = 188)	Insulin-Dependent Diabetics (n = 34)
(1) Fibrinolytic Activity (= 100/DBCLT)	0.28	0.20
(2) Platelet Adhesiveness (%)	44.3	46.5
(3) Fibrinogen (mg/dl)	282.5	305.6
(4) Factor V	127.5	135.6
(5) Factor VII	97.7	104.1
(6) Factor VIII	94.6	97.5

Summary

It seems that not all cardiac morbidity and mortality in diabetics in the age groups considered can be ascribed to atherosclerotic coronary disease. Nevertheless, young diabetic women probably have a substantially increased risk compared with non-diabetics, though not necessarily reaching that of male diabetics. Cardiac morbidity and mortality below the age of 50 years is still an uncommon event in female diabetics and, in terms of the whole community, does not contribute greatly to the sum of CHD. However, diabetics in this age group are characterised by a number of putative risk indices for CHD which may be related to the excess of CHD observed in older subjects.

References

Bradley, R.F. & Partamian, J.O. (1965) Coronary heart disease in the diabetic patient. *Medical Clinics of North America,* **49,** 1093-1104.

Garcia, M.J., McNamara, P.M., Gordon, T. & Kannell, W.B. (1974) Morbidity and mortality in diabetics in the Framingham population. *Diabetes,* **23,** 105-111.

Hamby, R.I., Zoneraich, S. & Sherman, L. (1974) Diabetic cardiomyopathy. *Journal of the American Medical Association,* **229,** 1749-1754.

Hayward, R.E. & Lucena, B.C. (1965) An investigation into the mortality of diabetics. *Journal of the Institute of Actuaries,* **91,** 286-336.

Jarrett, R.J. (1961) The immediate prognosis of myocardial infarction in diabetics. *Postgraduate Medical Journal,* **37,** 207-209.

Jarrett, R.J. (1977) Diabetes and the heart: Coronary Heart Disease. *Clinics in Endocrinology and Metabolism,* **6** (2).

Jarrett, R.J. & Keen, H. (1975) Diabetes and atherosclerosis. In *Complications of Diabetes,* ed. Keen, H. & Jarrett, J. Ch. 5, pp. 179-203. London: Arnold.

Kannel, W.B., Hjortland, M. & Castelli, W.P. (1974) Role of diabetes in congestive heart failure: the Framingham Study. *American Journal of Cardiology,* **34,** 29-34.

Kessler, I.I. (1971) Mortality experience of diabetic patients. *The American Journal of Medicine,* **51,** 715-724.

Królewski, A.S., Janeczo, D., Kobryn, A. & Puncewicz, B. (1975) Survival after myocardial infarction in diabetic patients. *Acta medica Polona,* **16,** 45-59.

Królewski, S., Czyzyk, A., Janeczko, D. & Kopczynski, J. (1977) Mortality from cardiovascular diseases among diabetics. *Diabetologia,* **13.** In Press.

Lloyd-Mostyn, R.H. & Watkins, P.J. (1975) Defective innervation of heart in diabetic autonomic neuropathy. *British Medical Journal,* **3,** 15-17.

Meade, T.W. (1973) The epidemiology of thrombosis. *Thrombosis et Diathesis Haemorrhagica,* Suppl. **54,** 317-320.

Ostrander, L.D., Francis, T., Hayner, N.S., Kjelsberg, M.O. & Epstein, F.H. (1965) The relationship of cardiovascular disease to hyperglycemia. *Annals of Internal Medicine,* **62,** 1188-1198.

Page, M. McB. & Watkins, P.J. (1977) Cardio-respiratory arrest in diabetic autonomic neuropathy. Paper presented at the Spring meeting of the Medical and Scientific Section of the British Diabetic Association.

Partamian, J.O. & Bradley, R.F. (1965) Acute myocardial infarction in 258 cases of diabetes: immediate mortality and five-year survival. *New England Journal of Medicine,* **273,** 455-461.

Rubler, S., Dlugash, J., Yuceoglu, Y.Z., Kumral, T., Branwood, A.W. & Grishman, A. (1972) New type of cardiomyopathy associated with diabetic glomerulosclerosis. *The American Journal of Cardiology,* **30,** 595-602.

Seneviratne, B.I.B. (1977) Diabetic cardiomyopathy: the preclinical phase. *British Medical Journal,* **1,** 1444-1446.

Discussion 4C

Mitchell (Nottingham)   How do you distinguish diabetes from what might be diabetes when patients are admitted to hospital with acute myocardial infarction?

Jarrett   Such patients have steroid-induced glucose intolerance or even hyperglycaemia, but it does not mean anything unless the hyperglycaemia is maintained 3-6 months later.

Spain (Brooklyn)   Were you implying that insulin might induce myocardial micro-angiopathy?

Jarrett   This kind of microangiopathy has only so far been reported in patients who developed diabetes either in adolescence or childhood, who are mostly insulin-dependent. After many years of insulin, a microangiopathy occurs affecting a number of systems, including the small vessels of the coronary circulation. It probably presents to cardiologists as an idiopathic cardiomyopathy.

Epstein (Zurich)   It is probably correct that diabetes does not contribute as a community problem to coronary heart disease either in young women or, for that matter, in middle-aged men. A different problem is whether latent chemical diabetes or hyperglycaemia is a risk factor and whether it is a risk factor independent of others contributing to genesis of the lesions over the years.

Jarrett   In our study of 18,000 people, we examined the relationship between blood sugar and the coronary heart disease mortality. It was difficult to separate blood sugar measured after glucose loads from other risk factors, but I do not think that it has a significant independent contribution on the community scale. Unfortunately, the Bedford study was carried out in 1962 and was a rather unsophisticated exercise which did not include measurements of plasma lipids. The average age of the newly found diabetics was 57 and the average age of the so-called borderline diabetics was 54. CHD mortality over 10 years in men was not significantly different in the chemical diabetics or borderline diabetics from the controls, but in women it was higher. So there was a sex difference, but in a much older age group.

16. Immunological mechanisms and coronary heart disease in young women

J.-L. BEAUMONT AND VIOLETTE BEAUMONT

The main cause of coronary artery disease is atherosclerosis, a slowly developing disease which is not observed in young women unless some special conditions may accelerate the atherogenic process, the first of which being an inborn error of lipoprotein metabolism.

Anyhow, several kinds of arterial lesions, in which immunological factors are involved, may induce coronary diseases. Coronary arteritis, true atherosclerosis and thrombosis were reported in Horton's disease, Takayasu's disease, panarteritis, rheumatoid arthritis, systemic lupus erythematosus, are all considered with growing evidence as auto-immune diseases. Some of them may affect young women.

Moreover, the wide use of contraceptive hormones is at present the first cause of arterial and coronary thrombosis in young women, for which an immunological mechanism can also be implicated.

Coronary arteritis

Takayasu's disease

Coronary arteritis, leading to coronary insufficiency, was reported in several cases of Takayasu's disease, a non specific fibrotic process, probably of allergic character, which involves the aorta and its main branches. The disease affects women predominantly. Coronary symptoms are often mentioned among the other manifestations of the disease (Rosen & Gaton, 1972); a case of myocardial infarction was reported in an 11 years Bantu girl.

According to Juzi (1967) obstructive changes in the coronary arteries are present in 30 per cent of the autopsied cases. The arterial lesions are characterized by granulomatous tissue, fibrosis and monocytic infiltrate, without atheroma. They resemble the experimental lesions typical of immunisation-induced arteriopathies (Minick & Murphy, 1973) and serum sickness. The mechanism of the early immunological lesion remains open to question. According to experimental findings, it might be related to an immune antigen-antibody complex filtration through the arterial wall (Cochrane, 1968).

Systemic lupus erythematosus

In SLE, cardiac symptoms are seen in 50 to 89 per cent of patients, usually in relation with pericarditis and myocarditis. However, death from myocardial infarction due to

* Unite de recherches sur l'Atherosclerose; INSERM 432 Hopital Henri Mon doz, Creteil 94010, France.

F

coronary occlusion, though infrequent, was reported by several authors, predominantly in young women: one 16 years-old, two, 24 and 25 years-old; one 29 years-old; one 35 years-old (Meller *et al*, 1975). In all cases, myocardial infarction was the cause of death. Several other cases, although no autopsy was available, were suspected on angina pectoris attacks.

There is little doubt that occlusion was due to the SLE disease, because the ischaemic disease appeared far below the usual age for women, and in the absence of other risk factors.

Autopsy findings showed widespread coronary arteritis with necrotizing and occlusive lesions. An antigen-antibody reaction was proposed as the pathogenesis of the lesion (Meller *et al*, 1975), but the antigen-antibody complexes were not found in the arterial wall as they were in the golmeruli.

Coronary atherosclerosis

True coronary atherosclerosis may be seen in immunological conditions.

Systemic lupus erythematosus

In SLE, typical occlusive atherosclerotic plaques, indistinguishable from ordinary atherosclerosis, were described (Meller *et al*, 1975), though it is known that the usual arteritis lesion contains no lipids.

Auto-immune hyperlipidemia

Atherosclerosis may also develop in relation with an immunologically induced risk factor, autoimmune hyperlipidemia (AIH).

AIH described in 1964-65 (Beaumont, 1965) is a metabolic disease in which lipoprotein lipolysis is inhibited by circulating autoantibodies. At present, several types of autoantibodies are known to induce hyperlipidemia (Beaumont & Beaumont, 1977) and, according to their specific action, 2 main types of AIH may be distinguished: (1) AIH with antilipoprotein antibodies, in which the inhibition of lipolysis is due to antibodies blocking on the surface of lipoproteins, sites necessary for a correct enzyme attack; (2) AIH with antienzyme antibodies in which the inhibition of lipolysis is due to antibodies which interfere with the lipase molecule or its production (antiheparin and antilipase antibodies).

AIH is the result of a disturbed immunoglobulin production of unknown mechanism. It may be either associated with myeloma, lymphoma, SLE and rheumatoid arthritis, or primary. No case was reported up to now in young women, but many cases of hyperlipidemia with ischaemic disease may be due to AIH and that in AIH associated with ischaemic disease, the age of onset is usually rather young.

The mechanism by which AIH induces atherosclerosis may be different in the antilipoprotein and antienzyme types. In both, hyperlipidemia is itself a factor. In antilipoprotein AIH, the circulating immunoglobulin-lipoprotein complexes may be harmful by themselves, inducing arterial damage and deposition of lipids and cholesterol.

Coronary thrombosis in oral contraceptive users

It is admitted at present that the use of oral contraceptive increases the risk of coronary heart disease. The first case was reported as early as 1963 in a 32 years-old woman who experienced myocardial infarction after six months of oral contraception, without any other risk factor. However, although epidemiological surveys soon indicated significant data for venous, pulmonary (Report from Boston Collaborative Surveillance Program, 1973) or cerebral (Collaborative Group for the Study of Stroke in Young Women, 1973) thrombosis, they were not conclusive for coronary diseases. Though such a correlation was suspected in women under 40, it was only in 1975 that morbidity for coronary heart diseases in pill users was shown to be increased 5.7 fold in the age 40-44, 2.7 fold in the age 30-39 (Mann et al, 1975). Only a few autopsy reports from cases of myocardial infarction in pill users are available. They indicate that atherosclerosis is rarely concerned and that the arterial lesions are characterised by endothelial proliferation, intimal thickening and fibrosis, and locally-formed, multilayered thrombi. Diffuse proliferative lesions, without thrombi, were also seen in the arteries and veins of 20 women with thromboembolic disease during oral contraception (Irey et al, 1970). They might represent the first step of an occlusive process.

These vascular lesions may not be different from those described in immunological conditions. The thrombogenic mechanism is still unclear despite documented studies of changes in haemostasis, coagulation and fibrinolysis and on the role of associated risk factors, hyperlipidemia, systolic blood pressure and tobacco smoking.

Immunological mechanisms

Arguments which are felt to be consistent with an immunological mechanism were found in a case of pulmonary artery thrombosis and monoclonal gammapathy in a 36 years-old woman on oral contraceptives (Beaumont & Lemort, 1976). Three features were of note in this case history: (1) the pulmonary thrombosis (or embolism) occurred abruptly in a healthy woman without signs of previous phlebitis. (2) she had been on oral contraceptives for 2½ years at a daily dose of 50 μg ethinyl-oestradiol. (3) electrophoretic patterns revealed a monoclonal IgG λ gammapathy of about 700 mg/100 ml.

Both diseases are rare in young women and this led to a search for antibody activity in the monoclonal protein. After appropriate purification (Beaumont & Lemort, 1976), the binding activity of the IgG λ was studied by Sephadex gel-filtration, ultra-centrifugation and dialysis equilibrium. An IgG λ-bound ethinyl-oestradiol was found with a valency of 2 and a K_a of 10^7 M^{-1}. This figure is much higher than the weak bonds usually found between hormones and many proteins including immunoglobulins. The binding was reversible and specific for ethinyl-oestradiol. According to these data, this monoclonal IgG λ behaves like an anti-ethinyl-oestradiol antibody. Since this time, we have found similar antibodies in several other cases.

As such an immunological reaction was felt possibly to be implicated in the thrombotic risk of contraceptive hormones, an epidemiological survey was started to detect immunoglobulin changes in several groups of women (Beaumont et al, to be published). A simplified test of serum immunoglobulin precipitability, derived

from the above study, was applied to 200 women distributed in 4 groups:
1. women who had never used oral contraceptives;
2. women on oral contraceptives;
3. women who had used oral contraceptives in the past;
4. women with vascular thrombosis during oral contraceptives.

Almost 100 per cent of women in group 4 had highly abnormal test values, as compared to group 1. In group 2, 2 populations could be distinguished: a non-reactive population with test values within the normal range even after years of oral contraception; and a reactive population with high values statistically different from the former.

These results support the hypothesis of an immunological mechanism for the unexplained thrombotic risk related to oral contraception. It is felt that the test of immunoglobulin precipitability might be an easy way to detect susceptible women.

As to the thrombogenic mechanism, it is conceivable on one hand that the antibodies may have something to do with the changes in haemostasis and coagulation; and on the other hand, that the immune complexes may be harmful to the vessel wall, as suggested by the diffuse vascular lesions.

References

Beaumont, J.L. (1965) L'hyperlipidémie par auto-anticorps anti-beta-lipoprotéines. Une nouvelle entité pathologique. *Comptes-Rendus des Seances de l'Academie des Sciences de Paris,* Série D, **261**, 4563-4566.

Beaumont, J.L. & Lemort, N. (1976) Oral contraceptive, pulmonary artery thrombosis and anti-ethinyl-oestradiol monoclonal IgG. *Clinical and Experimental Immunology,* **24**, 455-463.

Beaumont, J.L. & Beaumont, V. (1977) Autoimmune hyperlipidemia. *Atherosclerosis,* **26**, 405-418.

Beaumont, V., Lemort, N., Lorenzelli, L. & Beaumont, J.L. (To be published). Hormones contraceptives, risque vasculaire et précipitabilité anormale des gamma-globulines sériques.

Cochrane, C.G. (1968) The role of immune complexes and complement in tissue injury. *Journal of Allergy,* **42**, 113-129.

Irey, N.S., Manion, W.C. & Taylor, H.B. (1970) Vascular lesions in women taking oral contraceptives. *A.M.A. Archives of Pathology,* **89**, 1-8.

Juzi, U. (1967) Takayasusche Arteritis mit Herzinfarkt. *Schweizerische Medizinische Wochenschrift,* **13**, 397-405.

Report from the Boston Collaborative Drug Surveillance Program: Oral contraceptives and venous thromboembolic diseases, surgically confirmed gall bladder disease and breast tumors. *The Lancet,* (1973) **1**, 1399-1404.

Mann, J.I., Vessey, M.P., Thorogood, M. & Doll, R. (1975) Myocardial infarction in young women with special reference to oral contraceptive practice. *British Medical Journal,* **2**, 241-245.

Meller, J., Conde, C.A., Deppisch, L.M., Donoso, E. & Dack, S. (1975) Myocardial infarction due to coronary atherosclerosis in three young adults with systemic lupus erythematosus. *The American Journal of Cardiology,* **35**, 309-313.

Minick, C.R. & Murphy, G.E. (1973) Experimental induction of athero-arterio-sclerosis by the synergy of allergic injury to arteries and lipid-rich diet. II. Effect of repeatedly injected foreign protein in rabbits fed a lipid-rich, cholesterol-poor diet. *American Journal of Pathology,* **73**, 265-292.

Collaborative Group for the Study of Stroke in Young Women (1973) Oral contra-ception and increased risk of cerebral ischaemia or thrombosis. *The New England Journal of Medicine,* **228**, 871-878.

Rosen, N. & Gaton, E. (1972) Takayasu's arteritis of coronary arteries. *Archives of Pathology,* **94**, 225-229.

Discussion 4D

Spain (Brooklyn)   There was no evidence of any inflammatory process in the lesions described by Prof. Beaumont. He referred to findings in three groups of cases — those on sex steroids, those in the third trimester of pregnancy and those post-partum — and there were similar findings in all groups. I comment on this in relation to the fact that the antibodies may not occur only to administered oestradiol. They were also cases in which there was pulmonary thrombosis. The thrombi overlayed intimal proliferation which may be an 'itis' but in no case was there any inflammatory process present in these lesions. Pulmonary artery thrombosis is not the same as arterial thrombosis. It occurs in a low pressure system and local thrombi can form as in other venous systems. Another point is that the vascular changes illustrated were in an intramural coronary vessel and not in an epicardial major coronary artery. There was intimal proliferation but no thrombus. Binding may occur in relation to localised pre-existing atheroma.

Beaumont   Atheroma may develop on many kinds of injury. If injury occurs at a high pressure site on the vascular bed, then probably an arterial reaction will develop there. I prefer the idea that the injury was first, the atheroma second.

Fultòn (Glasgow)   Have you applied your technique to other patients who have developed cardiovascular disease? Might it reflect an immunological process in relation to some extraneous factor other than oestrogen.

Beaumont   We looked into the possibility of development of such antibodies in women taking other kinds of oestrogen. Mestranol has the same ability, but with the so-called natural hormones, up to now, we have not found any activity of this sort. The numbers are too small, however, to say that these natural hormones are inactive immunologically.

Baird (Edinburgh)   The affinity constants of your antibody are rather low in com-parison with most antibodies that are generated against steroids; experimentally. Oestradiol normally binds to sex hormone-binding globulin. During electrophoresis, does the antibody migrate solely with this globulin or is it distributed amongst other plasma proteins?

Beaumont   The affinities are not lower than those usually found for antibodies but they are lower than that of the serum binding globulin — in the 10^{-7} range.

Baird (Edinburgh)   There is biological significance when antibodies to steroids are
generated experimentally at 10^{-9} or 10^{-10}

Beaumont   This does not affect the reaction with the receptors. The pill is
active in inducing this reaction because binding activity is much less than the affinity
of the receptors.

Somerville (London)   Is there any marker, immunological or otherwise, that can
allow one to say which women will develop these antibodies? How is it possible that
such a small proportion react to the pill in this way?

Beaumont   It is possible with our tests to say, two months after beginning
the pill, if a woman is reactive or not. When she stops, it is also possible to say up to
3 years whether a reactive woman had taken an oral contraceptive. In the human
there are millions of different antibodies. An antibody is highly specific, there is
great specificity in the capacity of one human being to react to a given stimulation.
Thus only part of the population will respond. This response may be genetically
determined.

17. Thrombotic factors

A. S. DOUGLAS

This symposium is concerned with coronary heart disease in young women; while the emphasis will be placed on that aspect, this account necessarily deals with the broader issues of thrombotic factors in arterial vascular occlusion. The areas highlighted will be — use of the contraceptive pill, smoking and lipids (including diabetes).

While thrombotic factors may have their action simultaneously on the venous and arterial sides of the circulation, the emphasis clinically is usually on one or the other. Antithrombin III deficiency, for example, is predominantly a venous disease, but may have arterial involvement. Smoking influences the arterial side of the system rather than the venous.

Blood coagulation, fibrinolysis and platelets

At the outset it may be helpful to outline the current concepts of blood coagulation, the fibrinolytic enzyme system and the role of platelets — in haemostasis and thrombosis. It is probable that the events leading to thrombus formation are similar to those resulting in a haemostatic plug. Both involve platelet adhesion and aggregation followed by fibrin formation. Blood clotting is a consequence of thrombin production, fibrinolysis of plasmin formation. Adherent and aggregated platelets are a feature of the haemostatic plug or of parts of the thrombus.

Blood coagulation

Only when there is an explosive development of thrombin does fibrin formation occur; smaller amounts are neutralised rapidly by antithrombins. Prothrombin is present as an inert pro-enzyme capable of the production of thrombin. The various stages of the coagulation mechanism lead to the activation of prothrombin by factor Xa (see Fig.17.1). So long as blood remains in contact with healthy intact vascular endothelium it remains in a fluid state. Contact activation occurs when blood encounters other surfaces e.g. damaged endothelial cells or the tissue surface in exposed sub-endothelial tissue.

The mechanism for thrombin production with blood coagulation can follow two pathways (see Fig. 17.1). One of these involves constituents only within the blood (the intrinsic thromboplastin system). Another involves tissue damage (the extrinsic thromboplastin mechanism). Under either of these systems, acting alone or in conjunction, prothrombin (factor II) will be converted to the proteolytic enzyme thrombin. Thrombin cleaves fibrinopeptides A and B from fibrinogen and the fibrin monomers polymerize to produce fibrin.

BLOOD COAGULATION

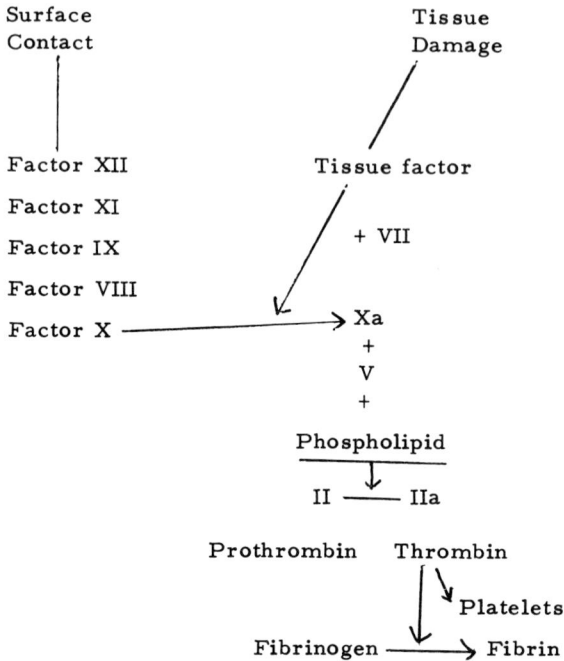

Surface   Tissue
Contact   Damage

Factor XII   Tissue factor

Factor XI

Factor IX   + VII

Factor VIII

Factor X ──────────→ Xa
                       +
                       V
                       +
           Phospholipid
           ───────────
             II ─── IIa

Prothrombin   Thrombin
                        ↘ Platelets
        Fibrinogen ────→ Fibrin

Fig. 17.1

Fibrinolysis (see Fig. 17.2)

Whenever fibrin is deposited there is plasminogen with it in sufficient quantity to ensure its subsequent lysis by the generation of the proteolytic enzyme plasmin. The activation can occur by a number of different routes. The response activity can arise from the blood itself; whether depressed blood fibrinolysis is thrombogenic is unproven. This occurs as pregnancy advances without a thrombotic problem most of the time. It is depressed in diabetes and in obesity and these patients have an increased risk of vascular disease.

Platelets

These participate in the arrest of bleeding by plugging the disrupted vessel wall or aggregate in the head of a thrombus. The platelets contain phospholipid which is an essential component of prothrombin conversion by the intrinsic route.

Platelets adhere to surfaces other than healthy intact vascular endothelium and to each other. The surface of the platelet contains receptors for thrombin, collagen, adenosine diphosphate (ADP), thromboxanes, adrenaline and serotonin; these agents lead to platelet aggregation.

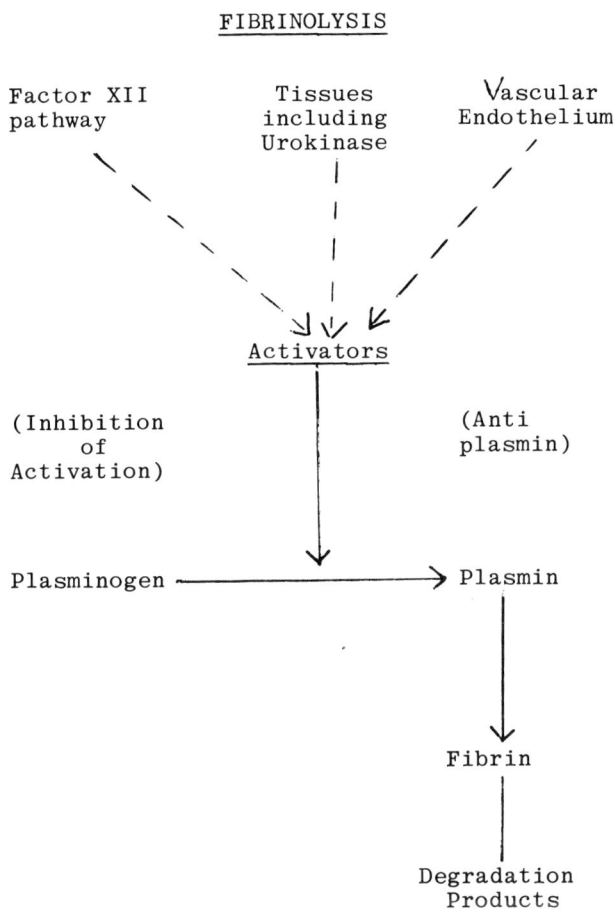

FIBRINOLYSIS

Factor XII
pathway

Tissues
including
Urokinase

Vascular
Endothelium

Activators

(Inhibition
of
Activation)

(Anti
plasmin)

Plasminogen ⟶ Plasmin

Fibrin

Degradation
Products

Fig. 17.2

The mechanism that enables platelets to stick to foreign surfaces or to one another, is unclear, but it may involve coagulation on the surface of the platelet with generation of thrombin which causes platelet aggregation. Adenosine diphosphate and thromboxanes may be generated from the platelets, providing the impetus for further events.

Platelets lose their discoid shape, adhere to other platelets and result in the formation of large aggregates.

The vessel wall

While this account is more concerned with blood constituents, there is some overlap with biochemical aspects of the vessel wall.

F*

The effect of microthrombi When an area of platelet/fibrin deposition has occurred on an arterial endothelial surface, there is then a stiffening of the vessel wall with consequential alteration of normal flow patterns. Endothelial cell loss or damage may be mechanical and particularly liable to occur in unsupported vessels at the sites of branchings, where there is loss of linear flow pattern (Duguid 1977). A rise in fibrinogen concentration causes a change in blood viscosity and thereby altered flow.

Thromboxanes and prostaglandin endoperoxides One of the fatty acids in our diet is arachidonic acid, and this is one of the biochemical components of platelets. From it, thromboxanes arise. These are released from platelets and have the action shown in Table 17.1 of promoting platelet aggregation and causing vasospasm.

Prostacyclines are also derived from arachidonic acid and are related to the platelet thromboxanes released from the vessel wall. They inhibit platelet aggregation and dilate arteries (Moncada *et al*, 1977). It is a theoretical possibility that under the influence of the contraceptive pill or of ageing that there is depletion of prostacyclines (It may be of therapeutic importance that aspirin blocks not only the release reaction from platelets but also the release of prostacyclines from the vessel wall. Information is needed whether the women who have suffered myocardial infarction were in fact chronic aspirin ingestors.)

Table 17.1

Thromboxanes	Prostaglandin Endoperoxides (Prostacyclines)
(only in platelets)	(only in vessel wall)
Promotes platelet aggregation Causes vasospasm	Inhibits platelet aggregation Dilates arteries

Heparans In the vessel wall there have been identified materials 'heparans' which are chemically related to heparin. If, for example, there is a small diminution in the concentration of antithrombin III this might become critical if at the same time there was also interference with the concentration of heparans in the vessel wall.

Virchow's Triad

According to Virchow's hypothesis thrombosis occurred because of:
1. A provocative lesion in the vessel wall
2. Changes in pattern of flow
3. Changes in the blood so as to render it 'hypercoagulable'.

The author is now satisfied that 'hypercoagulability' leading to thrombosis does occur; this conviction follows the study of a Hebridean family with inherited deficiency of antithrombin III; the affected family members had an impressive clinical record of venous thrombo-embolic disease and also (relevant to the topic of this symposium) one of the members, who died at the age of 29 years, had very aggressive atheroma and arterial occlusions. In this form of thrombophilia the antithrombin III is only 50 per cent deficient. Antithrombin III (a protease inhibitor) is one of several mechanisms for the destruction of thrombin; it also inhibits several other steps in the coagulation pathway − particularly activated factor X. It is the co-factor which enhances the action of heparin.

The concept of a system of 'checks and balances' influencing fibrin formation and dissolution and also platelets, has long been postulated. Many of the steps in blood clotting, fibrinolysis, and in platelets have their own controlling system. Antithrombin III deficiency is an example of the blood coagulation mechanism being off balance.

Hypercoagulability

Tullis (1976) quotes from the works of William Hewson, London, published by the Sydenham Society in 1846 'Believing it would be sufficient for this purpose to attend to the properties of the blood, as it flows at different times from an animal that is bleeding to death, I therefore went to that markets and attended the killing of sheep ..... and received the blood into cups ..... I observed that the blood which came immediately from the vessels ..... was about 2 minutes in beginning to coagulate; that taken as the animal became weaker coagulated in less and less time ..... till at last .... (it) had hardly been received into the cup before it congealed'.

This is the hypercoagulability of haemorrhagic shock. It is now known whether a simple quantitative increase in one of the clotting factors is sufficient to lead to an increased risk of thrombosis. For example, is the thrombocytosis of iron deficiency anaemia or the elevated factor VIII level of normal pregnancy to be considered 'thrombotic'? Is the raised concentration of factor X in pregnancy of importance? It is more likely that the presence of activated factor X is more important than the presence of increased concentration. Antithrombin III activity is concerned with the destruction of activated coagulation factors, not inactive forms.

Some would consider changes in pregnancy as physiological but nevertheless there is an increased risk of thrombosis in pregnancy.

Theoretically there are many changes which can be postulated.
1. Coagulation − increased concentration
   − increased reactivity
   − decreased inhibition
   − decreased body capacity to remove activated clotting factors

2. Fibrinolysis − reduction of activator
   − increased inhibition

3. Platelets − increased numbers
   − increased reactivity
      (e.g. adhesiveness or aggregating agents)

Alterations in molecular structure may lead to thrombosis. There are variants of the fibrinogen molecule which render it more readily susceptible to conversion to fibrin. Antithrombin III has been reported to occur as an inherited abnormality of the molecule rendering it less efficient.

Contraceptive pill

As is well established the synthetic oestrogens are incriminated in the thrombotic hazard of oral contraception. Natural oestrogens prepared from the horse still produce some changes in the coagulation and platelet parameters.

On the high oestrogen content pill the concentration of factors I (fibrinogen), II, VII and X increases. Factors VIII and IX increase in concentration but the rises are small and comparable with other clinical situations not recognised as 'thrombotic'. Antithrombin III levels are reduced. The reason for the deficiency is not known; the production may be reduced or the antithrombin III is consumed by intravascular fibrin formation.

The clinical vascular manifestations are similar to inherited AT III deficiency — e.g. mesenteric venous occlusion is a recognised feature of both situations.

At the end of pregnancy the antithrombin III level of the mother has fallen. Following placental delivery the antithrombin level rises rapidly; if however the mother is given oestrogen (e.g. for inhibition of lactation) then this rise of anti-thrombin III does not occur. This could correlate with an increased tendency to thrombosis in the puerperium, when oestrogens are given.

Plasminogen increases with oral contraception but the significance is uncertain; there is a rise in antiplasmin concentration. Any changes in fibrinolytic activator as a consequence of oestrogen administration are minor and inconsistent. This contrasts with pregnancy where there is diminishing plasminogen activation until delivery of the placenta when there is a rapid return of activator level to normal.

Fibrin (ogen) breakdown products (FDP) Evidence of the presence of intravascular coagulation or of excessive fibrinolysis would be the demonstration of raised fibrin (ogen) breakdown products in the serum. There have been sporadic reports of these being found in women on the high oestrogen content pill.

The molecular weight of fibrinogen is 330,000. After the release of fibrinopeptides A and B by thrombin, fibrinogen monomer is formed which polymerises to form fibrin. The proteolysis of fibrin by plasmin results in fibrin degradation products (F.D.P.); these complex with themselves or fibrinogen to produce complexes with a molecular weight of 450,000.

Plasmin is also proteolytic to fibrinogen and there results a derivative with a new molecular weight of 260,000.

There can be in circulation therefore
1. Fibrinogen polymer MW 450,000   2 per cent
2. Fibrinogen MW 330,000   82 per cent
3. Fibrinogen first derivative MW 260,000   16 per cent
  (a) If (1) rises and (3) falls — thrombus formation
  (b) If (1) falls and (3) rises — thrombus dissolution.
The first of these two patterns (a) is found in a quarter of women on the high oestrogen content pill.

Platelets One particular technique for studying platelets has been found to be very sensitive to platelet aggregation. Recalcified platelet rich plasma is rotated slowly in a continuous loop of plastic tubing. The time taken from recalcification to the appearance of platelet clumps is measured. It is shortened on the pill; this may be a manifestation of decreased antithrombin and is due therefore to the enhanced thrombin action on platelets.

This is probably the most sensitive of indicators of an action on the haemostatic parameters by oestrogens and can be found even in low dosage pills, and furthermore can be detected following at least one of the progestogens (this is the only reported abnormality following progestogen pills — Poller 1976).

Changes occur in particular aspects of platelet electrophoretic mobility as a consequence of women using the high oestrogen content pill.

It has been argued that the changes in these various parameters are not very different from those arising in pregnancy — usually a physiological situation. However, while some of the changes are similar, others are not. For a fuller account of the action of the contraceptive pill on haemostatic/thrombotic factors the account by Poller (1976) should be consulted.

Endothelial cells Endothelial cell proliferation and other changes can be seen on histological examination in patients on the contraceptive pill, when compared with controls (Irey, 1970).

Smoking Individuals studied immediately after smoking a cigarette show increased platelet aggregation and at a lower concentration of the challenging agent — e.g. A.D.P. The responsible factor is present in plasma. Nicotine releases serotonin from platelets — this causes platelet aggregation and vessel spasm.

Smoking raises the plasma levels of free fatty acids and of prebetalipoprotein and betalipoprotein. These are the same biochemical changes as are present in type IIA familial hyperbetalipoproteinaemia. The endothelial cells of the umbilical arteries of babies of smoking mothers show structural changes when compared with those of non-smoking mothers.

Lipids and lipoproteins

There is an extensive literature on 'thrombotic aspects', related to blood lipid change and it is not reviewed here. A limited number of personal observations are mentioned. Comparisons were made on plasma following high and low fat meals (Sweet *et al*, 1966; Dubber *et al*, 1967).

1. Fibrinolytic activity diminished — plasminogen activator was measured using the euglobulin lysis time (E.L.T.); this correlated with the dilute clot lysis time. The level was lowered by about one third after the high fat as compared with the low fat meal.
2. Thrombi were more resistant to lysis by streptokinase. Thrombi were made incorporating labelled fibrinogen and then the property of streptokinase to lyse these was studied. The thrombi made following high fat intake were more resistant to lysis by streptokinase than those following the low fat breakfast.

Clotting times using Russell Viper Venom (R.V.V.) This was markedly shortened in the plasma after the high fat breakfast in a comparison with the low fat meal — the test being carried out following removal of the platelets by centrifugation. This shortening could be correlated with the concentration of triglyceride. In separate investigations Sweet and colleagues (1966) found that the triglyceride level correlated with the inhibition of fibrinolysis.

In both R.V.V. time and E.L.T. measurements therefore the evidence is that the important lipid effect is mediated by triglyceride.

Diabetes

The Chandler tube technique shows accelerated platelet aggregation. The fibrinogen concentration is greater. The reactivity of platelets to aggregating agents is increased. Platelet turnover is greater. Factor VIII level and related antigen levels are raised in diabetics. There is depressed fibrinolysis. Diabetic premenopausal women have the same risk of myocardial infarction as diabetic men of the same age. The development of diabetes has removed the advantage of young women over young men.

Obesity

There is a very clear correlation between obesity and decreased fibrinolytic activator activity. It would be interesting to know whether the women on the pill, who developed a thrombotic event, were also obese.

Exercise

The effect of exercise on the haemostatic system has been investigated by Prentice *et al.* (1972).

The exercise was running as fast as possible over half a mile and the following changes were noted:

1. Factor VIII level rose by a factor of 2-3 times the resting value
2. Plasminogen activator level rose so that it was ten times greater than the pre-exercise value
3. The platelets were more active in aggregating to a standard challenge with ADP after exercise than before
4. Platelet adhesiveness to glass beads was increased immediately after exercise
5. Platelet phospholipid availability can be tested by clotting under the influence of Russell Viper Venom; in platelet-rich plasma the clotting time was shortened following exercise. This was also true for high spun, platelet free plasma and there was evidence of the release from platelets of micro-particulate material — possibly membrane complexes released from platelets.

Stress and adrenergic stimulation (See Fig. 17.3)

For 70 years it has been known that stimulation of the adrenal glands consistently shortens the clotting time of whole blood. Tissue extracts of the aortic endothelium have coagulant activity; this can be discharged by perfusion with adrenaline in experimental animals. Injection of adrenaline causes vesicle formation on the endothelium, with adherence of platelets and concurrent shortening of the plasma recalcification time. This may occur as a consequence of availability of platelet phospholipid as a consequence of platelets adhering and aggregating subsequent to endothelial change. These actions can be prevented by beta-adrenergic blockade.

Adrenaline injection causes an increase in platelet count possibly as a consequence of splenic contraction.

Stress releases adrenaline and noradrenaline. Adrenaline causes platelet aggregation in vitro and the release of free fatty acids from adipose tissue and these cause platelet aggregation.

STRESS

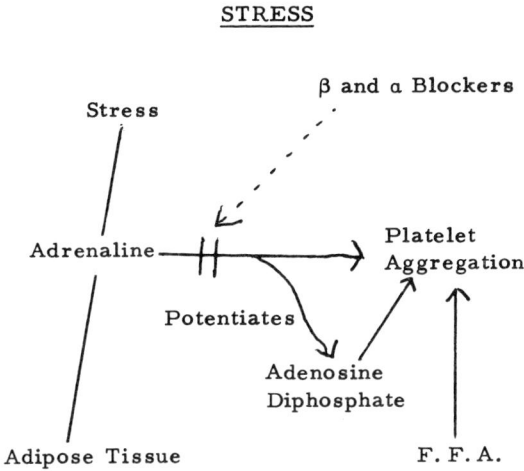

Fig. 17.3

Ageing

With ageing fibrinogen rises, factors V, VII and VIII rise, F.D.P's rise, platelet count rises, platelet turnover is faster, antithrombin III falls, fibrinolytic activator falls as does lipoprotein lipase. Also coagulation response to a standard coumarin drug challenge increases with age.

Defences against 'hypercoagulability'

Following trauma to the microcirculation it would be reasonable to find the haemostatic response reflected in the general circulation. The body however defends against this. With platelet aggregation A.D.P. and thromboxanes are generated in the platelets which inhibit extension of the aggregate. Histamine and serotonin are released and encourage further platelet aggregation at the same time cause local vasospasm to prevent spread of the process to the rest of the circulation. As fibrin is laid down it is lysed by plasmin. Fibrin degradation products are formed, which inhibit further platelet aggregation. Antithrombin III is very powerful and there is excess total antithrombin activity to neutralise potential thrombin. Any activated clotting factors which reach the systemic circulation are effectively inactivated during passage of blood through the liver. During work done by Professor Bonnar it was demonstrated that the clotting time of whole blood collected from the uterine vein during placental separation was very short but that this activation could not be found in blood taken simultaneously from a superficial arm vein.

References

Dubber, A.H.C., Rifkind, B., Gale, M., McNicol, G.P. and Douglas, A.S. (1967) The effect of fat feeding on fibrinolysis, 'stypven' time and platelet aggregation. *Journal of Atherosclerosis Research*, **7**, 225-235.

Duguid, J.B. (1977) *Dynamics of atherosclerosis.* Aberdeen University Press, page 68.

Irey, N.S., Manion, W.C., Taylor, M.B. (1970) Vascular lesions in women taking oral contraceptions. *Archives of Pathology*, **89**, 1-8.

Moncada, S., Higgs, E.A., Vane, J.R. (1977) Human arterial and venous tissues generate prostacycline (Prostaglandin X), a potent inhibitor of platelet aggregation. *Lancet*, **1**, 18-20.

Poller, L. (1976) *Stroke.* Gillingham, F.J., Mawdsley, C. and Willingas, A.E. (Eds). Churchill Livingstone, Edinburgh, London and New York, pages 317-346.

Prentice, C.R.M., Hassanein, A.A., McNicol, G.P. and Douglas, A.S. (1972) Studies on blood coagulation, fibrinolysis platelet function following exercise in normal and splenectomised people. *British Journal of Haematology*, **23**, 541-552.

Sweet, B., Rifkind, B.M. and McNicol, G.P. (1966) The relationship between blood lipids and the fibrinolytic enzyme system. *Journal of Atherosclerosis Research*, **6**, 359-367.

Tullis, J.L. (1976) *Clot.* Charles C. Thomas, Springfield, U.S.A. page 375.

Discussion 4E

Chaktabarti (London)   I would like to comment on the effects of age on two of the variables Prof. Douglas has discussed. First, fibrinogen rises steadily with age, at about the same rate in both men and women. Secondly, fibrinolytic activity falls with age in men up till the age of 50 after which it levels off, or even rises a little; so far our findings are based on cross sectional data, so the apparent rise at older ages could be due to a survivor effect.

Fuller (London)   In an earlier paper, Dr. Chakrabarti, you showed that women on the pill have increased fibrinolytic activity. Perhaps then the vascular risks on the pill occur in those women who do not increase their fibrinolytic activity sufficiently to overcome all other abnormalities mentioned.

Nordin (Leeds)   When one gives oestrogen preparations to post-menopausal women in the belief that one is replacing a deficiency, are you impressed by the changes reported in coagulation parameters? If so, do you think it has been shown that different oestrogens in these small doses have different effects?

Douglas   The use of oestrogens for any purpose increase the thrombotic risk, but this may be so small that it can be accepted. It has not been shown that different oestrogens have different effects.

Nordin (Leeds)   In practice, assuming one has not got your facilities available, what tests should or could be applied to select out people who are not suitable for oestrogen preparations?

Douglas   I do not know a reliable test.

Mitchell (Nottingham)   I think there are none because we do not know whether any of the tests described are predictive. I think it would be fair to say that measurements of platelet adhesiveness are hardly worth undertaking at present because of the intrinsic variabilities in techniques. This is a harsh truth. Until the answers come out from predictive studies, your question cannot be answered.

Potts (London)   Of the complex changes you talked about, are many of them time-related? As I understand the epidemiological evidence about pill-related thrombosis, duration of use does not make much difference but you implied, in relation to antithrombin III, that long-term oestrogens might have a cumulative effect.

Douglas   We do not know whether we are generating a group of women, now aged 45 to 50, who have been taking these pills for 20 years, with arteries looking like those of a 29 year old man.

Hazzard (Seattle)   Could you give us an idea of the variance in individual response in these parameters, and whether or not changes in one parameter would be inter-correlated with changes in another factor in a given person?

Douglas   There is unquestionably some individual variation in response and one will occasionally find women with extremely minimum changes, particularly in antithrombin III. Recovery is also variable over several months after the patient stops the pill. I think the so-called 'natural' oestrogens have fewer effects than the synthetic ones.

18. Hypertension and coronary heart disease in young women

J. J. BROWN, ALISON M. M. CUMMING, A. F. LEVER,
J. I. S. ROBERTSON AND R. J. WEIR

Although the incidence of coronary heart disease is very low in young women, it is clear from epidemiological studies that a raised blood pressure is a predisposing factor. Kannell (1977) has emphasised that the risk of myocardial infarction increases in proportion to the blood pressure, both systolic and diastolic, at any age and in either sex. Indeed, the mean systolic pressure at initial examination in women 30 to 49 years old, who subsequently developed coronary heart disease, was 146 mmHg, compared with a mean of 130 mmHg for those who did not (Kannell, 1977).

Furthermore, young women presenting with coronary heart disease often have a raised blood pressure. Thus, Oliver (1974) found a diastolic blood pressure greater than 100 mmHg in 34 per cent of a series of 150 women under the age of 45 who had symptoms and signs of ischaemic heart disease. Mann *et al* (1976) similarly reported on 77 women under the age of 45 who had suffered myocardial infarction, and compared them with control patients. It was found that eleven of the women with infarction (14.9 per cent) had received drug treatment for hypertension, as compared with six of 197 control patients (3.1 per cent), a highly significant difference ($p < 0.01$). In addition, previous treatment for pre-eclamptic toxaemia was reported by 21 of the 77 infarct patients (28.4 per cent) and by 22 of the controls (11.2 per cent), again a highly significant difference ($p < 0.01$).

The association between hypertension and coronary heart disease in young women becomes even more apparent when those presenting to a specialist hypertension centre are considered. Since 1972, 44 women aged 45 or younger have been admitted to the MRC Blood Pressure Unit, Glasgow, for the investigation and treatment of severe hypertension (diastolic pressure > 120 mmHg). Eighteen of these had angina pectoris or had suffered myocardial infarction.

Case history

A particularly striking instance was a woman who was admitted at the age of 37 with an arterial pressure of 230/140 mmHg, pulmonary oedema, congestive cardiac failure, proteinuria and bilateral papilloedema with extensive retinal haemorrhages and exudates (Weir & Willocks, 1976). She had never taken oral contraceptives, glucose tolerance was normal, and she had normal levels of serum cholesterol, triglycerides and lipoproteins. She smoked 20 cigarettes daily. Two pregnancies, respectively 11 and 8 years previously, had been complicated by hypertension and proteinuria in the last trimester, but on both occasions she had spontaneous uncomplicated vaginal deliveries. Hypertension and cardiac failure were controlled with a combination of bethanidine 200 mg daily, methyldopa 3 gm daily and frusemide 120 mg daily.

After treatment of the hypertension for one year, the retinal lesions had resolved, but she then developed angina, together with severe intermittent claudication in the right calf. Arteriography revealed extensive atheroma of the right common iliac artery, occlusion of the right main renal artery and possible slight narrowing at the origin of the left renal artery. Ureteric catheter studies showed normal function in the left kidney, but no urine flow on the right. Because of the severe claudication, a right aorto-femoral graft was inserted, the non-functioning right kidney being removed at the same operation. Claudication was relieved and for several months blood pressure was controlled with methyldopa alone. After six months, however, bendrofluazide and bethanidine had to be reintroduced.

Three years after her initial presentation with malignant hypertensions she again became pregnant and was anxious that the pregnancy should proceed. She was seen at 2-weekly intervals and blood pressure control became noticeably easier, treatment consisting of methyldopa alone from the second trimester. At 32 weeks she was admitted to hospital for closer observation, and at 36 weeks caesarian section was performed with the delivery of a healthy child who subsequently progressed normally. Two days after delivery, however, she developed a transmural anteroseptal myocardial infarction from which she made a good recovery. For the next two years she remained well and symptom-free, requiring only bendrofluazide 10 mg daily to control the blood pressure. She then had an anterior myocardial infarction from which she again made a good recovery. A further, fatal, myocardial infarction occurred six months later, that is 5 years after presenting in the malignant phase of hypertension and 2½ years after the birth of her third child.

Oral contraceptives and hypertension

The combined oestrogen/progestagen oral contraceptive pill is also a risk factor for coronary heart disease in young women. Radford and Oliver (1973), in a study of 22 women aged 31-45 with acute myocardial infarction, found a significantly greater prevalence of oral contraceptive use than in the general female population of similar age. Further, Mann et al (1975) found that in 63 women admitted to hospital with myocardial infarction, there had been significantly greater oral contraceptive use in the month before admission than in control women.

One way in which the oestrogen/progestagen oral contraceptive may predispose to coronary heart disease is by inducing a rise in arterial pressure. In some women the increase in blood pressure caused by oral contraceptive therapy is pronounced. Figure 18.1 summarises the findings in a series of 26 women aged 20-44 (mean 32 years) in whom marked elevation of blood pressure was caused by the oestrogen/ progestogen pill (the oestrogen content in all cases was 50 µg, while the progestogen content varied from 0.25 to 3.0 mg). All these women had been known to have arterial pressure below 140/90 mmHg before starting therapy (mean 118/79 $\pm$ 11/6 SD). While taking the oral contraceptive for 1 to 12 years (mean 4 years), blood pressure rose to a mean of 171/110 ($\pm$ 17/6 SD). 6 to 12 months after stopping the pill, blood pressure had fallen to a mean of 126/82 (SD 15/5). In only 2 women did significant

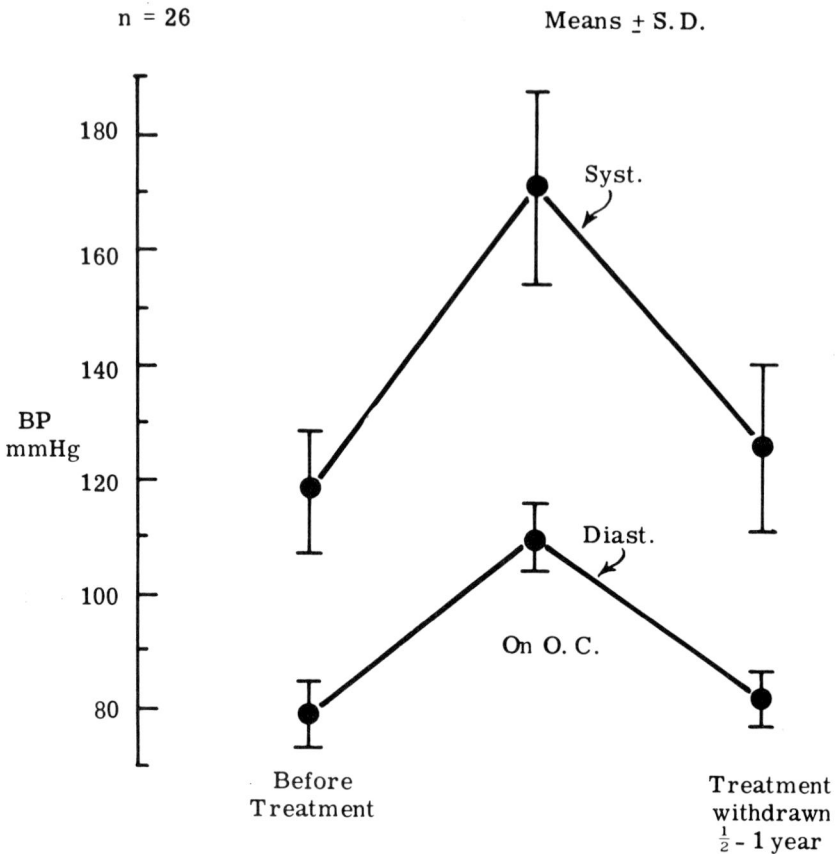

Fig. 18.1 Distinct hypertension induced in 26 initially normotensive women by oestrogen/progestagen oral contraceptives. Also shown is the fall in mean pressure when treatment stopped.

hypertension persist after one year (160/110 and 154/94 mmHg respectively). 14 of these 26 women had previously been pregnant; of these 7 gave a history of hypertension in pregnancy. 8 gave a history of urinary tract infection and one had had a renal stone. The family history included hypertension in 10, coronary heart disease in 9, and cerebrovascular disease in 3. Only 2 of the 26 women, however, showed electrocardiographic evidence of ischaemic heart disease and none had symptoms.

Distinct, but milder, elevation of arterial pressure is a very consistent feature of combined oestrogen/progestogen oral contraceptive therapy. In a prospective controlled study set up jointly by the MRC Blood Pressure Unit and the Glasgow Clinic of the Family Planning Association (Weir et al, 1974), mean systolic pressure had risen after 2 years by 10.2 mmHg ($^+$0.81 SEM) and mean diastolic by 6.0 mmHg ($^+$0.79 SEM) in 186 women on the pill. No significant change in pressure occurred in 60 control women employing mechanical methods of contraception. After 5 years blood pressure had risen in 13 out of 15 women taking oral contraceptives (mean systolic rise 12.3 mmHg; largest individual increase 41 mmHg; mean diastolic rise 8.8 mmHg; largest increase 34 mmHg). In this series the blood pressure changes were unrelated to changes in weight, to a past history of renal disease, a family history of hypertension, parity, social class or to cigarette smoking. Only one woman showing a rise of blood pressure while taking oral contraceptives gave a previous history of pregnancy hypertension. In 32 women who had taken oral contraceptives for between 1 and 3 years, blood pressure fell to pre-treatment levels within three months when the pill was discontinued.

Renin, angiotensin and myocardial lesions

Considerable interest has centred on whether renin (or more accurately, its peptide product, angiotensin II) has a vasculotoxic and cardiotoxic effect independently of its pressor action.

We reported five cases of severe hypertension (including 2 young women) known to have high circulating levels of angiotensin II, who had sudden, presumably cardiac, deaths, and who were found post mortem to have multifocal myocardial necroses in the absence of demonstrable lesions in the intra-myocardial arteries or arterioles (Gavras et al, 1975). Similar multifocal myocardial necroses were produced by the infusion of high doses of angiotensin II into rabbits, also in the absence of light-microscopic lesions in the cardiac arteries or arterioles (Gavras et al, 1975). Giacomelli et al (1976) confirmed in the rat that angiotensin II administration caused multifocal myocardial necroses. They found medial fragmentation and extensive vascular necrosis in the intra-myocardial, but not in epicardial, arteries, and suggested that increased permeability of epicardial arteries might be due to elevated pressure, while the vascular lesions of intra-myocardial arteries was more readily attributable to vasoconstriction. In our infused rabbits, there was a significant correlation between the severity of the cardiac abnormalities and the plasma concentration of angiotensin II achieved during the infusion ($r = +0.58$; $p < 0.001$). However, there was an even closer correlation between the blood pressure increment during angiotensin II administration and the cardiac lesion 'score' ($r = +0.82$; $n = 10$; $p < 0.01$). Thus neither in experimental animals nor in man can the cardiac necroses, on present evidence, be attributed to angiotensin II per se rather than to the severity of the hypertension. Nevertheless, these experiments demonstrate that myocardial necrosis can occur in the absence of structural occlusion of the coronary arteries.

Epidemiological studies of renin and cardiovascular disease

In a clinical report on 219 patients with essential hypertension, Brunner et al (1972) suggested that those with high plasma renin activity (and hence, by implication, high plasma angiotensin II) were prone to develop heart attacks and strokes, while those with low plasma renin were relatively immune to these complications. However, the study was open to several criticisms. The group with high plasma renin had a higher mean diastolic pressure, a higher mean blood urea and a greater incidence of retinal haemorrhages and exudates than the other groups. These are all features known to be associated with poor prognosis, irrespective of renin level. The racial compositions of the groups were dissimilar, so that ethnic or social factors could have influenced the results. Although the patients were followed for 10 years, no effect of treatment on plasma renin or on blood pressure was reported. In a further report on the same series, now expanded and followed for longer, Brunner et al (1975) found a roughly equal incidence of heart attacks and strokes in all three groups. Although this survey has aroused much interest it cannot, in our opinion, be regarded as supporting convincingly the concept of a vasculotoxic effect of renin independently of blood pressure.

Myocardial lesions and catecholamines

Rather similar myocardial lesions to those caused by angiotensin II administration can be produced in experimental animals by infusions of a variety of catecholamines, including adrenaline and noradrenaline, and are also found in patients with phaeochromocytoma dying after a hypertensive paroxysm (see Gavras et al, 1975). It remains uncertain whether these lesions also are a consequence of hypertension per se; other possibilities are myocardial cell anoxia due to an imbalance between oxygen need and availability, a thrombogenic effect of the platelet-aggregating properties of catecholamines or a direct action of catecholamines on vessel walls. Bagnall et al (1976) recently described a 31-year-old woman with bilateral intraadrenal phaeochromocytomata and hypertension, in whom extensive T-wave inversion developed on the electrocardiograph. This appearance (which resolved after removal of the tumours) was attributed to catecholamine-induced myocardial lesions.

Antihypertensive therapy and coronary heart disease

The treatment of severe hypertension which, as we have seen, is often accompanied by coronary artery disease, presents certain difficulties. Diazoxide is a potent and popular drug for both oral and intravenous use in severe hypertension. However, diazoxide causes an increase in heart rate and cardiac output and a rise in plasma renin and angiotensin II. O'Brien et al (1975) administered diazoxide by intravenous 300 mg bolus to 20 hypertensive patients who had been admitted with recent myocardial infarction. They found that electrocardiographic changes occurred in 9 cases immediately after the diazoxide administration which suggested an increase of myocardial injury. Several other reports have implicated diazoxide as provoking myocardial infarction in hypertensive patients (see Brown et al, 1977). Labetalol, a recently introduced drug which has both alpha and beta-adrenergic receptor blocking actions, contrasts with diazoxide in that it does not cause an increase in heart rate or cardiac output, and will also reduce raised levels of plasma angiotensin II (Brown et al, 1977). Figure 18.2 illustrates the use of graded infusions of labetalol intravenously to correct severe hypertension in a 16-year-old girl. Intravenous sodium nitroprusside, which is less prone than diazoxide to cause tachycardia, and which dilates the coronary arteries, might also be useful in such cases (Yeh et al, 1977).

Although long-term oral antihypertensive therapy has shown clear benefits in reducing the incidence of subsequent strokes, no comparable protection against myocardial infarction has yet been seen. However, there are suggestions that the

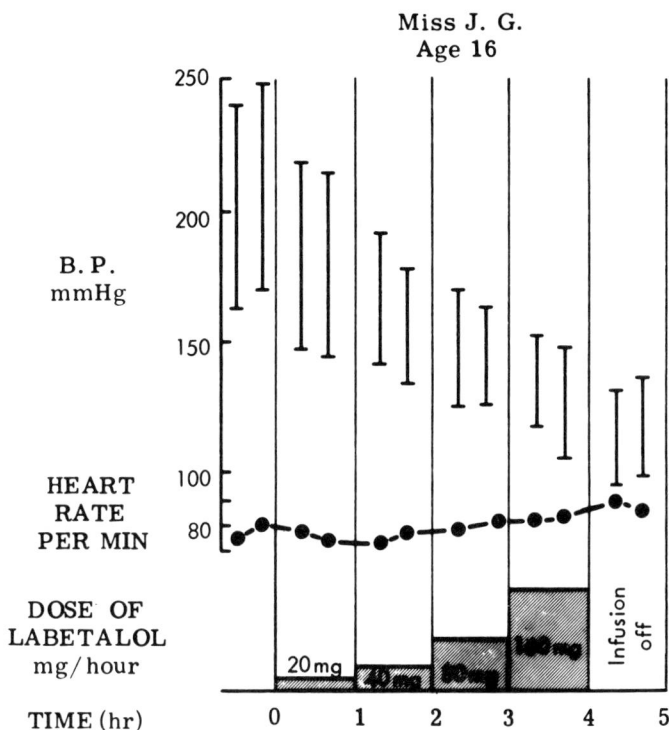

Fig. 18.2 Severe hypertension in a 16-year-old girl, reduced by graded infusion of labetalol intravenously. Blood pressure and heart rate values shown are means for each 30-minute period.

use of β-adrenergic receptor blocking drugs, probably because of actions additional to their antihypertensive effect, may minimize the risk of myocardial infarction in hypertensive patients. Lambert (1975) reported that when β-blockers were given long-term to patients with ischaemic heart disease the incidence of subsequent infarctions was significantly lower than in similar patients not given β-blocking drugs. The benefit was especially evident in those patients with blood pressure over 140/90 mmHg.

Stewart (1976), studying severely hypertensive patients without overt coronary artery disease, found that, despite comparable control of blood pressure, and similarity of other known risk factors, the incidence of first myocardial infarcts was significantly lower in patients treated with propranolol than in those not given a β-blocker.

Both of these studies were uncontrolled, however, and the apparent protective effect of β-adrenergic blocking drugs against myocardial infarction in hypertensive patients requires to be confirmed in a controlled clinical trial.

Summary

A raised blood pressure predisposes to coronary heart disease in young women, as in other groups. In young women with severe hypertension, coronary heart disease is common. Oral contraceptives induce a distinct, although usually mild, increase in arterial pressure in most women, and a marked elevation in some. Hypertension thus is one mechanism whereby oral contraceptives increase the risk. Infusions of angiotensin can induce myocardial necroses in rabbits and rats. However, epidemiological studies implicating renin, independently of the arterial pressure level, as a risk factor for myocardial infarction, are inconclusive. Infusions of catecholamines can also produce myocardial necroses, which are similarly observed in phaeochromocytoma. Diazoxide, given intravenously for hypertensive emergencies, may provoke or worsen myocardial ischaemia. Labetalol or nitroprusside seem safer alternatives. In the long-term treatment of hypertension, β-adrenergic blocking drugs may minimize the risk of myocardial infarction, although the initial observations require confirmation.

References

Bagnall, W.E., Salway, J.G. and Jackson, E.W. (1976) Phaeochromocytoma with myocarditis treated with alpha-methyl-p-tyrosine. *Postgraduate Medical Journal,* **52,** 653-656.

Brown, J.J., Lever, A.F., Cumming, A.M.M. and Robertson, J.I.S. (1977) Labetalol in hypertension. *Lancet,* **1,** 1147.

Brunner, H.R., Laragh, J.H., Baer, L., Newton, M.A., Goodwin, F.T., Krackoff, L.R., Bard, R.H. and Buhler, F.R. (1972) Essential hypertension: renin and aldosterone, heart attack and stroke. *New England Journal of Medicine,* **286,** 441-449.

Brunner, H.R., Gavras, H., Laragh, J.H., Marrus, G. and Sealey, J.E. (1975) The risk of low-renin hypertension: an updated analysis. Abstracts, 9th Annual Meeting of European *Society for Clinical Investigation.* Rotterdam, April 1975, p.53.

Gavras, H., Kremer, D., Brown, J.J., Gray, B., Lever, A.F., MacAdam, R.F., Medina, A., Morton, J.J. and Robertson, J.I.S. (1975) Angiotensin- and norepinephrine-induced myocardial lesions: experimental and clinical studies in rabbits and man. *American Heart Journal,* **89,** 321-332.

Giacomelli, F., Anversa, P. and Wiener, J. (1976) Effect of angiotensin-induced hypertension on rat coronary arteries and myocardium. *American Journal of Pathology,* **84,** 111-138.

Kannell, W.B. (1977) Importance of hypertension as a major risk factor in cardiovascular disease. In *Hypertension,* J. Genest, E. Koiw and O. Kuchel, (Eds) 888-910, McGraw-Hill, New York.

Lambert, D.M.D. (1975) Long-term survival on beta-receptor-blocking drugs in general practice – a three-year prospective study. In *Hypertension – its Nature and Treatment,* D.M. Burnley, G.F.B. Birdwood, J.H. Fryer and S.H. Taylor (Eds) 283-285, Ciba, Horsham, England.

Mann, J.I., Vessey, M.P., Thorogood, M. and Doll, R. (1975) Myocardial infarction in young women with special reference to oral contraceptive practice. *British Medical Journal,* **2**, 241-245.

Mann, J.I., Doll, R., Thorogood, M., Vessey, M.P. and Waters, W.E. (1976) Risk factors for myocardial infarction in young women. *British Journal of Preventive and Social Medicine,* **30**, 94-100.

O'Brien, K.P., Grigor, R.R. and Taylor, P.M. (1975) Intravenous diazoxide in treatment of hypertension associated with recent myocardial infarction. *British Medical Journal,* **4**, 74-77.

Oliver, M.F. (1974) Ischaemic heart disease in young women. *British Medical Journal,* **4**, 253-259.

Radford, D.J. and Oliver, M.F. (1973) Oral contraceptives and myocardial infarction. *British Medical Journal,* **3**, 428-430.

Stewart, I.McD.G. (1976) Compared incidence of first myocardial infarction in hypertensive patients under treatment containing propranolol or excluding beta-receptor blockade. *Clinical Science and Molecular Medicine,* **51**, Supplement 3, 509-511.

Weir, R.J., Briggs, E., Mack, A., Naismith, L., Taylor, L. and Wilson, E. (1974) Blood pressure in women taking oral contraceptives. *British Medical Journal,* **1**, 533-535.

Weir, R.J. and Willocks, J. (1976) A successful pregnancy following malignant phase hypertension. *British Journal of Obstetrics and Gynaecology,* **83**, 584-586.

Yeh, B.K., Gosselin, A.J., Swaye, P.S., Larsen, P.B., Gentsch, T.O., Traad, E.A. and Faraldo, A.R. (1977) Sodium nitroprusside as a coronary vasodilator in man. I. Effect of intracoronary sodium nitroprusside on coronary arteries, angina pectoris and coronary blood flow. *American Heart Journal,* **93**, 610-616.

Discussion 4F

Singh (Birmingham) How long did it take between starting the pill and the development of hypertension?

Weir (Glasgow) It varied from 6 months to 7 years.

Singh (Birmingham) How long did it take before they became normotensive again?

Robertson Between 6-12 months after the pill was stopped, although in 2 of the 26 women the blood pressure remained high.

Nordin (Leeds) Can you tell us from your experience whether you now think it is the oestrogen or progestogen in the pill that is the problem. If you think it is the oestrogen, is it dose-related? Finally, are there any changes in renin-angiotensin levels when you start on the pill?

Robertson The changes in renin-angiotensin on the pill are very consistent in our experience. Oestrogens cause a rise in the levels of renin substrate but in our patients the levels of angiotensin II are unremarkable. So we do not regard the rise in blood pressure either as due to a rise in angiotensin II, despite the rise in renin substrate, or to a disproportion between angiotensin and renin. Having said that, there is a contrary finding from Gast and his colleagues in the U.S. where they do find a rise in angiotensin II on the pill. There are a number of areas where we do not agree with their findings but this is an inter-laboratory dispute.

Weir (Glasgow) For the first two years of our prospective survey, the dose of oestrogen was 100 µg and then, after the Committee of Safety on Medicine's report, this was reduced to 50 µg. The prospective study is basically on 50 µg preparation. We found no difference between the results during the first year or two on the 100 µg with those for the 50 ug dose. Also, we found no difference in our prospective study between the rise in blood pressure in those taking a high dose of progestogen compared with a low dose. We have now taken these women off the combined pill. To some, we have given a 30 microgram oestrogen preparation and to others a progestogen preparation. The numbers are so far very small, but it seems that in some their blood pressure increases again whether on the progestogen-only preparation or on the 30 µg oestrogen preparation, although in others the blood pressure has remained normal.

Spain (Brooklyn) I challenge your concept that cardiogenic shock is synonymous with extensive heart failure. That is putting the cart before the horse. Cardiogenic shock occurs subsequent to myocardial necrosis and does not initiate the myocardial necrosis.

Somerville (London) In conjunction with Dr. Denis Noble of the Department of Physiology in Oxford, we have made observations on about 40 young people, of whom 38 are young men under the age of 35, practically all commercial airline pilots, RAF pilots or Army Officers. They had in common psychological qualities approximating closely to Rosenman and Friedman's Type A personality. They all had abnormal electrocardiograms, like the ones that you have shown as depicting catecholamine myocarditis, with inverted T waves in certain leads indistinguishable from those of myocardial ischaemia. All of them had unobstructed coronary arteries by arteriography. All of them had normal left ventriculograms. The ECG changes disappeared within a matter of an hour with an adequate dose of beta-adrenergic blocker, or overnight by a rest. When the electrocardiogram had been normal with big, upright T waves, the abnormalities could be induced again by intravenous adrenaline injections and were virtually dose related. When the infusion was stopped the ECG returned to normal. Paradoxically there is another group of individuals with T inversions which do not normalise with rest, but disappear with an intravenous infusion of adrenaline.

Oliver (Edinburgh) Of the 150 women I originally reported, one of those excluded had, by mistake, been given an i.v. injection of adrenaline. She was 26 and went to her family doctor in order to have her varicose veins treated and, instead of giving sodium morrhuate, he gave adrenaline. She had a transmural Q wave infarct with acute pulmonary oedema and was exceedingly ill. Subsequently coronary arteriography showed that she had normal coronary arteries. Some years ago, when we were enthusiastic for reasons which I find difficult to explain now about the giving of i.v. noradrenaline to patients with so-called cardiogenic shock, we found out of a group of 18 patients who died in cardiogenic shock, 8 in whom the pathologist demonstrated acute disseminated myocardial necrosis. He described this in considerable detail and related it to the myocarditis, described so clearly by Raab in 1962, as a catecholamine-induced myocarditis.

Mitchell (Nottingham)   Cardiologists over the years have used the word 'ischaemia' to describe changes in electrocardiograms when they really have not the faintest idea whether they are due to that. We should say 'The T waves are upside down and I do not know why'. The temptation is to write on the report, 'Ischaemic changes'.

General discussion

Mitchell (Nottingham)   Is there any way of identifying which women on the oral contraceptive are going to be at risk? Screening of all women going on the pill would be a formidable endeavour. How can we focus on a group who really ought to be screened in the complex ways that have been described?

Hazzard (Seattle)   Until I heard Professor Beaumont's presentation, I would have said there was no adequate way of predicting which woman might have a catastrophic event when she was placed on the pill. I would like to draw a contrast between young women — less than 25 or so — who have a catastrophic event and older women — 40-45 years of age. I think there may be quite different pathogenic mechanisms. With regard to the younger person with no other risk factors, I am impressed that there could be some sort of autoimmune idiosyncratic reaction, which may primarily involve the endothelium in its interaction with the blood coagulation system. At the other end of the spectrum, we have acceleration of the atherosclerotic process. In these other women we would look for universal responses. The one I would focus on is a change in lipoproteins. There is an increase in triglycerides, which may or may not be important, and low density lipoprotein cholesterol. There is a decrease in high density lipoproteins with oestrogens alone, although an increase with the oral contraceptive. I think this is an important difference. These changes would mostly accelerate the atherosclerotic process. In the blood coagulation system, there may be deleterious changes, not only with the formation of the thrombus, but the more important changes in platelet aggregation with release of factors which promote smooth muscle cell replication and possibly have some changes on the endothelium. While there may be the occasional woman who has a catastrophic rise in blood pressure, for most women it is a mild change which over the long run could contribute significantly to the burden of coronary heart disease. Altered carbohydrate tolerance also contributes in a subtle way. So, the oral contraceptive may in other women move her more towards the constellation of risk factors which would be characteristic of men of similar age and accelerated atherosclerosis.

Robertson   I think we can be more positive about what to do about blood pressure. In the Framingham study, those women between the age of 30 and 49 at presentation who went on to have a myocardial infarction in the next 20 year period, had a mean systolic pressure of 146 mmHg while those who had no CHD had a pressure of 130 mmHg. That is a mean difference of 16 mmHg and it is almost exactly the mean increment reported by Dr. Weir for patients on the oral contraceptives. Therefore, these degrees of blood pressure elevation produced by the pill may carry the same risk as in the Framingham study. I think women should have their blood pressure regularly checked when on the pill — say twice a year — and I think it is inappropriate for them to remain on the pill for more than 10 years.

Hazzard (Seattle)   Is there a strong correlation between blood pressure before going on the pill and the response during the pill? Does the initial value help to discriminate?

Robertson   I think not.

Weir (Glasgow)   There is one thing we can do as far as the blood pressure is concerned and this is to take a careful history. In the 26 women referred to me with marked hypertension on the pill, it was common to find a previous history of hypertension in pregnancy, or renal disease, or family history of hypertension or cardiovascular disease.

SESSION 5 Oral contraceptives and oestrogens

Chairman: D.T. Baird

19. Current practice

MALCOLM POTTS

Oral contraceptives are unusual drugs. They are given to healthy women for a long period, sometimes several years, in situations where there are no clinical indications for therapy. They are meeting a convenience of society and the medical profession has no consistent philosophy about their availability. Doctors often have rather conservative attitudes towards contraception, although they tend to be liberal in practice. As a result of these conflicts, the Pill has not been fitted into the mainstream of medicine and the prescription of oral contraceptives has become one of the very few items of service within the NHS for which individual payment is received.

In a sentence, the Pill is both inside and outside routine medical practice. To some doctors the Pill is an important part of preventive medicine, to others it is a symbol of the permissive society and for yet others part of their income.

Users

The 1976 value of the oral contraceptive market was estimated at £13,000,000 and the share of the market by competing brands is known in some detail. Since contraception became part of the Health Service, prescription records have been published in *Health and Personal Social Service Statistics for England* (1976). The age, marital status and parity of oral contraceptive users is not regularly monitored on a sample basis nationwide, but is known from a number of family planning surveys.

Numbers

In 1964 approximately half a million women took oral contraceptives, by 1968 the number exceeded one million and then grew to 1.5 million in 1970, 2.8 million in 1975 and jumped to an estimated 3.2 million by April 1977. One projection of use in 1980 is for 3.7 million users. By 1974 the bulk of oral contraceptives being prescribed were those with 50 μg or less of oestrogen and the predominate oestrogen was ethinyl oestradiol. The leading share of the market in that year went to Minovlar (19 per cent), Gynovlar 21 (16 per cent), and Minilyn (11.5 per cent). Today, 40 per cent of Pills prescribed contain less than 50 μg of oestrogen, 57 per cent are at the 50 μg level, only 1.6 per cent contained over 50 μg.

The record of Pill use derived from the industry suggests that one third of women at risk for pregnancy now use oral contraceptives. The big rise in recent years is consistent with the observed improvement in use of contraception.

Over the past four years *both* the birth rate and the legal abortion rate have declined. It also received independent confirmation from records of prescriptions (Table 19.1).

Table 19.1 Oral contraceptive prescriptions written by general practitioners. United Kingdom 1973-77.

Year	Number of prescriptions x 1000
1973	4.009
1974	4.645
1975	6.389
1976	7.500
1977 (April)	8.017

Note prescriptions are usually given for several cycles at a time and the record indicates trends not absolute figures. The records only cover general practitioners and it should be noted that the proportion of women receiving the Pill from family planning clinics fell during this interval.

It is important to note that there has been a very significant rise in oral contraceptive users in the past four years — a rise which exceeds the total number of users at the time when some of the key epidemiological dissertations on Pill use were made.

Perhaps it is useful to fit these figures first into the framework of family planning and then into the context of medical practice. It is not always generally realised that, as a method of family planning, the Pill was until very recently in the third rank, after the use of condoms and *coitus interruptus.* Even for couples marrying in 1965 and later, Woolf (1971) found the current or last used method of birth control in 41 percent of her sample was the condom, in 29 percent *coitus interruptus* and in only 24 percent oral contraceptives. Estimates of current prescription practices would suggest that the Pill now enjoys a more commanding position among the reversible methods, although it is by no means in an unrivalled position, even for young couples. Among marriages taking place in 1971, 53 percent of those using a contraceptive within a year of marriage (88 percent) chose the Pill (Peel and Carr, 1975).

The Pill, of course, is the method most often discussed with doctors. As far back as 1967-68 Langford (1976) found that reference to oral contraceptives occurred in 58.9 percent of cases when contraception was discussed with a professional person, and when a professional person suggested a method of birth control the Pill was mentioned in 51.9 percent of cases. Today these figures would be higher.

In 1975, 280 million prescriptions were issued in England. The largest single group was for tranquillizers, totalling over 20 million. Oestrogen-progestagen combinations accounted for 3.5 million prescriptions. In other words, prescriptions for the Pill are a significant part of general practitioners' work, but by no means the largest item. The recent survey of use of medicines in general practice by Skegg, Doll and Perry (1977) based on a thorough analysis of prescriptions issued by 19 general practitioners found that oral contraceptives made up 4.6 percent of all prescriptions, falling a long way behind psychotropic drugs which made up 17.4 percent of the total. Drugs for the treatment of rheumatic diseases were prescribed as frequently as the Pill.

In 1976 the average principal in general practice had an income of £14,500 and in that year contraceptive fees only represented 0.89 percent of the average income (although it should be noted that the calculation was based on less than a full year's experience and the percentage is probably higher now) Hansard (1976). At that time, it was comparable to the income derived from night visits and less than a third of the income derived from maternity fees. The Royal College of General Practitioners estimates that the total recurrent costs of maintaining one doctor in general practice, including prescription costs, hospital referrals etc., is about £43,000 a year, so that contraceptives and their costs are a small proportion of the whole. Out of a total drug bill of more than £260 million for Area Health Authorities in England in 1975, £4.3 million were spent on oral contraceptives.

Monthly records of pill sales have been published for 1965 to 1971 (Office of Health Economics, 1972) and reveal the effect of publicity on use. The Papal Encyclical in 1968 caused only a slight dip in sales and certainly less than that resulting from series of press reports on oral contraceptive related deaths in late 1966. The biggest dip in use came at the end of 1969 when a Committee for the Safety of Drugs statement on low dose pills was misinterpreted as a threat, rather than the step forward in reducing risks which it actually represented.

Characteristics of users

Younger women have grown up with the option of oral contraceptives and the method has been available during their years of highest fertility and maximum sexual activity, so it is not surprising that, while for marriages contracted in the years 1941-50 only 6 percent of women were using the Pill by 1967/68, for those contracted in 1961/65, 31.3 percent had adopted the method (Langford 1976) and those in 1971, 53 percent (Peel and Carr, 1975). It is also the pre-eminent method among those who have premarital intercourse and 9 percent of single women were using the Pill in 1970 (Bone, 1975).

It is suspected that some oral contraceptive side effects, for example the risk of liver tumours and certain metabolic changes, may be related to duration of use. In practice Pill use is often relatively brief. Peel and Carr (1975) looked at the sequence of contraceptive techniques adopted in their national sample of 2,160 women who married between January and March 1971. Thirtyone percent of Pill users discontinued the method within 12 months of their first prescription, partly because they planned a pregnancy, but more frequently because they were dissatisfied with the technique. Most Pill users switched to condoms, but there was also a large group who began with the condom and changed to the Pill. For 45 percent of couples the Pill was the second choice and this group included many taking up the Pill for a second time.

Clinical practice

Except for a trivial number brought in from abroad by airhostesses and other travellers, and manufacturers' samples which doctors sometimes give to their wives, the Pill in Britain is only obtained in response to a doctor's prescription. What in theory should doctors do before prescribing the Pill, what in practice do they do and could any changes be made?

The theory of prescribing

Most instructions, from manufacturers' packet inserts to documents by expert committees and individual textbooks, mix preventive medicine, reasonable deduction from epidemiological studies of the Pill and biological speculations. They usually suggest that active or recent history of liver disease and a past history of deep vein thrombosis or pulmonary embolism are absolute contraindications to use. Most texts also refer to rare hereditary diseases of the liver, although many doctors will never meet them in clinical practice. Neoplasms of various organs are commonly listed as contraindications, but the *FPA Clinic Handbook* (1970) provides a more liberal approach and suggests the Pill should not be prescribed in cases of breast cancer unless there has been discussion with the woman's general practitioner and the consultant responsible for the treatment of her cancer.

On the whole, I suspect that most doctors are aware of and follow these contra-indications. If anything, I would guess that doctors are too mechanical in their interpretation of the situation. They will often forbid the Pill for mild varicose veins or a previous history of superficial thrombosis, although a few are beginning to rethink the problem and will prescribe the Pill in selected cases with a previous history of deep vein thrombosis, especially if former disposing factors, such as obesity or smoking, have been eliminated.

The IPPF Medical Committee (1970) summarised the possible reasons for withdrawing the Pill as.

> '(a) cramps, pain or oedema of the legs, (b) sudden severe migraine or unusual headache, (c) sudden onset of severe chest pain, (d) visual disturbances'.

— and probably most doctors would respond to these problems by discontinuing use. In addition, there is an awareness that the Pill may need to be withdrawn before elective surgery.

There are some areas where texts recommend caution but in a real doctor/patient situation it is unlikely that such caution would be exercised. For example, the *FPA Clinic Handbook* under its absolute contraindications to the Pill says, 'where diseases of the pituitary are recognised' or, even more vaguely, under probable contraindications it speaks of headaches which 'should not be immediately dismissed'.

It needs to be emphasised that all the above items arise from the woman's history. The only physical examination which is likely to be directly relevant to the initiation and continued use of the Pill is the recording of the blood pressure.

In the clinic

Huber (1973) reviewed the clinical care received by 51 women who attended a specialised family planning clinic adhering to the policies outlined in the *FPA Clinic Handbook*, but whose request for oral contraceptives was refused because the prescribing doctor felt contraindications to use existed. The 51 cases came from a sequence of 1,527 women attending the clinic in question, of whom 1,021 sought the Pill. The five percent who were refused at the first visit were matched with 51 women given the Pill at the first visit.

In no case was the Pill refused because of findings on pelvic examination. In 6 cases the refusal was related to blood pressure recording. Most of the women refused were young, nulliparous and only five were over 30. Twenty cases had been given the Pill elsewhere at an earlier stage in life and 25 were subsequently given the Pill when they visited the *same* clinic on a later occasion. No consistent pattern emerged concerning those refused a prescription on the first visit and those given the Pill later. Seventy eight percent of the women refused the Pill stopped attending the clinic in the next two years and probably some of these then obtained the Pill elsewhere (Table 19.2).

Table 19.2 Oral contraceptive refusal in clinic practice

Reason for denial	Never given o.c.s	Refused o.c.s first time, given later
Family history diabetes or heart diseases	5	6
Menstrual irregularities	6	5
Personal history of heart disease	1	1
Personal history of jaundice	1	1
Personal history epilepsy fibroids, anorexia nervosa	3	0
History hypertension	0	1
Hypertensive on *examination*	2	4
Breast tender on *examination*	0	1
Miscellaneous	8	6

After Huber and Huber (1975)

Overall, the clinic doctors seem to have taken care to record the general history, but less than half took a gynaecological history. The blood pressure was not taken in 16 cases refused the Pill and in 4 who were given it.

Cartwright (1970) also reviewed clinic procedures in her 1967/68 survey. She found that 94 percent of women receiving the Pill from a family planning clinic were given a vaginal examination, 69 percent had their breasts examined, but the blood pressure was only taken in just over half the cases (Table 19.3).

Table 19.3 Prescribing practices

Examination	Performed in general practice % of cases	Performed in family planning clinic % of cases
Blood pressure	19	57
Breast	15	69
Vaginal	29	94

After Cartwright, 1970.

In general practice

Cartwright (1970) interviewed over 1,500 women and men in 1967/68 about their family planning experiences. The commonest response of the general practitioner to a request for family planning advice was to prescribe the Pill. 'General practitioners', writes Cartwright, 'were not always as meticulous about examining their patients or taking a history when they first prescribed the Pill as doctors at family planning clinics'. But the more cavalier attitude was not necessarily bad and there were no more side effects or discontinuations among the GP-prescribed cases than the clinic.

Only 29 percent of GPs did a vaginal examination and 15 percent a breast examination. 19 percent took the blood pressure. Those who had a physical examination were less likely to develop problems and had a better continuation rate than those who did not, although whether this was a result of the reassurance given, or the doctor selecting potential problem cases forestalling future difficulties is impossible to determine.

The problem and an alternative approach

It is interesting that the least relevant examination, the vaginal, seems to be performed consistently, while the blood pressure recording, which is probably the most useful, is taken irregularly. The caution over younger rather than older women may also be the reverse of what might be the most useful. Finally, follow-up may be more important than initial examination in the overall care of women. There is also a strong indication that the Pill is the first, and sometimes the only, option a busy doctor puts before a woman seeking family planning advice. But it is unfortunate if one method of birth control is considered in isolation from others. The persistent importance of condoms and *coitus interruptus* as reversible methods of contraception has been noted. Sterilisation is increasingly available and sought in Britain and, when the known hazards are amortized against the number of years protection normally given, tubal ligation and, most especially, vasectomy represent very acceptable choices.

But the surprising element in the total fertility control picture is that of abortion. Over the last decade a previously unforeseen string of complications attending Pill and IUD use have been uncovered, but in the case of abortion, at least when performed early in pregnancy, observation has revealed a previously unsuspected safety and relative freedom from side effects. The mortality amongst over three quarters of a million legal abortions performed during the first 8 weeks of pregnancy in the USA was 0.4/100,000 operations — considerably less than the risk attending use of the Pill over one year.

It must be recognised that the combination of a mechanical method of contraception and legal early abortion, should the contraceptive fail, is much safer than use of the Pill or IUD alone. For older women the differential is particularly marked. Although it might be unaesthetic, and some people would say ethically questionable, in terms of risk to life of the user, if a woman over thirty threw all methods of contraception away and just relied on repeated early abortions she would still be better off than she would taking the Pill.

To return to the realities of Pill prescribing, oral contraceptives entered wide-spread use after most doctors now in practice left medical school. The low dose Pills are an even more recent development. Something is known about the diffusion of knowledge related to other drugs which may be relevant. Coleman and his co-workers (1959) followed the spread of a new antibiotic in the USA. Over 16 months, 9 out of 10 doctors came to prescribe the new drug, but use overlapped with, rather than excluded, similar pre-existing drugs and this trend would probably apply to the use of low dose oral contraception pills. Specialists adopted the antibiotic more rapidly than general practitioners. Predictably, the innovators were those who read most journals, attended most scientific meetings and were in practice with others. In the case of the Pill, the spotlight of lay publicity and the recommendations of the Committee of Safety of Drugs probably accelerated the diffusion of knowledge. Coleman found that the advice of colleagues was particularly important in ambiguous situations and this may apply to choices between brands of Pill.

It is likely, if only for reasons of medical politics and income, that doctors will continue to prescribe the Pill. But in 1974, a group of specialists, taking their clue from a Statement by the Central Medical Committee of the IPPF in 1973, suggested, 'it would be a responsible and constructive step forward in medical practice to widen the range of those empowered to dispense oral contraceptives to include state regist-ered nurses, midwives and health visitors'. They did not imply that the Pill was without risks, but that the little objective screening that is possible could be taught to others. *A Report by the Joint Working Group on Oral Contraceptives* (1976) that the DHSS set up in response to this idea endorsed the suggestion. It concluded 'it is not desirable in present circumstances to make oral contraceptives available other than on prescription, but we do not regard it as necessary to restrict authority to issue prescriptions for oral contraceptives to doctors'. They believed that 'nurses, midwives, health visitors and pharmacists had the relevant skills and knowledge which would enable them to be trained'. This option for future development remains open and the analysis of current practice suggests it is a reasonable one.

Conclusion

In summary, Pill use is widespread and apparently still increasing, but prescription practices contain some paradoxes. Theoretical medical standards in this field are some times unrealistic. There is a degree of arbitrariness in the groups of women refused the Pill and some evidence that, at least until recently, doctors are more reluctant to give the Pill to young than older women.

However, in practice theoretical standards are rarely upheld and if one doctor refused the Pill another may well give it. Users often adopt the Pill for relatively short intervals. Demand is greatest among young women and so in a way the user safeguards her own interests.

It is concluded that a simplification of Pill prescribing techniques and delegation to other than medical practitioners could be a constructive step forward.

References

Bone, M. (1973) *Family Planning Services in England and Wales,* HMSO, London.

Cartwright, A. (1970) *Parents and Family Planning Services.* Routledge and Kegan Paul, London.

Coleman, J., Menzel, H. and Katz, E. (1959) Social Processes in Physicians' adoption of a new drug. *J. Chronic Dis.* **9**, 1-19.

Family Planning Association Clinic Handbook (1970 updated), Graphic, London.

Family Planning in Britain (1972) Office of Health Economics, London.

Health and Social Service Statistics for England 1976, HMSO, London.

Huber, D.H. (1973) *Health Aspects of Oral Contraceptive Use*, MSc thesis, London School of Hygiene and Tropical Medicine.

Huber, D.H. and Huber, S.L. (1975) Screening oral contraceptive candidates and inconsequential pelvic examination. *Studies in Family Planning,* **6**, 106-208.

IPPF (1970) *Comments on Steroidal Contraception.* Ed. R.L. Kleinman, IPPF, London.

Langford, C.M. (1976) *Birth Control Practice and Marital Fertility in Great Britain.* Population Investigation Committee, London.

Peel, J. and Carr, G. (1975) *Contraception and Family Design,* Churchill Livingstone, Edinburgh.

Report of the Joint Working Group on Oral Contraceptives (1976) HMSO, London.

Retail Business (1975) April **210**, 16.

Skegg, D.C.G., Doll, R. and Perry, J. (1977) Use of medicines in general practice. *Brit. Med. J.* **11**, 1561-1563.

Smith, K. and Kane, P. (1975) *The Pill off Prescription.* Birth Control Trust, London.

Woolf, M. (1971) *Family Intentions.* HMSO, London.

Discussion 5A

Mann (Oxford) What proportion of women are using a pill containing less than 50 micrograms of oestrogen?

Potts These figures came from the Family Planning Association (FPA) and they obtained them from a variety of manufacturers: 40% of pills prescribed contained less than 50 micrograms, 57% at the 50 microgram level, and the rest were over 50 micrograms. The data was assembled in April, 1977.

Julian (Newcastle) Can you tell us about patient compliance. One assumes it is very good.

Potts I do not have the data at my fingertips, but it is good.

Vessey (Oxford) I think that this shift to the 30 microgram pill is very encouraging. The time has surely come for us to regard the 50 microgram pill as hazardous. The Advisory Panel to the FPA have officially recommended that 50 microgram pills should now merely be regarded as approved but that 30 microgram pills should be regarded as approved and preferred. I think now that a practitioner who prescribes the 50 microgram pill for a new patient is making an error of judgement. Virtually all the epidemiological data we have relates to 50 or 100 microgram pills. It will be some time before we can possibly evaluate data on the 30 microgram pill.

Potts   In a way we are in a more academically insecure situation than we were in the late 1960s because we have more new people using new pills about which we do not yet have epidemiological information.

Loudon (Edinburgh)   In clinical practice in Australia, at least 60 percent of women are now on the 30 microgram pill and it is standard practice where possible to change all women on 50 microgram pills to 30 microgram.

Slack (London)   Would Dr. Potts give us some idea of what guidelines are given to the doctors in the FPA clinics with regard to the risks that they should look for before they prescribe the pill. I am particularly interested in whether they have any instructions about prescribing the pill in people who have a family history familial hypercholesterolaemia?

Potts   I think Dr. Loudon could answer that question.

Loudon (Edinburgh)   If we find somebody with such a history we would certainly screen them closely. May I ask Dr. Potts what information he hopes will diffuse through to the doctors who prescribe the pill in family planning clinics?

Potts   We consider a previous history of venous thrombosis to be important. I do not think people are taking the age factor quite as seriously as they should. I also do not think that most general practitioners are looking at any of the metabolic effects which have been discussed, because they really have no adequate way of viewing this. One of the main problems is propagating new information on the pill to those who are prescribing it in our clinics.

20. Oral contraceptives and the cardiovascular risk

J. I. MANN

Introduction

The situation before 1975

Early papers concerning the relationship between myocardial infarction and oral contraceptives were inconclusive. Case reports describing small numbers of patients who developed the disease while using oral contraceptives did no more than provide a suggestion that such an association might exist. In their study of deaths from thromboembolic disease occurring in 1966, Inman and Vessey found that women who died from coronary thrombosis in the absence of predisposing factors had been using oral contraceptives more frequently than would have been expected from the experience of the control group. (Inman and Vessey, 1968). Statistically significant differences between the infarction and control patients were apparent, however, only when patients with hypertension, diabetes and obesity were excluded (relative risk approximately 2). On the other hand, a Danish study of fatal myocardial infarction suggested that oral contraceptive use before death from this cause was not different from that in the general population of the same age group.(Fischer and Mosbech, 1970).

In their early study of non-fatal thromboembolic disease, Vessey and Doll were able to include only 17 cases of non-fatal myocardial infarction; they confined their attention, however, to idiopathic disease. (Vessey and Doll, 1969). With so few cases no conclusions could be drawn. Oliver reported on an appreciable number of cases under the age of 45 years. Of those admitted to hospital during the years 1964-72 (during which time use of oral contraceptives was widespread) 52 per cent were taking the preparations. (Oliver, 1974). This proportion was thought to be greater than might have been expected. However, since there was no difference in the prevalence of major risk factors for ischaemic heart disease among those women taking oral contraceptives in comparison with those not doing so, Oliver concluded that the preparations only increased the risk of myocardial infarction in the presence of one of the major risk factors. Inman *et al* in 1970 reviewed the reports of thromboembolism occurring between 1965-1969 received by the drug safety committees in the United Kingdom, Sweden and Denmark, and were able to show an increased risk of myocardial infarction in connection with the use of preparations containing larger amounts of mestranol, and a similar trend was apparent when comparing the two dosages of ethinyloestradiol used at that time. (Inman *et al*, 1970).

It was against this background and in the knowledge that the ongoing cohort studies of women using oral contraceptives were unlikely to provide a definitive answer with regard to myocardial infarction within a reasonable period of time (because of the infrequency of this disease in young women) that we commenced our two case-control studies.

A study of non-fatal myocardial infarction

Procedure

Data were obtained concerning non-fatal myocardial infarction by investigating women under the age of 45 years who were discharged from the major hospitals in three regions in England and Wales during the years 1968-72. (Mann *et al*, 1975; Mann *et al*, 1975; Mann and Thorogood, 1975; Mann *et al*, 1976). In the great majority of cases information concerning oral contraceptive practice and other risk factors was obtained during an interview in the patients' homes. When this could not be arranged, a postal questionnaire was completed or the required information was obtained from the general practitioner. Three control patients were selected to match each patient with infarction with respect to age, marital status and hospital and year of admission. They were selected at random from lists of patients admitted with a wide range of acute medical and surgical conditions, and for certain elective surgical procedures and were investigated in the same manner as the infarction patients. Blood samples were collected from as manh as possible of the infarction patients and controls.

Results

Table 20.1 shows that the proportion of patients who used oral contraceptives during the month before admission to hospital was substantially higher in the infarction than in the control group. The relative risk of developing myocardial infarction, compared

Table 20.1   Oral contraceptive practice amongst myocardial infarction and control patients

Oral contraceptive practice	No. (%) of M.I. patients		No. (%) of controls	
Never used	44	(61.1)	150	(78.9)
Used during month before admission	20	(27.8)	16	(8.4)*
Used only more than one month before admission	8	(11.1)	24	(12.6)
Used any time before admission	28	(38.9)	40	(21.0)**
TOTAL	72	(100)	190	(100)

* Comparison between proportions of patients using oral contraceptives during the month before admission:
$$X^2_{(1)} = 13.3, P < 0.001$$

** Comparison between proportions of patients using oral contraceptives at any time before admission:
$$X^2_{(1)} = 7.5, p < 0.01$$

G*

with that in women who had never used oral contraceptives, is estimated from these figures to be 4.3 to 1 (95 per cent confidence limits 1.7 to 10.4) for women who had used them during the month before admission and 1.1 to 1 for women who had stopped using them more than a month previously. Table 20.2 shows that, even when allowing for the effect of all the other risk factors measured, a statistically significant increase in risk remained. Diabetes was not considered in this analysis, because only four patients were known to have the disease and none was using oral contraceptives.

Neither bias nor chance is likely to account for these findings, but in view of their importance and because criticisms have been made of the published data, we have carried out further analyses to examine whether some confounding factor might explain the association between oral contraceptive use and non-fatal myocardial infarction. A spurious association could have arisen if women with hypertension, diabetes or hyperlipidaemia (all important risk factors for coronary heart disease) had been prescribed the preparations more frequently than other women because they were considered to be at great risk from the complications of pregnancy and were therefore thought to require the most effective method of contraception available. That this is not so is shown by the fact that 27 per cent of the infarction patients known to have one or more of these risk factors before their index hospital admission were using oral contraceptives, a proportion identical to that in the whole series of patients with infarction. Furthermore, the six hypertensive patients and one diabetic in the control series had never used these preparations.

Cigarette smoking could be of greater importance since it is the most frequently occurring risk factor for coronary heart disease and is the one, which, after standardisation caused the greatest reduction in the relative risk of myocardial infarction attributable to oral contraceptives. (Table 20.2). A very striking association was apparent between myocardial infarction and cigarette smoking. (Table 20.3). In comparison with non-smokers and ex-smokers, the relative risk increased from 1.9 to 1 in women smoking fewer than 15 cigarettes a day, to 4.4 to 1 in women smoking 15-24 a day, and 19.1 to 1 in women smoking 25 or more a day.

Table 20.2 Estimated relative risk of myocardial infarction in patients currently using oral contraceptive preparations after standardisation for possible confounding variables. (Data based on the study of survivors of myocardial infarction).

Variable standardised	Relative risk Estimate	x^2	Significance level
None	4.3	13.3	P <0.001
Cigarette smoking	3.2	6.6	P <0.01
Pre-eclamptic toxaemia or hypertension	3.8	10.1	P <0.001
Type II hyperlipo- proteinaemia	3.6	8.3	P <0.01
All above variables simultaneously	3.1	5.5	P <0.05

Table 20.3 Cigarette smoking habits of myocardial infarction (M.I.) and control patients

No. of cigarettes smoked per day	% of M.I. patients N = 72	% of controls N = 181	Relative risk of M.I.
Never or ex-smoker	20.9	48.6	1.0
1 - 14	23.6	29.3	1.9
15 - 24	37.5	19.8	4.4
25+	18.1	2.2	19.1
TOTAL	100	100	100

Test for linear trend amongst all smoking categories: X_1^2 = 35.9, P 0.001

Women with hypertension, diabetes and hyperlipidaemic have been excluded from the infarction and control groups in each smoking category shown in Table 20.4. The proportion of women currently using oral contraceptives is higher in the infarction group than amongst the controls in each smoking category. In non-smokers there is a 1.8 fold increase in risk associated with oral contraceptive use and amongst smokers the risk in users as compared with non-users is 4.8:1. These data suggest a strong interaction between oral contraceptives and cigarette smoking. The number of non-smokers is small and the confidence limits for the risk such that it is possible that chance could explain the increased risk attributable to oral contraceptives in this group.

Table 20.4 Oral contraceptive practice of myocardial infarction and control patients not known to be hypertensive, diabetic or hyperlipidaemic at time of index admission

No. of cigarettes smoked daily at onset of episode	No. (%) of patients using oral contraceptives at onset of episode		Total	
	M.I. patients	Controls	M.I. patients	Controls
None	2 (16.7)	9 (10.1)	12	89
1 - 14	2 (20.0)	2 (4.4)	10	46
15 or more	11 (33.3)	5 (13)	33	38
TOTAL	15	16	55	173

Our data are too few to enable us to establish the quantitative effect of other combinations of risk factors. To do so would require very large numbers of infarction patients and controls. However, the data in Table 20.5 show the proportions of patients known to have had various numbers of risk factors, those who had only one risk factor being subdivided according to the nature of the factor. Information on the presence of one or more factors was not obtained for a few patients, and lipid analyses were carried out on only 70 per cent of the patients with infarction, so that the number who had one risk factor or none at all is likely to have been smaller than appears from the Table. It should also be noted that hypertension and diabetes were recorded only when the patient had been treated for these conditions before the infarction occurred. The risk estimates derived from the data in Table 20.5

Table 20.5 Risk factors in myocardial infarction and control patients.

	No. (%) of M.I. patients		No. (%) of controls	
No risk factor	14	(18.9)	128	(64.0)
One risk factor:				
Current oral contraceptive use	4	(5.4)	9	(4.5)
Type II hyperlipoproteinaemia	4	(5.4)	1	(0.5)
Diabetes	1	(1.4)	0	
Cigarette smoking (15 or more daily)	12	(16.2)	33	(16.5)
Hypertension or pre-eclamptic				
toxaemia	5	(6.8)	19	(9.5)
Two risk factors	20	(27.0)	9	(4.5)
Three or more risk factors	14	(18.9)	1	(0.5)
TOTAL	74	(100.0)	200	(100.0)

nevertheless strongly suggest that the combined effect of the factors is synergistic. In comparison with patients not known to have any risk factors, the relative risk increased from 4:1 in women with one factor to 20:1 in women with two factors and 128:1 in women with three or more factors.

Of particular relevance to the present discussion is the fact that none of the risk factors, except perhaps type II hyperlipoproteinaemia, appeared to exert a strong effect when present on its own. Only four of the infarction patients studied had experienced an acute myocardial infarction while using oral contraceptives in the absence of other risk factors. I shall return to these data when I attempt to consider further the clinical application of these findings.

Studies of fatal myocardial infarction

Procedure

In 1973 Inman and I obtained transcripts of all death certificates relating to women under the age of 50 years who died in England and Wales and which had been coded to rubric 410 according to the eighth revision of the International Classification of Diseases (myocardial infarction and synonomous terms). (Mann and Inman, 1975; Mann and Inman, 1976). Initially we investigated all the deaths under 40 years of age and a random sample of those in the older age groups (40 - 49 years). (Mann and Inman, 1975). Information concerning drug use was obtained chiefly from the patients' general practitioners, who were also asked to provide control information by selecting at random from their files women who matched each fatal case with regard to age and marital status. Later, because very few women aged 40 - 44 in either the infarction or the control groups had been current users of oral contraceptives, we obtained data concerning the deaths not previously studied occurring in this age group. (Mann and Inman, 1976). Twenty-three per cent of the patients selected for study could not be investigated because their general practitioners could not be traced, their records had been lost, or the general practitioner could not be interviewed. The data presented in this paper are based on those cases in whom the diagnosis was substantiated by postmortem findings or by a history of chest pain together with electrocardiographic or enzymatic confirmation as defined by the World Health Organization.

Results

The frequency of use of oral contraceptives during the month before death (current users) was significantly higher in the group with infarction than during the same month in the control group (see Table 20.6) and the average duration of treatment was also longer. In an investigation of fatal cases it was clearly not possible to get detailed information concerning other risk factors, but the data in Table 20.7 suggest that the association between myocardial infarction and oral contraceptives could not be explained by an association between them of these preparations and diabetes or hypertension (defined in this study as previous medical treatment for these conditions). No information was available concerning cigarette smoking habits or cholesterol levels.

Table 20.6 Oral contraceptive practice of women dying from myocardial infarction (M.I.) and their controls.

Age (Years)	Group	Total number	% of total women currently using oral contraceptives	Relative risk of M.I. in current oral contraceptive users
< 40	M.I.	47	44.7	2.8
	Control	76	22.4	(1.2-6.5)*
40 - 44	M.I.	106	17.0	2.8
	Control	102	6.9	(1.2-7.2)*

* 95% confidence limits.

Table 20.7 Estimated relative risk of death from myocardial infarction in patients aged 40-44 years currently using oral contraceptive preparations after standardisation for possible confounding variables.

Variable standardised	Relative risk estimate	x^2	Significance level
None	2.8	3.9	$P < 0.05$
Hypertension	2.7	3.8	$P < 0.05$
Diabetes	2.8	3.8	$P < 0.05$
Both variables simultaneously	2.7	3.8	$P < 0.05$

Clinical application of these studies

Our investigations were carried out to study the epidemiology of myocardial infarction in young women. It is extremely difficult to use the data to make definitive recommendations concerning groups of women for whom oral contraceptives should not be prescribed. The data given in Table 20.8 are derived from the study of fatal cases, information concerning the structure of the female population of England and Wales, and the total number of deaths from myocardial infarction given in the report of the Registrar General for 1973. Despite the fact that the relative risk is identical in the two age groups considered, the attributable mortality is appreciably greater in the older group. These estimates of attributable mortality do not however

Table 20.8 Oral contraceptive practice and mortality from myocardial infarction

	Mortality from myocardial infarction per 100,000 women	
	Aged 30 - 39 years	Aged 40 - 44 years
Women currently using oral contraceptives	5.4	32.0
Women not currently using oral contraceptives	1.9	12.0
Mortality attributable to oral contraceptives	3.5	20.0

take into account the synergistic effect apparent when more than one risk factor for coronary heart disease is present in the same individual. It has already been mentioned that our data are too few to provide accurate risk estimates for individual combinations of risk factors since the confidence limits are wide.

It is however possible to make a *very crude* estimate of the risks of oral contraceptives when used by women with and without predisposing conditions for myocardial infarction. The best relative risk estimates for oral contraceptive use in the presence and absence of one predisposing factor are those derived from Table 20.4. The predisposing cause under consideration is cigarette smoking, and the relative risk estimates of 5 and 2 in smokers and non-smokers respectively may not necessarily apply to the other risk factors. However, using these estimates and information given in Table 20.5 (viz. approximately one-fifth of patients with infarction and two-thirds of controls, representing the population from which the cases were drawn have no risk factors for coronary heart disease — for the purpose of this calculation oral contraceptive use is of course not regarded as a risk factor), it is possible to derive estimates of attributable risk in women with and without predisposing conditions for myocardial infarction. (Table 20.9). The figures in the first column are based on the assumption that two-thirds of women in the general population do not have predisposing conditions and those in the second column that one-fifth of women dying from infarction have no predisposing condition. The estimated death rates in users of oral contraceptives have been calculated using the relative risk estimates of 5 and 2 respectively for women with and without predisposing causes. The estimates are crude for a number of reasons; risk estimates collected in a study of non fatal cases have been applied to mortality statistics, the interaction between cigarette smoking and oral contraceptives may not be the same as for the other risk factors (diabetes, hypertension and hyperlipidaemia), but the calculations do suggest that the risk of myocardial infarction, attributable to oral contraceptive use might be appreciably reduced if the preparations were not prescribed for women with existing risk factors. Furthermore, our results should not be extrapolated without qualification to populations where the prevalence of risk factors (including cigarette smoking) is very low.

Prospective studies

It is difficult to study a relatively infrequent disease prospectively. However, data from the two British prospective studies of oral contraceptive use provide supportive

Table 20.9 Mortality from myocardial infarction attributable to oral contraceptive use in women with and without other risk factors for this disease

Age	Population of England & Wales in 1973 (in thousands)	No. of deaths in 1973	Death rate per 100,000	Estimated death rate in users of oral contraceptives	Estimated death rate attributable to oral contraceptive use
All women					
30-39	2830.3	65	2		
40-44	1424.1	184	13		
Women with predisposing conditions					
30-39	943.3	52	6	30	24
40-44	474.7	147	31	155	124
Women without predisposing conditions					
30-39	1886.9	13	0.7	1.4	0.7
40-44	949.4	37	3.9	7.8	3.9

Table 20.10 Coronary heart disease in the Royal College of Practitioners' Study

	Oral contraceptive users		Controls		
	Observed number	Standardised rate **	Observed number	Standardised rate **	Relative risk
Acute myocardial infarction (410)*	5	0.13	1	0.02	5.2
Acute and subacute ischaemic heart disease (411)*	1	0.08	2	0.03	2.5
Chronic ischaemic heart disease (412)*	3	0.09	1	0.03	3.5

* Numbers in brackets indicate ICD categories
** Standardised rate per thousand woman years

Table 20.11 Deaths from coronary heart disease in the Oxford/Family Planning Association Prospective Study of Contraceptive Use

	Method of contraception in use on admission			
	Oral	Diaphragm	I.U.D.	Total
Number of deaths	4	0	0	4
Number of person years of observation	46,600	21,700	15,200	83,500

evidence for the retrospective case-control studies I have described above. The published material from the Royal College of General Practitioners' Study (1974) and unpublished data from the Oxford University/Family Planning Association Investigation (Vessey, Personal Communication, 1977) are shown in Tables 20.10 and 20.11. The fact that in both the studies the oral contraceptive users were at the outset healthier than the controls (users of other methods or no method in the R.C.G.P. study) strengthens the evidence for an association between myocardial infarction and oral contraceptive use. The magnitude of the increased risk and the precise effect of interaction of risk factors remain to be confirmed in larger case-control studies at present being conducted in the United States.

Finally, with regard to the interpretation of the data I have presented, it should be remembered that all the investigations were carried out before the widespread introduction of oral contraceptives containing 30 µg of oestrogen. The data of Inman *et al* (1970) would suggest that these preparations may be associated with a reduced risk of myocardial infarction.

References

Fischer, A.J. & Mosbech, J. (1970) Mortaliteten af koronarokklusion hos yugre kvinder med henblik pa p-pillen som en mulig aetiologisk faktor. *Ugeskrift for Laeger,* **132,** 2480-2482.

Inman, W.H.W. & Vessey, M.P. (1968) Investigation of deaths from pulmonary, coronary, and cerebral thrombosis and embolism in women of child-bearing age. *British Medical Journal,* **2,** 193-199.

Inman, W.H.W., Vessey, M.P., Westerhold, B. & Engelund, A. (1970) Thrombo-embolic disease and the steroid content of oral contraceptives. A report to the Committee on Safety of Drugs. *British Medical Journal,* **2,** 203-209.

Mann, J.I., Vessey, M.P., Thorogood, M. & Doll, R. (1975) Myocardial infarction in young women with special reference to oral contraceptive practice. *British Medical Journal,* **2,** 241-245.

Mann, J.I., Thorogood, M., Waters, W.E. & Powell, C. (1975) Oral contraceptives and myocardial infarction in young women: a further report. *British Medical Journal,* **3,** 631-632.

Mann, J.I. & Thorogood, M. (1975) Serum lipids in young female survivors of myocardial infarction. *British Heart Journal,* 790-794.

Mann, J.I. & Inman, W.H.W. (1975) Oral contraceptives and death from myocardial infarction. *British Medical Journal,* **2,** 245-248.

Mann, J.I., Doll, R., Thorogood, M., Vessey, M.P. & Waters, W.E. (1976) Risk factors for myocardial infarction in young women. *British Journal of Preventive and Social Medicine,* **30,** 94-100.

Mann, J.I. & Inman, W.H.W. (1976) Oral contraceptive use in older women and fatal myocardial infarction. *British Medical Journal,* **2,** 445-447.

Oliver, M.F. (1974) Ischaemic heart disease in young women. *British Medical Journal,* **4,** 253-259.

Royal College of General Practitioners: Oral contraceptives and health: A preliminary report. (1974) Pitman. New York City.

Vessey, M.P. & Doll, R. (1969) Investigation of relation between use of oral contraceptives and thromboembolic disease. A further report. *British Medical Journal,* **2**, 651-657.

Vessey, M.P. (1977) Personal communication.

Discussion 5B

Mitchell (Nottingham) You were able to exclude Type 2 hyperlipidaemia by blood tests. This is not necessarily practicable when first prescribing. We need to answer Dr. Slack's question as to how one can screen for hyperlipidaemia without taking a blood sample.

Mann   There are two issues here. One is the issue of people with familial hypercholesterolaemia who undoubtedly have a risk factor for coronary heart disease and the pill, by giving them a further risk factor, increases their overall risk. I think these may be different from the group of women who get metabolic abnormalities as a result of the oral contraceptive. These abnormalities are not identical with familial Type 2 hypercholesterolaemia. There may be two different situations.

Mitchell (Nottingham) If you have histories available, as well as blood samples, could you have 'screened' as effectively by selected questions as by blood samples?

Mann   In our data we obviously asked about the family history and a family history of vascular disease was not predictive. Admittedly the question was not carefully phrased, and we did not ask 'At what age did this occur?' We are at the moment constructing a study where we are looking at just how predictive the family history is for cholesterol levels.

Slack (London) It would not be strongly predictive but undoubtedly by taking the family history and taking early coronary deaths, you will focus on a high risk group.

Mann   Will this pick up all those people who have familial hypercholesterol-aemia?

Slack (London) It should pick up half of them, because half of the affected parents will be fathers and they would have a high risk of having died early.

Mitchell (Nottingham) In medical student training, a family history is often given that 'parent died of heart disease'. Half of everybody's parents die of heart disease at some age, and so the discriminatory value presumably comes in with age of death.

Oliver (Edinburgh) In a series I reported some time ago, we tried to score family history, not only on the age of death but also on the age on onset of symptoms — not necessarily the same thing. The age at which a patient has a myocardial infarct is more relevant than the age of death. We found that lipid abnormalities were of more importance in those patients having a myocardial infarction at an early age.

Hazzard (Seattle) I think it is reasonable to point out that Type II hyperlipo-proteinaemia as used by Dr. Mann and familial hypercholesterolaemia as used by Dr. Slack are far from synonymous. Of those with Type II hyperlipoproteinaemia, only one in 25 will turn out to have familial hypercholesterolaemia.

Mann I confused the situation by starting the discussion by talking about familial hypercholesterolaemia. Of those in the series with Type II hyperlipoprotein-aemia, there were few with familial hypercholesterolaemia, as one might have expected.

Beaumont (Paris) I understand that you cannot give any figures to evaluate the risks of the 30 microgram pill, but are you aware of any cardiovascular events seen with this pill?

Mann I know of two cases of women who have been on the 30 microgram pill who have had a coronary. One might expect the 30 microgram pill to have a much lower risk, but as yet we have no reliable data.

Beaumont (Paris) We have also seen 2 cases with the 30 microgram pill.

Julian (Newcastle) Why do some women take the pill rather than use other forms of contraception? Presumably there are important psychological factors, and for example, type A and B personalities may be relevant.

Mann We have not been able to include that sort of data in our study, and I personally would view it in small print.

Julian (Newcastle) Women who take the pill may well be different from those who do not take it?

Mann (Oxford) We know that.

Venning (High Wycombe) Professor Rose pointed out that the apparent risk factor of smoking for subsequent coronary mortality was explainable entirely by social class differences. Did you look at this aspect in your study? Another question I want to ask is that you said very firmly that you had absolutely no information on the risk with the 30 microgram pill, but Prof. Vessey said it was improper for people not to use them. Are these two statements compatible?

Rose (London) In our Civil Servant study the excess coronary mortality risk in men who said they inhaled their cigarette smoke was largely accounted for by the concentration of those inhaling in the lower social classes. There are social class related factors that have a major bearing on coronary risk which we cannot yet measure, and it is quite possible that the excess coronary risk associated with pill takers might be a coincidental association and not a causal one.

Mann   We did get information on social class from the husband's occupation. This is the only sort of classification that we have. There was no association at all in our data between social class and myocardial infarction which is surprising. Admittedly social class is difficult to classify in this sort of study, but for what it is worth, using the Registrar General's grading in our data, social class did not appear to be a factor. To answer Dr. Venning's point, if one has an overall risk estimate for cigarette smoking as compared to not smoking, the relative risk in our data, for what it is worth, was five. That risk estimate is not appreciably altered by other risk factors though, of course, it is slightly increased, as one might expect, by oral contraceptives.

Wald (Oxford)   On the data available from the Tobacco Research Council, the social class differences in cigarette consumption are proportionate with the numbers of smokers in the different social classes.

Hazzard (Seattle)   Do you have any information on blood pressure in your data?

Mann (Oxford)   Our study was a classical case-control type study, data being collected after they had a coronary. The only objective measurement that we had was lipid concentrations. These were analysed at least 6 months after the acute event. We did not have blood pressure readings. We simply had, in some, a history of having been treated for hypertension. Very few of the pill users were also hypertensive, but of those that were most had been treated.

Chakrabarti (London)   In younger women especially, we have found higher levels of triglycerides, cholesterol and factor VII in those on oral contraceptives, compared with those who are not; fibrinolytic activity is also higher in women on oral contraceptives, and this may be a protective response to changes possibly favouring thrombogenesis, such as the increase in factor VII. However, this rise in fibrinolytic activity is largely offset by smoking.

21. Cardiovascular disease and non-contraceptive oestrogen therapy

BRIAN MacMAHON

This paper deals with the risk of cardiovascular disease among women taking oestrogens for other than contraceptive purposes. Usually, these drugs are being taken for replacement or supplementation of natural sources in the peri- or post-menopausal years. The literature on this subject is far scantier than that on the oral contraceptives. It seems, in addition, more difficult to interpret – for reasons which will be outlined.

Hoover and Gray (1977) have extended the follow-up of a cohort of 1891 oestrogen users, originally assembled for the evaluation of cancer risk (Hoover *et al*, 1976), to include mortality from all causes. They have kindly permitted me to use some of the preliminary data from the extended follow-up for this presentation. I must, however, stress the preliminary nature of the findings – observed and expected values may change slightly as the follow-up is completed.

Methodologic problems

Evaluation of the health effects of non-contraceptive oestrogen therapy is about as difficult an epidemiologic task as one could devise. There is bias in the selection of women who receive the therapy, severe confounding by factors of relevance to many parameters of health and bias in the observation of outcome in exposed and non-exposed women. The direction and magnitude of all these sources of bias must be estimated to interpret the meaning of any empirically observed association.

Bias in selection seems to be of particular importance in the context of possible effects on the cardiovascular system. Among its most obvious sources is the fact that oestrogens are frequently used as replacement therapy following surgical removal of the ovaries. In such instances the odds are high that the patient was initially a good surgical risk – a judgement in which her cardiovascular state would play a major part. Even without surgery – when oestrogens are being used for supplementation rather than replacement – some physicians would tend not to prescribe these drugs for patients with cardiovascular disease, particularly hypertension

Somewhat arbitrarily, I distinguish confounding from selection bias in referring to confounding as the situation in which differences between exposed and non-exposed groups are introduced indirectly and not by direct selection in terms of the outcomes to be evaluated. In the present context, oestrogen users differ from non-users in respect to such characteristics as age and socioeconomic status (which can usually be accommodated in the analysis), and access to and perceptions of the utility of medical care (which usually cannot be accommodated in the analysis). These characteristics are important determinants of the frequency of cardiovascular disease and/or its diagnosis. Furthermore, the very diseases for which oestrogen is prescribed may influence the health outcomes to be assessed. This is certainly true, for example, for diseases treated by hysterectomy and oophorectomy if the outcome of interest is cancer and it may well be true that such procedures also influence the subsequent occurrence of cardiovascular disease (Oliver and Boyd, 1959; Higano, Robinson and Cohen, 1963).

The data of Hoover and Gray (1977) illustrate what are probably to a considerable extent the results of selection bias and confounding. Total deaths from all causes in the cohort, followed for an average of 12 years, were only 40 percent of the number expected on the basis of age-specific rates in the general population. This ratio increased from 20 percent in the first five years after initiation of therapy to 70 percent after fifteen or more years of follow-up. The increase from 20 to 70 percent probably reflects selection bias, since such bias is strongest in the years after initiation of therapy and decreases with the passage of time; any true protective effect of the oestrogen therapy would be expected to produce a trend in the opposite direction. The fact that 15 years and more after initiation of therapy the observed deaths are still significantly below expectation, may reflect persistence of the selection bias, confounding by factors associated with low mortality, observation bias (see below) or all three. As expected, the deficit of deaths is larger among patients having surgery prior to initiation of therapy but it exists also among those who did not — the ratio of observed to expected is 0.4 in the first 15 years of follow-up and 0.8 thereafter among the non-surgical patients. A similar overall deficiency of total deaths (observed/expected = 0.4) is reported by Burch, Byrd and Vaughn (1975) in a study of 735 oestrogen users followed over an average of 15 years. The data of Burch *et al.* are not given by duration of follow-up and do not permit comparison of surgical and non-surgical cases since all patients were hysterectomized.

Observation bias has several forms. There is, to begin with, our old friend 'loss to follow-up'. This may be particularly troublesome in studies of oestrogen users in that many of them are in age groups when mortality rates are high. Thus, the follow-up rate in the study of Hoover and Gray was over 90 percent, but there were still 186 patients (of 1891) whose status was unknown. If most of these were dead — in Florida, Arizona or other salubrious places — the difference between observed and expected deaths, particularly in the long duration of follow-up categories, might be eliminated. Burch *et al.* report a 100 percent follow-up, but this figure is difficult to interpret, since to become eligible for inclusion in the series a woman had to *either* develop a 'complication of any kind' after three or more months of oestrogen therapy *or* have 5 years of oestrogen use. This is clearly a group of patients in which the criteria of long-term use and the occurrence of complications introduce additional selective factors.

Another form of observation bias stems from the fact that oestrogen users are more likely to be under medical supervision than are non-users. This problem has been stressed particularly in interpreting the association of endometrial cancer with oestrogen use, but we cannot exclude the possibility that it might have some application to the observation and diagnosis of the various forms of cardiovascular disease.

The above difficulties have been described as they are seen in cohort studies — that is, studies in which exposed individuals are followed, either retrospectively or prospectively, and their experience compared with that of an unexposed cohort or with the general population. However, with the exception of the problem of loss to follow-up, the same difficulties, in somewhat different format, affect the interpretation of case-control studies. Case-control studies have two additional problems — uncertainty as to the reliability of histories of exposure obtained from affected and unaffected women and low sensitivity if the cases in which the exposure forms part of the etiologic complex comprise only a small proportion of all cases of the disease under study.

This formidable list of sources of bias and error is not intended to discourage the assembly and presentation of epidemiologic data on oestrogen users. It is intended only to stress the care with which we must move from observed association to causal inference in this context.

Arteriosclerotic heart disease (ASHD)

In both of the cohort studies referred to earlier, a marked deficit of deaths from arteriosclerotic heart disease was observed. In the data of Burch *et al.* the relative risk of death from 'heart disease' (presumably mostly arteriosclerotic) was 0.4 and in those of Hoover and Gray the relative risk of arteriosclerotic heart disease was 0.3. In discussing this observation, Burch (1974, 1975) makes it clear that he considers a protective effect of oestrogen a likely explanation. However, in the data of Hoover and Gray there is a strong trend with duration of follow-up, there being no deaths (14.8 expected) in the first five years and the relative risk 15 or more years after initiation of therapy being 0.8 — not significantly different from unity. Furthermore, a consistent dose-response relationship is not evident. These features suggest that the association results from selection bias rather than from a protective effect of the oestrogens.

This suggestion is strengthened by a case-control study of Rosenberg, Armstrong and Jick (1975) of cases and comparison patients from two multipurpose surveys of hospitalized patients. The cases were post-menopausal women, aged 40 to 75 years of age, with non-fatal, acute myocardial infarction. Although the crude relative risk associated with oestrogen use was 0.47, this increased to 0.97 (confidence limits 0.48 to 1.95) after adjustment according to a multivariate risk score based on age, past history of myocardial infarction, angina, diabetes, hypertension and other risk factors.

As already noted, case-control studies will be insensitive if the proportion of all cases in which the exposure of interest is implicated is small. The proportion of oestrogen users in the study of Rosenberg *et al*, (5 percent among the comparison patients) is sufficiently small and the frequency of myocardial infarction sufficiently high that lack of sufficient sensitivity to detect a real effect must certainly be considered. Nevertheless, the results are consistent with the suggestion that the low rate of ASHD deaths in the two reported cohort studies results from selection and/or confounding, rather than from a protective effect of oestrogens.

Stroke

The two major cohort studies are again consistent in reporting a substantially higher risk of death from stroke than from ASHD. In both, the relative risk for death from stroke is 0.8. Furthermore, in the data of Hoover and Gray the relative risk after 15 years of follow-up is 1.7, although numbers are small and the excess not statistically significant. The highest risk is among women taking the larger doses of oestrogen, but numbers are small for this analysis and too small to examine the effects of dose level and duration of follow-up simultaneously.

In a case-control study of 210 stroke patients, whose mean age was 75 years, there was no overall association between oestrogen use and stroke (relative risk 1.12), but in the age group in which the largest numbers occurred (ages 70-79) there was a significantly increased risk for users (relative risk among non-diabetics 1.74, confidence limits 1.09 - 2.75) (Pfeffer and Van Den Noort, 1976). Most of the excess risk appeared to operate through an association between oestrogen use and hypertension. There was no association between oestrogen use and stroke in normotensive women. More than half of the oestrogen prescriptions filled by women in this study were for doses of 0.625 or 1.25 mgm.

Hypertension

The most convincing evidence for a relationship between oestrogen use and hypertension comes from the case-control study just quoted, although the cases were selected in terms of having had a stroke (Pfeffer and Van Den Noort, 1976). In that group, the relative risk of hypertension (including borderline hypertension) for oestrogen users was 2.4. In a random sample of women, 35 to 59 years of age, in three Northern California communities, blood pressures were higher for oestrogen users than for non-users, but not so high for users of medications containing oestrogen alone as for users of oestrogen-progestogen (contraceptive) compounds (Stern et al, 1976). Spellacy and Birk (1972) made serial blood pressure measurements on 415 volunteers and noted that oestrogens tended to elevate while progestogens lowered blood pressure.

Pulmonary embolism

The most striking known adverse effect of oral contraceptives is pulmonary embolism. The fact that risk of this complication increases with increase in oestrogen content of the medication (Inman et al, 1970) suggests rather strongly that unopposed oestrogen should also be associated with increased risk of pulmonary embolism. There are, however, few data bearing on this question directly. The Boston Collaborative Drug Surveillance Program (1974) reported a statistically non-significant increase of post-menopausal oestrogen users among cases of idiopathic venous thromboembolism relative to other patients (14 percent compared to 8 percent) but the study included only 18 cases of idiopathic embolism. In the cohort of Hoover and Gray only two deaths from pulmonary embolus, one of them post-operative, were recorded. None are reported by Burch et al (1975).

Man and other species

In this paper I have concentrated on epidemiologic data and not broached the considerable literature on the effects of oestrogens on the health of men and even lower species. Since men may be closer to women than are members of some other species, I should at least make reference to the observations linking large oestrogen doses to a variety of cardiovascular disorders in that animal.

I have tried to discern a pattern of cardiovascular disorders among men taking large doses of oestrogen, but without success. Myocardial infarction appears to have been the primary reason for termination of the high (5 mgm/day) oestrogen group in the Coronary Drug Project, although pulmonary embolism was relatively even more frequent in this than in the placebo group (Coronary Drug Project Research Group, 1970). In the low oestrogen dose group (2.5 mgm/day), the excess of thrombophlebitis and pulmonary embolism predominated, with no indication of excess rates of myocardial infarction or other cardiovascular problem (Coronary Drug Project Research Group, 1973). In men treated with oestrogens for cancer of the prostate at doses of 5 mgm/day, both 'heart disease' and cerebrovascular accidents have occurred excessively, with the latter predominating (Veterans Administration Cooperative Urological Research Group, 1967). In patients with cerebrovascular disease, persons treated with 1.25 mgm Premarin per day had a considerable excess of both stroke and myocardial infarction relative to controls, but no excess of pulmonary embolism (McDowell, Louis and McDevitt, 1967). On the other hand, no excess of either 'cardiovascular' death (type unspecified) or of total deaths has occurred among men with prostate cancer treated with 0.2 or 1.0 mgm of diethylstilboestrol per day (Byar, 1973).

While these observations strengthen the inference that oestrogens have adverse effects on the cardiovascular system, they do not seem to clarify the mechanisms or the nature of the disorders produced.

Conclusions

Review of the epidemiologic evidence to date leads me to believe that:
1. Use of oestrogens in replacement or supplementation therapy is associated with increased risk of hypertension and, probably thereby, of cerebrovascular accident.
2. Doses of the order used in such therapy probably do not increase the prevalence of atherosclerotic heart disease or the incidence of myocardial infarction. However, the deficit of deaths from these causes among cohorts of treated women should not be interpreted as suggesting that oestrogens protect against these disorders.
3. Existing data are inadequate to evaluate the risk of pulmonary embolism associated with use of unopposed oestrogens in the doses commonly employed in supplementation or replacement therapy.

References

Boston Collaborative Drug Surveillance Program (1974) Surgically confirmed gallbladder disease, venous thromboembolism, and breast tumors in relation to postmenopausal estrogen therapy. *New England Journal of Medicine,* **290,** 15-19.

Burch, J.D. (1974) Discussion of The effects of long-term estrogen on hysterecto-mized women. *American Journal of Obstetrics and Gynecology,* **118**, 782.

Burch, J.D. (1975) Discussion of Burch *et al.* (1975) In *Estrogens in the Post-Menopause.* Basel: Karger.

Burch, J.D., Byrd, B.F. & Vaughn, W.K. (1975) The effects of long-term estrogen administration to women following hysterectomy. In *Estrogens in the Post-Menopause.* Basel: Karger.

Byar, D.P. (1973) The Veterans Administration Cooperative Urological Research Group's studies of cancer of the prostate. *Cancer,* **32**, 1126-1130.

Coronary Drug Project Research Group (1970) The coronary drug project: initial findings leading to modifications of its research protocol. *Journal of the American Medical Association,* **214**, 1303-1313.

Coronary Drug Project Research Group (1973) The coronary drug project: findings leading to discontinuation of the 2.5 mg/day estrogen group. *Journal of the American Medical Association,* **226**, 652-657.

Higano, N., Robinson, R.W. & Cohen, W.D. (1963) Increased incidence of cardio-vascular disease in castrated women: two-year follow-up study. *New England Journal of Medicine,* **268**, 1123-1125.

Hoover, R. & Gray, L.A. Sr. (1977) Personal communication.

Hoover, R., Gray, L.A. Sr., Cole, P. *et al.* (1976) Menopausal estrogens and breast cancer. *New England Journal of Medicine,* **295**, 401-405.

Inman, W.H.W., Vessey, M.P., Westerholm, B. *et al.* (1970) Thromboembolic disease and the steroidal content of oral contraceptives: a report to the Committee on Safety of Drugs. *British Medical Journal,* **2**, 203-209.

McDowell, F., Louis, S. & McDevitt, E. (1967) A clinical trial of premarin in cere-brovascular disease. *Journal of Chronic Diseases,* **20**, 679-684.

Oliver, M.F. & Boyd, G.S. (1959) Effect of bilateral ovariectomy on coronary artery disease and serum lipid levels. *Lancet,* **2**, 690.

Pfeffer, R.I. & Van Den Noort, S. (1976) Estrogen use and stroke risk in post-menopausal women. *American Journal of Epidemiology,* **103**, 445-456.

Rosenberg, L., Armstrong, B. & Jick, H. (1976) Myocardial infarction and estrogen therapy in post-menopausal women. *New England Journal of Medicine,* **294**, 1256-1259.

Spellacy, W.N. & Birk, S.A. (1972) The effect of intrauterine devices, oral contra-ceptives, estrogens, and progestrogens on blood pressure. *Gynecology,* **112**, 912-919.

Stern, M.P., Brown, B.W., Jr., Haskell, W.L. *et al.* (1976) Cardiovascular risk and use of estrogens or estrogen-progestogen combinations. Stanford three-community study. *Journal of the American Medical Association,* **235**, 811-815.

Veterans Administration Cooperative Urological Research Group (1967) Treatment and survival of patients with cancer of the prostate. *Surgery, Gynecology and Obstetrics,* **124**, 1011-1017.

Discussion 5C

Nordin (Leeds) An alternative explanation for this rise in the relative risk from 0.2 to 0.7 could relate to the follow-up period. If you follow up this series long enough, there will eventually be 100 percent mortality. I would have expected that the longer you go on with hormonal therapy, the less difference there will ultimately be in mortality between the treated and untreated groups.

MacMahon Theoretically you may be right but not in practice. The cohort will all eventually have to die. I cannot believe however that this will produce over a 15 year period, a difference between 0.2 and 0.7. If we had followed this cohort till they were 90, or some such age, your argument may apply.

Nordin (Leeds) A 15 year follow up takes many of these people into the 65/70/75 year age group, when deaths from all causes are rising very steeply.

MacMahon It is true the mortality is rising steeply, but at the age of 70 the median age of death for American women is still not reached.

Nordin (Leeds) No, you may not have reached the value of unity, but it is 0.7.

MacMahon I accept that ultimately your mechanism will come into play.

Gordon (Bethesda) You have told us about observed and expected mortality rates. How did you calculate the expected mortality rates?

MacMahon These are based on 5 year, age specific, total United States rates for whites. They were changed when we used rates for Kentucky which were slightly different.

Gordon (Bethesda) Why would that be the expected death rate for this particular group? They may be far healthier than the general population.

MacMahon This is a technical use of the word 'expected'. It is the application of the general population rates to this cohort. Frankly, I do not expect them to die at the same rate as the general population.

Gordon (Bethesda) What you are saying is that you are dealing with a selected group and a reference set of mortality figures inappropriate to the particular population.

MacMahon The expected value is simply saying 'How many deaths would this cohort have experienced if they had the same death rate as the general population?' The fact that they do not have the same death rate may be due to something causally related to their exposure to oestrogen. This is a highly selected group in terms of both medical and demographic characteristics.

Baird (Edinburgh) I think you should preface your remarks by saying that these were the results of a single practitioner's practice. By definition, this must be a selected group.

Doll (Oxford) I have had experience of following up records from an individual clinic or from an individual clinician and much the more likely explanation, to my mind, would be that the records of the patients who died have become differentially lost in the records of the clinic. I would make the prediction that in the follow up of this cohort from 1969/1977 their observed mortality rate will be just about the same as the expected rate, and that this an artefact due to the differential loss of women who died in the early years and whose records have been omitted.

MacMahon What is your evidence that, in the situation that you describe, it would be differential loss rather than selection that led to that observation?

Doll (Oxford) The evidence is that having obtained records, no matter how long they had been under observation in the past, their subsequent mortality immediately becomes equal to the expected mortality.

Wynn (London) The problem of what happens to women who are given medication from a single practitioner applies not only to this type of study, but as far as I know, it applies to a great many studies and Professor Doll has outlined some of the problems. When you have an enthusiastic prescriber, his results are usually better no matter which disease he is treating. It would be interesting to know the medico-legal implications for that particular prescriber if the results showed a high excess mortality amongst his patients.

MacMahon This cohort was assembled for a study of breast cancer and, indeed, there is a significant excess of breast cancer among those women followed up for 15 years or more. To return to Professor Doll's point, if there had been any differential loss of information it would have been on those who developed breast cancer.

Vessey (Oxford) The breast cancer risk may be even greater since it is against such a low background of mortality.

Lewis (London) What dosage of oestrogen was used?

MacMahon In about half of the patients it was replacement therapy. The modal dose of Premarin was 0.625 mg, some lower, a few higher.

Hazzard (Seattle) The gynaecologists in our institution say that the equivalent dose of 50 micrograms of ethinyl oestradiol was 0.5 mg. Premarin using the endometrium or the vaginal epithelium as end organs. Is this valid? If it is valid, is one of the reasons why there is a contrast between oral contraceptives and post-menopausal oestrogen replacement therapy one of dose?

Nordin (Leeds)   We have done a comparison of vaginal smears using various oestrogens of different doses. Premarin 0.625 mg is indistinguishable in its effect on the vaginal smear from 25 µg oestradiol.

Wynn (London)   It is the coronary artery that is subject to lipid changes. The vagina is quite irrelevant. Oestrogens are capable of inducing enzyme changes in a whole variety of tissues. Oestrogen receptors in the vagina are not the same as oestrogen receptors in the liver and pancreas.

Horton (Edinburgh)   This is a fundamental problem. We are talking about different substances and different tissues and trying to equate them. This is something you cannot do in many cases because the quality is often different and there is usually a quantitative difference on the particular test organ. At least the vagina is a recognised test for oestrogenic activity, but it may not be this activity in which we are interested.

Baird (Edinburgh)   It is extremely important that one has some kind of estimate of potency of compounds being compared. For example, the effects on carbohydrate metabolism of one oestrogenic preparation versus another.

Nordin (Leeds)   Professor Rose yesterday made the fundamental point that individual studies on smoking can be criticised in various ways but when you take the overall picture it all points on a common sense basis towards a positive relationship between smoking and cardiovascular disease. I think as yet we have insufficient studies on oestrogen replacement therapy, but I think one cannot ignore the fact that there appears to be an increased risk of breast cancer in this group. There would also appear to be a reduction of deaths from all causes, except breast cancer. While more studies are needed these two studies show extraordinary similarities and they really cannot be ignored.

General discussion

Doll (Oxford)   I would like to obtain some kind of estimate as to what the actual risks are for women taking the oral contraceptive in terms of rates per 100,000 women at risk in the different age groups. Also, by what factor are we increasing that risk by prescribing a 50 microgram pill?

Mann (Oxford)   I think the most reliable estimates we can make is from overall mortality in users and non-users of the oral contraceptives. The 'risk' is fairly low until the 40-45 age group.

Baird (Edinburgh)   We appear to have a dilemma. Older women on the oral contraceptive have an increased risk of cardiovascular disease. But Professor MacMahon quotes a series using compounds which are not identical, but have the same biological effect, and, if anything, the risk appears to be reduced. What is the explanation for this?

Mann (Oxford) We are dealing with two different situations. In the pre-menopausal woman, who is given the pill, some of her own ovarian activity is suppressed. In the post-menopausal woman, who has little ovarian activity, an entirely different preparation is given. Are the situations comparable?

Baird (Edinburgh) I would have thought that the bulk of the circulating oestrogens in either case would be comparable.

Beaumont (Paris) One must consider whether the compounds are immunologically different. This may be very important.

Baird (Edinburgh) Are we quite clear that ethinyl oestradiol increases the risk factor and Premarin decreases it?

Nordin (Leeds) Not only are the compounds different, but so are the doses. 0.625 mg Premarin is equivalent to 25 mg of ethinyl oestradiol, and in the study quoted 50 mg of ethinyl oestradiol was used. Perhaps the simplest explanation of the dilemma is the difference in dose.

Wynn (London) There is no such preparation as a 50 microgram oestrogen pill. It does not exist. We forget progestogen. The interaction between progestogen and oestrogen may be the vital factor.

Jarrett (London) I believe that Professor MacMahon's results cannot be interpreted. It is a nonsense to use indices of mortality from a totally different population, particularly as one population is highly selected and the other population is totally unselected. Another possible explanation is that the effect of oestrogens may well be different with age. We have had some evidence for this from the studies of Dr. Chakrabarti.

Lewis (London) I would define oestrogens as substances which stimulate development of secondary sex characteristics in women. However, we must remember that we are talking about the effect of oestrogen on platelets, vascular endothelium, on hepatic mechanisms synthesising lipoproteins to name just a few. With this in mind it is hardly surprising to find apparent differences between pre- and post-menopausal women taking oestrogen.

Venning (High Wycombe) I would like to give some information about the relative doses of these compounds. One can say with a good deal of confidence that if similar doses of oestrone sulphate were used in oral contraceptives as found, for example, in Premarin there would be a large number of pregnancies! The equivalent dose of ethinyl oestradiol in relation to replacement therapy for the treatment of menopausal symptoms would probably be between 1 and 10 micrograms, rather than 25 or 50.

Nordin (Leeds) I disagree. Using the vaginal smear, 0.625 mg of Premarin is equivalent to 25 micrograms of ethinyl oestradiol. They give an equivalent maturation value on vaginal smear.

Baird (Edinburgh) I agree with Dr. Venning. There are many post-menopausal women who will have satisfactory control of oestrogen deficient symptoms, that is flushing and vaginal atrophy, on doses of ethinyl oestradiol which are much lower than 25 micrograms per day.

Nordin (Leeds) And also on less than 0.625 mg of Premarin. When you define equivalents, you have to define them in terms of one particular test. That is what I have done.

Bonnar (Dublin) We do not yet have a system for assaying potency of oestrogens. In fact, the immature mouse uterus is what has been accepted as the biological test. I do not accept Professor Nordin's statement that the vagina of post-menopausal women is the best biological assay. Has he done tests on the effects of 10 micrograms of ethinyl oestradiol?

Nordin (Leeds) Yes, I have. The vagina may not be the best biological assay, but the one that I have used for my data.

Baird (Edinburgh) We ought to bear in mind that Premarin is not a uniform compound. It is a mixture of at least two, probably more, oestrogens. The manufacturers provide no evidence to show that the ratio of the various oestrogens within Premarin is constant from batch to batch and I think this is another major complication in interpreting any results involving the use of this drug.

SESSION 6 Coronary heart disease

Chairman: M.P. Vessey

H•

22. Coronary heart disease in young women

D. MORRIS, J. WILLIS HURST AND SPENCER B. KING

Any review of coronary heart disease in young women should acknowledge that the disease is relatively uncommon in this particular population. The Vital Statistics of the United States for 1973 reveal that only 1,102 women between 20 and 39 years of age died of coronary heart disease. On the other hand, coronary heart disease is now third among the natural causes of death in this population and has steadily climbed from a position of thirteen among natural causes of death for the same group in 1940. This increase in the significance of coronary heart disease as a cause of death in young women reflects both an increase in the actual number of deaths from this cause and a reduction of deaths from such causes as tuberculosis, pneumonia, kidney disease, and the complications of pregnancy.

Methods

At Emory University Hospitals, Atlanta, Georgia, we have attempted to look at coronary heart disease in young women through two different approaches. As previously reported (Morris, Hurst, Logue, 1976), we initially reviewed all the cases of myocardial infarction in women under 40 years of age admitted to Emory University Hospitals between January, 1968, and January, 1975. To the initial 24 patients, four additional patients have been added by continuing our review until May, 1977. Our methods for establishing the presence of both the myocardial infarction and risk factors (hyperlipidemia, hypertension, smoking, family history of coronary heart disease, diabetes, and oral contraceptives) were outlined in our previous report. Since this initial publication each of the patients has been followed up by personal contact or, in the deceased, by a review of their final hospitalisation. Secondly, we have maintained an ongoing prospective analysis of all women less than 45 years of age undergoing coronary angiography at Emory University Hospitals. The presence or absence of hypertension (diastolic >100 mmHg by history or examination), diabetes (persistently abnormal blood glucose requiring dietary or insulin therapy), smoking (greater than 5-year history of smoking one pack of cigarettes daily), hypercholesterolemia (cholesterol greater than 7.3 mmol/l), and family history (parent or sibling experiencing myocardial infarction before age 55 years) was established prior to angiography. Significant coronary atherosclerosis is then interpreted as 75 percent or greater angiographic obstruction in any one of the three major coronary arteries.

Etiology

Atherosclerotic coronary occlusion

In our retrospective analysis of young women with myocardial infarction, fourteen were documented by either post mortem examination or coronary angiography to have atherosclerotic coronary occlusion. Another nine patients were assumed to have atherosclerosis on the basis of a compatible history and lack of evidence suggesting another etiology. Myocardial infarction was thus concluded to be secondary to atherosclerosis in 82 percent of this portion of our population. (Fig. 22.1)

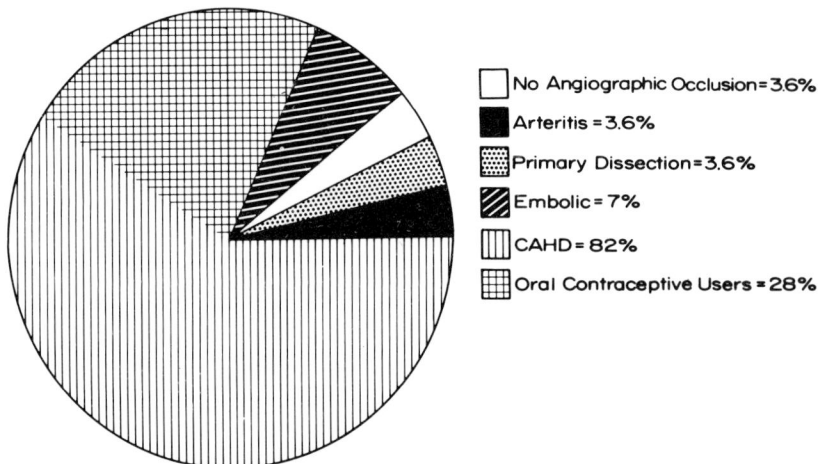

OCCLUSIVE PROCESS IN CORONARY ARTERIES OF YOUNG WOMEN WITH MYOCARDIAL INFARCTION

No Angiographic Occlusion = 3.6%
Arteritis = 3.6%
Primary Dissection = 3.6%
Embolic = 7%
CAHD = 82%
Oral Contraceptive Users = 28%

Fig. 22.1

Nonatherosclerotic coronary occlusion

The nonatherosclerotic occlusive process in the remaining 18 percent was embolic in two instances, arteritis in another, and a single example of primary dissection of a coronary artery. (Fig. 22.1)

Associated conditions While in each of these four cases the exact nature of the coronary occlusion was established at post mortem examination; in retrospect, certain features of the clinical presentation had suggested a nonatherosclerotic etiology. None of these patients exhibited any risk factors for coronary atherosclerosis and, in each instance, there was no history of pre-infarction angina so typical of atherosclerotic occlusion. Moreover, each patient manifest a pre-existing condition which suggested another likely etiology for the coronary occlusion. In the two patients with embolic occlusion, rheumatic valvulitis existed in one and marantic endocarditis in the other. While the marantic endocarditis had not been diagnosed pre-mortem; the predisposing condition, adenocarcinoma of the pancreas, was recognised. Previous reviews of coronary embolism (Wenger and Bauer, 1958;

Shrader, Bawell, and Moragues, 1956) have established bacterial endocarditis as the condition most often associated with this event. Since the publication of these reviews, prosthetic valves have arisen as another commonly associated condition.

Coronary vasculitis, as in our patient with systemic lupus erythematosus, is usually associated with a collagen vascular disease. The particular disease most commonly involved is polyarteritis nodosa, while vasculitis resulting in sufficient myocardial necrosis to be of clinical importance is quite unusual in systemic lupus. A previous post-mortem study examining the cardiac changes accompanying systemic lupus erythematosus (Brigden, Bywater, Lessof, and Ross, 1960) found only two hearts among the group of 27 with extensive myocardial damage due to widespread arterial occlusion.

Dissecting aneurysm of the coronary artery is a cause of myocardial infarction occurring predominantly in young women. The dissecting aneurysm is characterised by the presence of a hematoma within, and limited to, the media of the coronary artery. The hematoma, in turn, produces the luminal narrowing. A review of the 43 previously reported cases (Smith, 1975) noted that 32 of the patients were women, including 19 less than 40 years of age; 12 of these patients were in the peripartal period. Except for the pregnant or postpartum state, no other associated conditions have been identified. Hypertension does not appear to play a role. Although our patient was not peripartal, she had been receiving large doses of oestrogens by pellet implantation. A possible contribution of oestrogen is suggested by an oestrogen induced generalised loosening of the ground substance of connective tissue in guinea pigs, (Perl and Catchpole, 1950).

The most perplexing condition encountered in our retrospective analysis was the enigma of myocardial infarction occurring in a 36 year old woman who subsequently exhibited normal coronary angiograms. The existence of this paradoxic condition is substantiated by three patients encountered during our prospective angiographic study. Each of these patients had documented evolutionary electrocardiographic changes of an anterior myocardial infarction and, on susbequent cardiac catheterisation, demonstrated a segmental contraction abnormality of the anterior left ventricular wall but normal coronary arteriograms. These angiograms were performed two to sixteen weeks following the myocardial infarction. Interestingly, in these patients, as in most of the patients reported in the literature, there was no associated lipid abnormalities or glucose intolerance. The condition appears to occur most commonly in the group in question, young women.

Associated conditions predisposing to premature atherosclerosis

A comparison between the thirty-four women less than 46 years of age with significant coronary obstruction on angiography and the eighty-one subjects with normal coronary arteriograms revealed significant differences ($P < .01$ from Chi-squared test) between the two groups in the incidence of smoking, diabetes, hypercholesterolemia, and a family history of coronary heart disease. (Table 22.1) Furthermore, there was not a single example of significant coronary obstruction in a woman without one of these four pre-existing conditions. The significance of these four conditions as precursors for premature coronary atherosclerosis was substantiated in the study of young women with myocardial infarction. All of these women, with one exception,

H

Table 22.1 Risk factors — women < 45 years of age

	CHD(34)	NCA(81)
Smoking	85%	42%
Diabetes	23.5%	1.2%
Hypertension	20.6%	19%
Lipids	53%	4%
Family history	62.5%	31%

CHD — Greater than 75% angiographic obstruction of at least one coronary artery.

NCA — Normal coronary arteriogram

exhibited one of these four conditions. The single exception was a 38 year old woman with no evidence of hyperlipidemia, diabetes, or a positive family history, but in whom a history with regards to smoking was not obtained.

Another condition often mentioned as a risk factor for coronary atherosclerosis is hypertension. This condition could not be confirmed by either of our studies as a precursor for severe coronary atherosclerosis in young women. Among the women evaluated by coronary angiography, there was essentially no difference in the occurrence of hypertension between the normal subjects (19 percent) and those with significant coronary atherosclerosis (20.6 percent). Since the U.S. National Health Examination Survey reports a 2.3 percent incidence of hypertension in white women and an 8.6 percent incidence in black women between ages 25 and 34, this similarity in the incidence of hypertension for the two groups might reflect an inordinately high incidence for both groups and does not exclude hypertension as a risk factor. The 4 percent incidence (a single patient) in our retrospective analysis of women with myocardial infarction, however, approximates these national averages and does not support the concept of hypertension as a risk factor in young women.

Relationship to extent of disease The significant contribution of 'risk factors' (smoking, hypertension, hypercholesterolemia, diabetes, and family history)to the development of premature atherosclerosis is also suggested by the finding of an inverse relationship between the number of coronary arteries demonstrating significant angiographic obstruction and the percentage of women in each group (single, double, or triple vessel disease) exhibiting only one risk factor. Forty-five percent (5/11) of those patients with isolated coronary disease (significant obstruction in one vessel without any other disease in the coronary system) had a single risk factor, while 29 percent of all patients with single vessel disease (significant obstruction in one vessel may or may not have another insignificant obstruction) had only one risk factor. Eighteen percent and 0 percent of double and triple vessel disease respectively had a single risk factor. (Fig. 22.2) Excluding hypertension did not change these percentages, while the exclusion of any of the other four conditions did make a difference. Two other interesting observations are that all patients with multiple vessel disease smoked, and the three women with juvenile onset diabetes had involvement of more than one vessel. These patients had each developed their diabetes relatively early in life, in their preteen years, and two had retinopathy.

RISK FACTORS (n)

TOTAL GROUP (34)   **SINGLE VESSEL (17)**

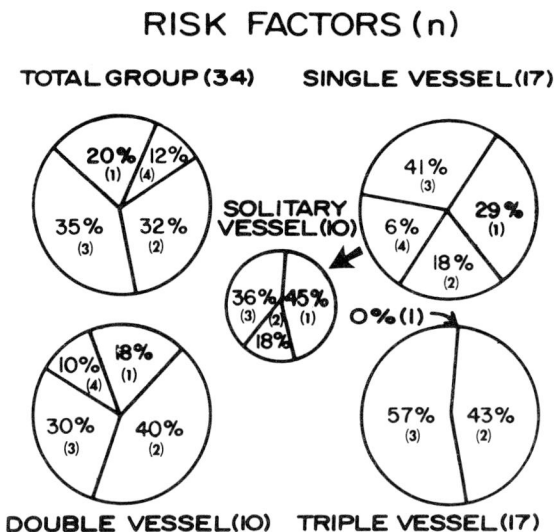

SOLITARY VESSEL (10)

DOUBLE VESSEL (10)   TRIPLE VESSEL (17)

"Vessel" refers to number of coronary arteries with >75% angiographic obstruction.

"Solitary vessel" refers to those patients with single vessel disease who had no other coronary disease (even insignificant) on angiography.

Fig. 22.2

Oral contraceptive agents Eight patients (28 percent) were using oral contraceptives at the time or shortly before their myocardial infarction. Two interesting features of the coronary occlusive disease in these particular women should be noted. First, each of the three women from this group who underwent coronary angiography had segmental obstruction of their proximal left anterior descending artery and minimal or no disease elsewhere. Similarly, eight of the nine patients reported in the literature who experienced a myocardial infarction while on oral contraceptives and subsequently underwent angiogrpahy had an identical finding. (Morris, Hurst, Logue, 1976) Secondly, all of the women in our study who had a myocardial infarction while on oral contraceptives had an additional risk factor for developing premature coronary atherosclerosis. This observation has been emphasised in previous reports on the subject. (Radford and Oliver, 1973; Mann, Vessey, Thorogood, and Doll, 1975) The use of oral contraceptives was not included in our prospective analysis of patients undergoing coronary angiography.

Extent of disease

The percentage of young women with single, double, and triple vessel disease on coronary angiography were compared with our entire population of patients having significant coronary obstruction on coronary angiography performed in the last five years. (1955 patients) The suggestion has previously been made that young women with clinically apparent coronary atherosclerosis have less widespread disease than older or male patients. Fifty percent of the young women had single vessel disease while only 18 percent had triple vessel disease; conversely, 35 percent of the entire population had single vessel disease and 33 percent displayed triple vessel disease. (Fig. 22.3) While the atherosclerotic process does appear to be more diffuse in the entire coronary disease population, the distribution of disease, (the sites most commonly involved) is very similar in the two groups. (Fig. 22.3)

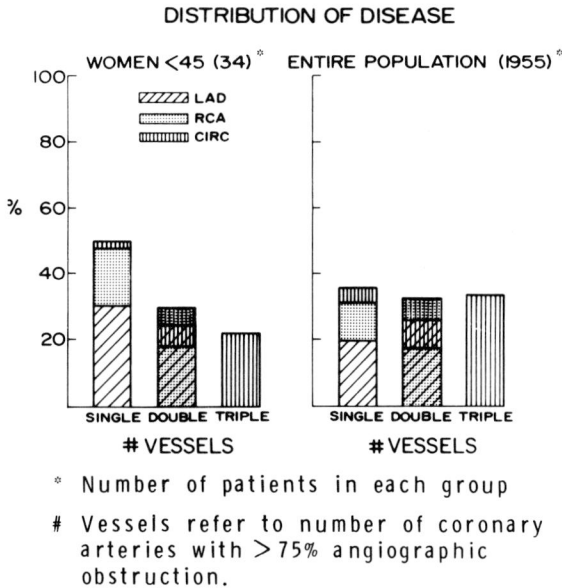

DISTRIBUTION OF DISEASE

* Number of patients in each group

Vessels refer to number of coronary arteries with >75% angiographic obstruction.

Fig. 22.3

Prognosis of coronary heart disease in young women

The 2-9 year follow-up of young women experiencing a myocardial infarction revealed that three of the five patients with an anterior myocardial infarction were dead. (Fig. 22.4) Two died suddenly, and one presented in the emergency room with ventricular tachycardia and could not be resuscitated. Among the patients with an inferior myocardial infarction, there has been only one death. This patient died following triple by-pass surgery. (Fig. 22.4) One patient in each of the two groups is surviving following by-pass surgery and the remainder are living and relatively free of chest pain without medications. Two patients had inferiolateral myocardial infarctions. One of these died suddenly, and the other is loss to follow-up.

We also examined the prognosis of these patients in terms of the number of coronary arteries involved on coronary angiography. All give patients with single vessel disease are alive. Three of these patients including the only one who had

WOMEN < 40 WITH MYOCARDIAL INFARCTION

Followup 2-9 Years

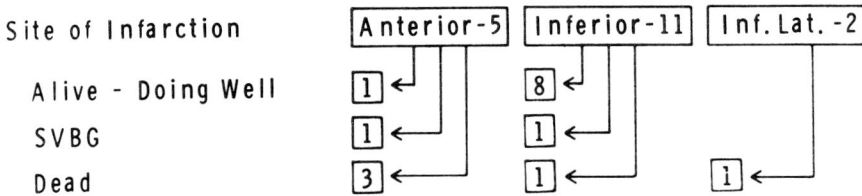

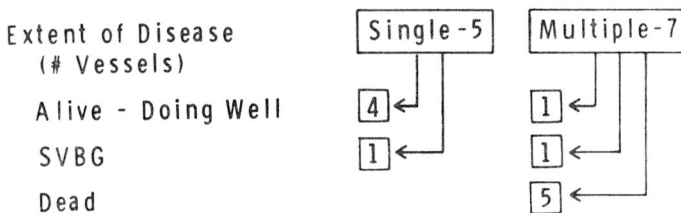

Site of Infarction	Anterior-5	Inferior-11	Inf. Lat. -2
Alive - Doing Well	1	8	
SVBG	1	1	
Dead	3	1	1

SVBG - Patient has received saphenous vein bypass graft to coronary artery

Fig. 22.4

saphenous vein by-pass surgery are completely free of pain and the other two have infrequent chest pain. Five of the seven patients with multiple vessel disease are deceased, one has undergone saphenous vein by-pass surgery, and the final one is alive and has infrequent chest pain. (Fig. 22.5) These data are in substantial agreement with previous information indicating that the prognosis of ischaemic heart disease is closely related to the extent of arterial involvement. (Reeves, Oberman, Jones, and Sheffield, 1974)

WOMEN < 40 WITH MYOCARDIAL INFARCTION

Followup 2-9 Years

Extent of Disease (# Vessels)	Single-5	Multiple-7
Alive - Doing Well	4	1
SVBG	1	1
Dead		5

(#vessels) - Number of coronary arteries with >75% angiographic obstruction.

SVBG - Patient has received saphenous vein bypass graft.

Fig. 22.5

Clinical application of data

Coronary occlusion in young women, as in other segments of the population, is usually secondary to coronary atherosclerosis. In that small percentage of young women with nonatherosclerotic coronary occlusion, the correct etiology is frequently clinically apparent by the development of a catastrophic coronary event without prodroma and by the presence of a condition predisposing to sudden arterial occlusion.

Atherosclerotic coronary occlusion rarely, if ever, occurs in the young woman in the absence of hyperlipidemia, smoking, diabetes, or a family history of coronary heart disease. In fact, these four conditions appear to be the best available predictive indices for the existence of significant coronary atherosclerosis in young women. Chest pain typical of angina pectoris is not very reliable as a predictive index of significant coronary disease. In a prospective analysis of the 641 women with chest pain undergoing coronary angiography in the last 4 years, 59 percent of those with symptoms typical of stable angina pectoris had no significant coronary obstruction, while only 41 percent had significant obstruction. (Douglas, King, Magill, Nathan, and George, 1977) Furthermore, exercise electrocardiography has proven inconsistent in diagnosing women with significant coronary obstruction. (Sketch, Mohiuddin, Lynch, Zencka, Runco, 1975) Recognition that coronary heart disease in young women is unlikely in the absence of a history of one of these four 'risk factors' should significantly improve the reliability of both the clinical history and the graded exercise test.

The medical management of the young woman experiencing a myocardial infarction should also be improved with the recognition of the extremely good prognosis of those with inferior myocardial infarction versus the poor prognosis in those with anterior myocardial infarction and the greater likelihood that those women with multiple risk factors will have multiple vessel disease. The young woman with an inferior myocardial infarction and only one risk factor is likely to have a good prognosis and might be managed without coronary angiography while angiography would seem to be definitely indicated in all other young women experiencing a myocardial infarction. The extremely poor prognosis (71 percent mortality in less than 8 years) in young women with multiple vessel disease indicates a need for a comparative analysis of this group with a similar group undergoing coronary by-pass surgery.

References

Douglas, J.S., King, S.B., Magill, D.H., *et al. Limitations of the history in the diagnosis of obstructive coronary atherosclerotic heart disease in women.* Submitted for publication.

Mann, J.D., Vessey, M.P., Thorogood, M., *et al.* (1975) Myocardial infarction in young women with special reference to oral contraceptive practice. *British Medical Journal, 2,* 241-245.

Morris, D.C., Hurst, J.W. & Logue, R.B. (1976) Myocardial infarction in young women. *American Journal of Cardiography, 38,* 299-304.

Perl, E. & Catchpole, H.R. (1950) Changes induced in the connective tissue of the symphysis pubis of the guinea pig with estrogen and relaxin. *Archives of Pathology,* **50,** 233-239.

Radford, D.J. & Oliver, M.F. (1973) Oral contraceptives and myocardial infarction. *British Medical Journal,* **3,** 428-430.

Reeves, T.J., Oberman, A., Jones, W.B. *et al.* (1974) Natural history of angina pectoris. *American Journal of Cardiology,* **33,** 423-430.

Shrader, E.L., Bawell, M.B., Moragues, V. (1956) Coronary embolism. *Circulation,* **14,** 1159-1163.

Sketch, M.H., Mohiuddin, S.M., Lynch, J.D., *et al.* (1975) Significant sex differences in the correlation of electrocardiographic testing and coronary arteriograms. *American Journal of Cardiology,* **36,** 169-173.

Smith, J.C. (1975) Dissecting aneurysm of coronary arteries. *Archives of Pathology,* **99,** 117-121.

Wenger, N.K. & Bauer, S. (1958) Coronary embolism. Review of literature and presentation of fifteen cases. *American Journal of Medicine,* **25,** 549-557.

Discussion 6A

Vessey (Oxford)   The figures you gave for hypertension are surprising. Another thing is the value that you give in your discriminant analysis for smoking. This raises the question of whether 'pack years' is, in fact an appropriate measurement of smoking.

Morris   Is the number of 'pack years' really reliable? Is it the duration or is it the quantity smoked that is significant? I do not have an answer for that and like you, I am a little surprised.

Lewis (London)   What proportion of risk factors did you find in those with triple vessel disease?

Morris   The question I was really studying was the association of coronary artery disease of those with single versus multiple risk factors. Those patients that had triple vessel disease, *all* had more than one risk factor. There were none that had a single risk factor. The incidence of a single risk factor was 18 percent for those with 2 vessel disease, 29 percent with single vessel disease, and 45 percent for those with 'isolated' solitary lesions. It looks like these are not only predictive indices as to the existence of disease, but they also give us some index of the severity or diffuseness of the disease.

Mitchell (Nottingham)   What is BCP?

Morris   It is the United States version of birth control pill.

Mitchell (Nottingham)   You quote a figure of 78 percent for those with atherosclerotic disease. Did that overlap with those on the birth control pill?

Morris   Yes. 78 percent included 20 percent for those on oral contraceptives. We do not yet know if this is the same disease but there are differences in the groups, in that there is a higher percentage of this 'isolated' disease apparent in the contraceptive group versus the other patients.

Jarrett (London)   Could I ask whether the diagnosis of diabetes in these people was made as a result of glucose tolerance testing after the development of cardiac pain, or was it diagnosed before?

Morris   It was diagnosed before.

23. Clinical characteristics and prognosis of angina and myocardial infarction in young women

M. F. OLIVER

Summary

The basis of this report is 150 women who developed symptoms and signs of coronary heart disease (CHD) under the age of 45. There were 81 who presented with myocardial infarction and 64 with angina; there was a definite nonathero-sclerotic cause for the premature onset of C.H.D. in the remaining 5 patients.

Hypercholesterolaemia, hypertension, or excessive cigarette smoking each occurred in a large minority, and more than one of these major risk factors was present in most patients. Hypercholesterolaemia was the commonest and in those in whom lipoprotein typing was undertaken, the type II pattern was more frequent than type IV. The prevalence of hypercholesterolaemia and hypertension was the same in those with myocardial infarction and in those with angina.

Excessive cigarette smoking was more common in women with myocardial infarction than in those with angina. The latter did not differ in their cigarette smoking habits from the normal population.

A premature menopause had occurred in 20 percent of these women, but there was no relation between the early onset of C.H.D. with age of menarche, parity, or the incidence of abortion.

Oral contraceptives increased the risk of myocardial infarction most when one of the major risk factors was also present.

Altogether 75 percent of patients with angina or myocardial infarction survived 12 years. Coexisting hypertension worsened the prognosis. The prognosis after myocardial infarction was similar in these women to that previously described for men under the age of 40.

Introduction

The clinical survey of coronary heart disease (CHD) in young women which comprises this report represents the experience of one physician over 20 years. While its strengths are the correlation of many cases and the length of follow-up, its weaknesses are its selective nature and that a considerable number of women did not have what would today be regarded as mandatory investigations.

Subjects

The study took place over a period of 18 years (1953-70), and there was a minimum of 2 and maximum of 20 years follow-up. In the 18 years there were 192 women who developed clinical features of C.H.D. under the age of 45 years and were seen by me in the Department of Cardiology in the Royal Infirmary of Edinburgh. There were seven other patients who presented with angina and were found to have valvular heart disease — four had clinical features of aortic stenosis and three had mitral valve disease — who were excluded from this series.

From these 192 women 150 were accepted for this clinical survey which had already been reported in detail (Oliver, 1974). The basis for acceptance was defined electrocardiographic abnormalities. The remaining 42 women had either no electrocardiographic signs to support a clinical diagnosis of myocardial infarction or angina or their features were insufficient to fulfil the defined criteria. The criteria for patients with myocardial infarction were Q wave electrocardiographic features sufficient to warrant classification as 1.1 or 1.2 using the Minnesota code. Patients accepted into the study with a clinical diagnosis of angina had either to have electrocardiographic abnormalities codable as 4.1 (S-T depression >1 mm) or 5.1 (T-inversion >5 mm) at rest or, in the absence of one of these, an abnormal exercise tolerance test result codable as 11.1 or 12.1 (these indicate a change from no codable item at rest to S-T depression >1 mm or T-inversion >5 mm). The criteria of abnormality in the resting electrocardiogram was based on an orthodox 12-lead record. The post-exercise abnormalities were based during the earlier years of this study on the results of a Master 2-step test and during the years 1968-70 on a bicycle ergometry with submaximal testing using W.H.O. standards.

Of the 150 women, 85 satisfied the criteria for myocardial infarction and 65 the criteria for angina (Table 23.1a). Five of the women (four with myocardial infarction

Table 23.1a The Study Group

Diagnosis	Numbers	Mean age (years)
Myocardial infarction*	81	40
Angina with positive ECG at rest or after exercise	64	41
Non-atherosclerotic I.H.D.	5	37
Study group: 2-20 years follow-up	145	40

*Minnesota code = 1:1, 1:2

Table 23.1b

Age	Presentation	Diagnosis	Outcome
26	M.I.	Fulminating acute myocarditis	Died - autopsy
26	Angina	Extreme anaemia	Well 15 years later
34	M.I.	Accidental — I.V. adrenaline	Well 16 years later
38	M.I.	Systemic lupus erythematosis	Died - autopsy
39	M.I.	Syphilis and gross A.I.	Angina — died 8 years later

and one with angina) were considered to have nonatherosclerotic causes for the premature development of C.H.D. These five women had a mean age of 37 years. The remaining 81 patients with myocardial infarction and 64 with angina had mean ages of 40 and 41 respectively. The study group, which was followed up from two to 20 years, comprised these 145 women with a mean age of 40 years. None of the women had had previous myocardial infarction.

The details of the 5 women whose clinical features were thought not to be due to coronary atherosclerosis are shown in Table 23.1b. In the four women, who presented with myocardial infarction there was a definite cause other than athero- sclerosis. In the fifth, angina was associated with haemoglobin levels in the region of 4 g/100 ml, and with correction of the anaemia and angina disappeared and the electrocardiogram returned to normal.

Methods

All patients had a physical, electrocardiographic and radiological examination. Blood pressure was recorded in the semi-recumbent position in the right arm and the lowest reading of three was taken over a period of 10 minutes and was the figure registered for the study. Patients under treatment for hypertension and those with diastolic blood pressure of 100 mm Hg or more when first seen or within one year of myo- cardial infarction were recorded as having hypertension.

Serum cholesterol was initially measured by the method of Jurand and Albert- Recht (1962), a modification of the Kendall-Abel method, and more recently by a Technicon Auto-Analyzer method. Serum triglycerides were initially measured by the glyceride-glycerol method of Carlson (1963) and more recently by a Technicon Auto-Analyzer method. Blood glucose was estimated by a glucose oxidase method. Lipoprotein phenotyping was undertaken on polyacrylamide gel.

Results

Risk factors

Major risk factors were defined as a serum cholesterol level of 270 mg/100 ml or more, diastolic hypertension of 100 mm Hg or more, and a consumption of 20 or more cigarettes daily.

One major risk factor was present in 74 percent of patients (Table 23.2a). Hyper- cholesterolaemia was the most common and was present in 46 percent of the group. Diastolic hypertension occurred in 34 percent. Excessive cigarette smoking was also common but more so in those with myocardial infarction than in those with angina.

A number of minor risk factors were also identified (Table 23.2b). The commonest was a premature menopause. Diabetes was not common in these young women but because it has in the past been thought to be important an oral glucose tolerance test was undertaken in 94 of the 145 women. This comprised an oral load of 75 g glucose with half-hourly blood sampling. Four of the 94 women had abnormal glucose tolerance which had not previously been known and five had flat glucose tolerance curves.

There was no statistically significant difference with regard to any predisposing factor (major and minor) between the myocardial infarction and angina groups,

Table 23.2a Major risk factors

	M.I.	Angina	Total
Numbers	81	64	145
Mean age (yrs)	40	41	40
	%	%	%
Hypercholesterolemia ($\geqslant$270 mg/100 ml)	48	44	46
Diastolic hypertension ($\geqslant$100 mm/Hg)	39	28	34
Cigarettes 20 or more/day	43	19	32
No major risk factor	21	31	26

Table 23.2b Minor risk factors

	M.I.	Angina	Total
Total group	81	64	145
	%	%	%
Premature menopause	22	17	20
Oral contraceptive	14	2	8
Obesity alone >15%	4	6	5
Diabetes mellitus	2	3	3
Abnormal oral G.T.T.	2	2	2*
No evident predisposing factor	14	27	19

*adjusted figures: G.T.T. done in 94 patients

with the exception of cigarette smoking which was more common in women with myocardial infarction. Only 11 percent of the total group did not have some evident associated risk factor.

Hyperlipidaemia

In 56 women, serum triglycerides were measured as well as serum cholesterol. The level above which serum triglycerides were considered to be raised was 200 mg/100 ml. Abnormal plasma lipid concentrations were present in 78 percent of the 56 women and the most common single abnormality was raised serum cholesterol.

Of the 145 women in the series, 42 had at some time either a serum cholesterol of 350 mg/100 ml or more or a serum triglyceride concentration of 200 mg/100 ml or more. Phenotyping of the lipoprotein classes was undertaken in 34 of these 42 women (Table 23.3). This survey was conducted from 1953-70 when phenotyping of lipoproteins was mostly not available. Many patients were receiving treatment and accurate assessment of the prevalence of lipoprotein abnormalities was not possible, though the commonest phenotype was type IIa.

Table 23.3 Hyperlipoproteinaemia (numbers)

Total group	M.I. 81	Angina 64	Total 145	
Se. cholest. 350 mg/100 ml	19	10	29	(20%)
Se. triglycerides				
200 mg/100 ml	9	4	13	(9%)
Lipoprotein type:				
II A	14	7	21	(14%)
II B	2	0	2	
III	0	1	1	
IV	7	3	10	(7%)
Not known	5	3	8	
Xanthomata	14	7	21	

Diastolic hypertension

Most women classified as having diastolic hypertension also had left ventricular hypertrophy. The most common associated finding was a history of hypertension during a previous pregnancy and not infrequently that of toxaemia of pregnancy. A history of C.H.D. in first degree relatives and the presence of significant obesity were common in these women.

Excessive cigarette smoking

There were significantly more smokers and more who smoked greater than 15 cigarettes daily among patients with myocardial infarction than among those with angina pectoris (Table 23.4). There was no significant difference in the prevalence of cigarette smoking in women with angina compared with that of women of similar age in the U.K. population (Todd, 1972).

Table 23.4 Smoking habits

	M.I.	Angina	U.K. Population* Women (30-45 yrs)
Total group	81	64	-
	%	%	%
Non-smokers	12	39	51
1-14/day	41	34	23
15-24/day	32	23	19
25 and more/day	15	3	7

*Estimated from Tobacco Research Council
 P 0.01 for non-smokers and 15 or more between MI and angina

Reliance had to be placed on the cigarette smoking habits of women before they presented with C.H.D. since most, particularly those who had myocardial infarction, reduced their smoking or discontinued it completely. Thus, it was impossible to relate prognosis to cigarette smoking with any accuracy.

Premature menopause

Menstruation had stopped in 29 (20 percent) of these women. The estimated prevalence in women aged 40 of a premature menopause is 3-5 percent. Amenorrhoea resulted from operative or radiation treatment for ovarian conditions in 18 and was spontaneous in 11. Most of those with a premature menopause had hyperlipidaemia.

Oral contraceptives

Most of these women were first seen before the widespread introduction of oral contraceptives. At the time of their presentation with C.H.D. only 12 (8 percent) — 10 of whom presented with myocardial infarction — had been taking oral contraceptives.

Parity

There was no significant difference in the numbers of children born to these women when compared with the expected, nor was there an excess miscarriage rate. Twelve spontaneous miscarriages occurred in the 108 married women who could recall clearly their gynaecological experiences.

Menarche

The age of the onset of menstruation was recorded in 122 of the 145 women. The median was 13.9 years with a mean of 14.4 years and a range of 11-17 years. This was not different from the expected.

Family history of C.H.D.

A history of C.H.D. in first degree relatives was recorded in about half of these women. It is difficult to quantify this but there was no significant difference in the importance of family history between patients with myocardial infarction and those with angina. A family history of C.H.D. was present in 16 (11 percent) of those without a major risk factor and in 92 (64 percent) of those with one or more major risk factors.

Obesity

While 21 percent of all patients with C.H.D. under 45 were obese to an extent of 15 percent or more above their standard weight, obesity alone (i.e. without other associated risk factors) occurred in only 5 percent of the whole group.

Hirsutism

Six of these young women had excess hair on the upper lip or below the chin and one shaved regularly.

Radiology

Coronary angiograms were not done in most of the women since the technique was developed several years after most women were admitted to the study and after some had died. Coronary angiograms were made in only 22 women; 8 had triple vessel disease, 6 had two coronary arteries with extensive atheroma, and 8 had more than 75 percent stenosis of one coronary artery.

Prognosis

Life tables were constructed to determine prognosis (Figs. 23.1 and 23.2). The follow-up was conducted at annual or occasionally biennial intervals. At each examination, a clinical history was taken and an electrocardiogram and radiological examination of the heart were made.

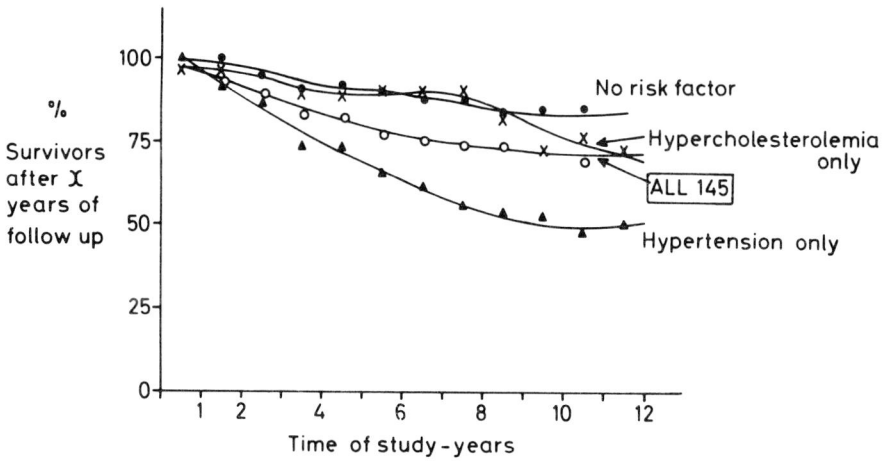

Fig. 23.1 The prognosis of women under 45 years (this series) with myocardial infarction or angina. There were too few deaths amongst those who smoked more than 20 cigarettes a day to plot a survival curve for this as a single risk factor.

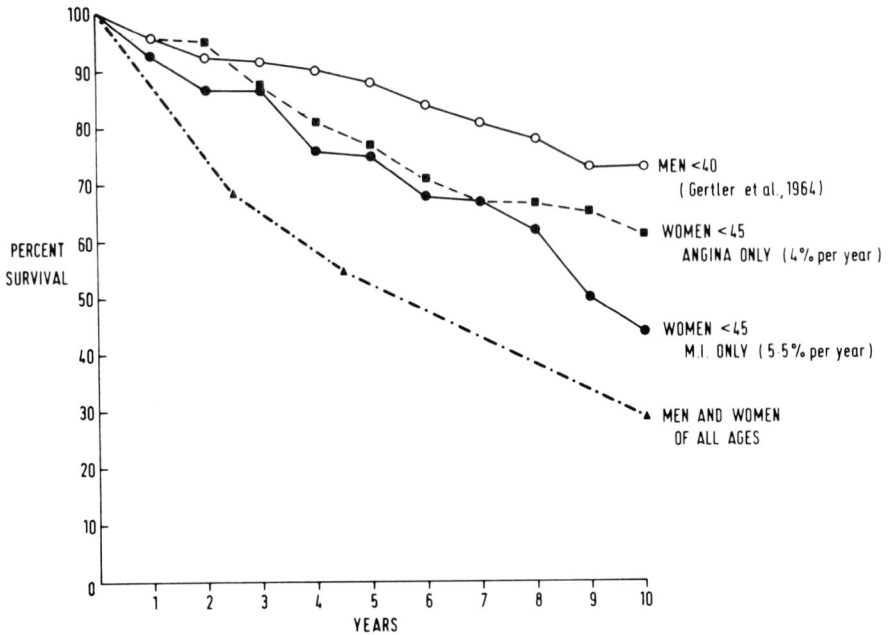

Fig. 23.2 Prognosis of ischaemic heart disease in patients with ischaemic heart disease. The young women referred to represent this series. A composite figure for men and women of all ages are derived from the Mayo Clinic experience.

The prognosis for young women with myocardial infarction was best if there were no associated major risk factors (Fig. 23.1). The presence of hypertension carried a worse prognosis than that of hypercholesterolaemia. It is possible to compare the prognosis of young women with myocardial infarction with that of young men with myocardial infarction and in Figure 23.2 the 12-year survival figures reported for 91 men under the age of 40 are contrasted with the findings of this study from 81 women under the age of 45 (Gertler *et al.*, 1964). Disregarding the presence of risk factors the overall prognosis of both sexes is similar, though perhaps a little worse for young women. The prognosis of these young patients is, as expected, better than older patients. Hypertension is also the risk factor of most importance in determining the poor prognosis in patients with angina pectoris (Oliver, 1974). There were no deaths over the 12-year period in the 28 women with associated hypercholesterolaemia, and only one death in the 13 women who smoked 20 or more cigarettes daily.

Discussion

There were several inherent difficulties in reporting this series of 150 women under 45 years who developed C.H.D. It only represents the experience of one cardiologist working for 20 years in a major university hospital serving a city of 450,000 with a surrounding population of about 1 million.

No conclusions can be reached concerning the prevalence of C.H.D. in young women, since unknown selection factors may have operated to provide such a large individual experience. Nor can reliance be given to the relative proportions presenting with angina or myocardial infarction.

Some of these women may have been referred to the Department of Cardiology in the Royal Infirmary because physicians in the community knew of my interest in C.H.D. and some bias may have operated to refer to me patients with an unrepresentative prevalence of risk factors. This is unlikely to have been a major influence, however, since all the women (96 patients) who were referred during the years 1953-64 by general practitioners were referred for a consultative opinion and not specifically to me though they were all seen by me either initially or within a few months of referral. There were 52 women with myocardial infarction and 44 with angina before 1965 and 33 and 21 respectively during 1965-70. The slight proportionate increase in those with myocardial infarction was probably due to the establishment in 1964 of a coronary care unit in the Royal Infirmary. Selective referral of patients from a distance can be excluded since only one lived outside a 50-mile radius from the centre of the city of Edinburgh.

The duration of the survey also led to problems since diagnostic methods change over a period of 18 years. Thus, lipoprotein typing was done in only one-third of patients and coronary arteriograms were undertaken in only 22 women. On the other hand, a smaller number studied more intensively would not necessarily have yielded more information.

A further weakness is that the prevalence of the major risk factors is not known for healthy women in the same community.

Hypercholesterolaemia was more common than hypertriglyceridaemia. Type IIa hyperlipoproteinaemia was the commonest of the abnormal phenotypes. While the numbers were small, this finding has been confirmed by Mann & Thorogood, 1975. A preponderance of type IIa has also been observed in women aged 40-49 (Wood *et al.*, 1972) and in older women with C.H.D. Presumably this reflects a major genetic component in the development of premature C.H.D. in these young women. The pattern differs from that observed in men.

The occurrence of left ventricular hypertrophy in most women with diastolic hypertension indicates its serious nature. Pregnancy hypertension or toxaemia were common precursors in those with hypertension. It has proved impossible to record with any consistency whether the blood pressure remained raised between the time of the pregnancy or of pre-eclamptic toxaemia and the onset of C.H.D.

A history of coronary heart disease was recorded frequently in first degree relatives of those who presented with hyperlipidaemia and in those with hypertension. This is consistent with the familial expression of hyperlipidaemia and hypertension.

There were fewer non-smokers among those with myocardial infarction compared with those who presented with angina pectoris and with the reported prevalence in the U.K. population (Todd 1972), and those with myocardial infarction smoked more than those with angina pectoris and the general population. These results are in keeping with those reported by Bengtsson (1973) for 47 women under the age of 60 years. A similar difference in cigarette smoking habits between patients who develop myocardial infarction and those who have angina has previously been reported in men (Doyle *et al.*, 1964). The rapid rise in mortality from C.H.D. in young women during recent years may be related in part to the striking increase in cigarette smoking which has occurred in women in their 20s and 30s over much the same period (Todd, 1972).

The relationship between premature cessation of ovarian function and the premature onset of C.H.D. has been described previously on the basis of surveys of women who developed a spontaneous premature menopause or had bilateral oophorectomy (Table 23.5) (Oliver and Boyd, 1959; Sznajderman and Oliver, 1963). The finding in this series that 20 percent of all women with C.H.D. under 44 years had already had a menopause confirms this association, and an additional 16 percent of women had had infrequent or very irregular menstruation during three months before the onset of angina or myocardial infarction. Further support can be derived from a recent Swedish survey (Bengtsson, 1973).

Table 23.5 Effect of ovarian failure on C.H.D.

	Nos.	Mean age (yrs)	I.H.D. (%)
Bilateral ovariectomy * <35 yrs	36	51	25.0
Spontaneous premature menopause ** <40 yrs	35	45	14.5
Unilateral ovariectomy *	31	52	3.0
Edinburgh population	1125	40	1.6
samples	951	50	3.1
Framingham Study	1000	40-49	2.0
(Standardised incidence)	1000	50-59	6.7

*   Oliver and Boyd (1959)
** Sznajderman and Oliver (1963)

Our earlier reports (Oliver, 1970; Radford & Oliver, 1973) suggested that oral contraceptives increase the risk of C.H.D., mostly in women already at risk, and that the risk is for myocardial infarction and not angina. This has been amply confirmed with the emphasis on women that the risk increases nearing the end of their reproductive life and in cigarette smokers (Royal College of General Practitioners, 1974; Mann *et al.*, 1975; Mann & Inman, 1975). Many of these women who developed myocardial infarction had been receiving high dose oestrogens — greater than 50 μg and even greater than 100 μg. Now that these have been withdrawn it is possible that the risk of myocardial infarction is less.

Diabetes mellitus was uncommon and only four out of 94 women had an abnormal glucose tolerance test result. Diabetes has frequently been suggested as an important explanation of the premature development of C.H.D. This was not so in these women and it was not more common in those with myocardial infarction than in those with angina.

The diagnosis of angina is not always easy to make in young women. Changes suggestive of myocardial ischaemia can occur in the post-exercise electrocardiogram in 10-26 percent of apparently normal women (Cumming et al., 1973). Taking this into account, an error in diagnosis might have been introduced into this series though it is likely to have been less since the women reported here also had symptoms of angina. Angina with electrocardiographic evidence of myocardial ischaemia may occur in some young women in the absence of demonstrable atherosclerotic occlusion of large coronary arteries. There is insufficient data to allow any conclusions about the incidence of this and much depends on the adequacy of the coronary angiograms. Most of the women reported in this series did not have coronary angiograms and so no comment can be made about the proportion that might have little or no disease in their coronary arteries. An ischaemic basis may exist, however, since infarction has occurred in such patients and increased lactate concentrations can occur in the coronary sinus blood. There is no satisfactory explanation for the occurrence in these women of myocardial ischaemia in the absence of coronary artery disease, though it could be due to undetectable small-vessel disease, coronary arterial spasm, a major thrombotic tendency, or an abnormal haemoglobin-oxygen dissociation curve. The most striking feature was that most of the 145 women with myocardial ischaemia or infarction had evident predisposing factor: 74 percent either had hypercholesterolaemia, diastolic hypertension, or smoked more than 20 cigarettes daily and one-third showed two or more of these major risk factors. In other words, young women who develop C.H.D. usually have one of the risk factors commonly associated with its premature development in men.

A contribution to our knowledge about C.H.D. in women is made by this study as a result of the long follow up. Many of the women were seen annually over periods of 15 or even 20 years. and 50 percent of the survivors were followed for 12 years. The prognosis of young patients with angina pectoris is better than that for those with myocardial infarction, the prognosis of whom is comparable to that reported previously for men with myocardial infarction under the age of 40. In both forms of C.H.D. co-existent hypertension carried a worse prognosis. The good prognosis of young women with angina should be noted with regard to the current uncertainty about the benefit which saphenous vein by-pass surgery may have on prognosis.

References

Bengtsson, C. (1973) Ischaemic heart disease in women a study based on a randomized population sample of women and women with myocardial infarction in Goteborg, Sweden. *Acta Medica Scandinavica Suppl.* No. **549**.

Carlson, L.A. (1963) Determination of serum triglycerides. *Journal of Atherosclerosis Research*, **3**, 334-36.

Cumming, G.R., Dufresne, C., Kich, L., Samm, J. (1973) Exercise electrocardiogram patterns in normal women. *British Heart Journal,* **35**, 1055-61.

Doyle, J.T., Dawber, T.R., Kannel, W.B., Kinch, S.H., Kahn, H.A. (1964) The relationship of cigarette smoking to coronary heart disease. *Journal of the American Medical Association,* **190**, 886-90.

Gertler, M.M., White, P.D., Simon, R. (1964) Long-term follow-up study of young coronary patients. *American Journal of Medical Science,* **247**, 145-55.

Jurand, J., Albert-Recht, F. (1962) The estimation of serum cholesterol. *Clinica Chimica Acta,* **I**, 522-28.

Mann, J.I., Inman, W.H.W. (1975) Oral contraceptives and death from myocardial infarction. *British Medical Journal,* **2**, 245-48.

Mann, J.I., Thorogood, M. (1975) Serum lipids in young female survivors of myocardial infarction. *British Heart Journal,* **37**, 790-94.

Mann, J.I., Vessey, M.P., Thorogood, M., Doll, R. (1975) Myocardial infarction in young women with special reference to oral contraceptive practice. *British Medical Journal,* **2**, 241-45.

Oliver, M.F., and Boyd, G.S. (1959) Effect of bilateral ovariectomy on coronary artery disease and serum lipid levels. *Lancet,* **2**, 690.

Oliver, M.F. (1970) Oral contraceptives and myocardial infarction. *British Medical Journal,* **2**, 210.

Oliver, M.F. (1974) Ischaemic heart disease in young women. *British Medical Journal,* **4**, 253-59.

Radford, D.J., Oliver, M.F. (1973) Oral contraceptives and myocardial infarction. *British Medical Journal,* **3**, 428-30.

Royal College of General Practitioners (1974) *Oral contraceptives and Health.* London, Pitman.

Sznajderman, M., and Oliver, M.F. (1963) Spontaneous premature menopause, ischaemic heart disease and serum lipids. *Lancet,* **1**, 962.

Todd, G.F. (editor) (1972) *Statistics of smoking in the United Kingdom.* London, Tobacco Research Council.

Wood, P.O.S., Stern, M.P., Silvers, A. (1972) Prevalence of plasma lipoprotein abnormalities in a free-living population of Central Valley, California. *Circulation,* **45**, 114-26.

Discussion 6B

Vessey (Oxford) Were all these women from the Edinburgh area or from a much wider district? What is the population of Edinburgh?

Oliver They all came from the Edinburgh area representing about 1.2 million.

Vessey (Oxford) It is really quite a small population and it is a remarkable collection of cases.

Somerville (London) What about the very large number of people who appear with typical prolonged myocardial ischaemic pain, and end up with an electrocardiogram that does not fit into any of the Minnesota codes that you mention? Do they have coronary disease or not.

Oliver They have been excluded because I felt the same doubt as you imply in your question. Do they have coronary disease or not? I was endeavouring to get as firm a diagnosis as I could. There are, in this series, 28 others who would fit into the category you describe but they were not included because I did not know how to categorise them. I suspect that there are more angina patients, as has been implied, and that the proportions of 81/64 are misleading. From 1964 every young woman who came to the coronary unit was included and so there would be preferential selection of women with myocardial infarction.

Rose (London) I would like to query your use of the term 'no evident predisposing factor' for those of your patients who did not have a single factor above a particular cutting point. The indication is that their occurrence was a complete mystery and I think that may not be so. We know from the epidemiological data that plasma cholesterol does not have to reach 270 mg/100 ml before it contributes to risk and that a combination of slight or moderate elevation of several factors in the same person can lead to just the same risk as a single factor that is very high. I wonder whether, before you imply that this proportion is unexplained, you might not look to see whether they did not include the association in the same woman of slight elevation of several factors.

Oliver The categories defined were mutually exclusive but I agree that a congruence of minor factors will have been overlooked. Furthermore, because of the time span of the study that triglycerides were not available as an estimate before about 1967 and fraction ion of lipoproteins until 1971. It is true that I have used an arbitrary cut of 270 mg/100 ml. I take your point and should say 'less' evident predisposing factors.

Bonnar (Dublin) Women who may benefit from oestrogen therapy are those who are subject to premature menopause or ovarian removal, say at the age of 35. Did any of your women who had removal of their ovaries or cessation of ovarian function receive oestrogen therapy? Have you any evidence that women who had ovariectomy and received oestrogen therapy were less subject to ischaemic heart disease?

Oliver The group with bilateral ovariectomy was not the group of women with coronary heart disease which I described. None of these received ostrogen therapy in the earlier retrospective survey and none had replacement therapy.

Bonnar (Dublin) Have you any evidence that women subject to premature menopause or ovariectomy given oestrogen are protected?

Oliver No, I cannot comment on that.

J

24. Coronary heart disease during the menopause

CALLE BENGTSSON AND OLOF LINDQUIST

There are diverging opinions as to whether there is an association between precocious menopause and coronary heart disease in women. Oliver and Boyd (1959) reported on such an association and the results from the majority of studies later on but not all agree with their results as reviewed e.g. by Bengtsson (1973), Blanc *et al.* (1977), Kannel *et al.* (1976).

An increased incidence of coronary heart disease might be caused by the early menopause *per se*. It might also be secondary to differences in risk factors for coronary heart disease between women with precocious menopause and other women. The purpose of the present communication is mainly to describe and evaluate such differences.

Material and methods

A population study of women in Göteborg, Sweden was carried out in 1968-1969 (Bengtsson *et al.* 1973). Women in five age strata between 38 and 60 years were studied. The sampling was made in such a way as to assure that the women were representative of the general population of women in the age strata studied. A high participation rate (90 percent) was a further guarantee for such a representativeness. Altogether 1462 women participated. Of these 29 women reported symptoms of angina pectoris as defined by Rose (1962).

Premenopausal women were defined as those who had been menstruating during the last month, while postmenopausal women were defined as those who had not had any menstruations since six months or longer. Women who had not menstruated since 2-5 months (n = 30) were excluded. Women who had had hysterectomy (n = 19) were excluded, while those with bilateral oophorectomy (n = 13) were included in the material. Studies of risk factors for ischaemic heart disease is in the present communication confined to 50-year old women, in all 398, in whom the numbers of premenopausal and postmenopausal women were similar.

The population sample of women was re-studied during 1974-1975. Altogether 1302 women participated in this follow-up study (89 percent of those studied 1968-1969). During the period between the two studied nine women had a myocardial infarct, and 42 women, who did not report symptoms of angina pectoris 1968-1969, reported such symptoms 1974-1975.

As a complement to the population studies, all women aged 57 years or younger in Göteborg who had myocardial infarction during the years 1968-1970 were studied according to the same principles as the women in the population sample. A case control study could thus be carried out, in which the women with myocardial infarction were compared with the participants in the population sample. The comparison was made with the women aged 50 and 54 years, who were of similar age as the women with myocardial infarction and the women with symptoms of angina pectoris (Bengtsson 1973).

Blood sampling was performed with the subjects fasting. Serum cholesterol was determined according to Levine and Zak (1964) and serum triglycerides according to Loftland (1964). Blood pressures measured with the subjects in the seated position are presented. Further details about material and methods have been given elsewhere (Bengtsson 1973, Bengtsson et al. 1973).

Statistical methods Conventional methods were used for calculation of mean values and standard deviations. Significance of differences between mean values was estimated with Student's t-test. The hypothesis of differences in frequencies between groups was tested by means of the chi-squared test. The differences were considered statistically significant for $p < 0.05$.

Results

Occurrence of coronary heart disease in relation to menopausal age

Table 24.1 shows the numbers of women who had the menopause at the age of 45 years or earlier in the series of women from the total population who had myocardial infarction and were included in the case control study and among those women in the population sample who reported symptoms of angina pectoris in the study carried out 1968-1969. Table 24.1 also presents data concerning menopausal state

Table 24.1 Number of women with menopause at the age of 45 years or earlier as found from a case control study (women with myocardial infarction and women with angina pectoris) and from a prospective study (initially symptomless women who had myocardial infarction or symptoms or angina pectoris during the 6-year interval between the two studies of the population sample) compared to women in the population sample of similar age.

	Women with myocardial infarction		Women with angina pectoris		Reference group of women	
	n	%	n	%	n	%
Case control study	10/46*	22	5/28	18	67/578	12
Prospective study	3/9	33	15/42***	35	67/578	12

*   Statistically different from the reference group, p < 0.05
*** Statistically different from the recerence group, p < 0.001

at the age of 45 years in those women in the population sample who had myocardial infarction during the interval between the two studies 1968-1969 and 1974-1975 or who had symptoms of angina pectoris in the second study but no such symptoms in the first study (a prospective study). A comparison is made with the women in the total population sample who were of similar age (women aged 50-54 years during the study 1968-1969). It is seen that early menopause (here arbitrarily defined as menopause at the age of 45 years or earlier), was more common in women with coronary heart disease. The results from the case control study and the prospective study are in agreement with each other.

Possible risk factors for coronary heart disease in premenopausal and postmenopausal women

Serum cholesterol Serum cholesterol values were higher in 50-year old postmenopausal women than in 50-year old women who still menstruated (Table 24.2). There was also a tendency towards higher serum cholesterol values in those 50-year old women who had been postmenopausal during the longest period as seen from the left part of Table 24.3.

Table 24.2 Serum cholesterol (mmol/l), serum triglycerides (mmol/l) and arterial blood pressure (mm Hg) in premenopausal (n = 175) and postmenopausal (n = 173) 50-year old women

| | Premenopausal women | | Postmenopausal women | | Significance |
	Mean	S.D.	Mean	S.D.	of difference
Serum cholesterol	6.96	0.99	7.43	1.20	$p < 0.001$
Serum triglycerides	1.17	0.49	1.35	0.64	$p < 0.001$
Systolic blood pressure	140	22	135	21	$p < 0.05$
Diastolic blood pressure	88	10	88	11	N.S.

N.S. = no statistical significance

Table 24.3 Means of serum cholesterol and the serum triglyceride values (mmol/l) in 50-year-old women in relation to the interval between the time of the examination and the time of the menopause (women examined after or before the menopause)

| | After menopause | | | | Before menopause | | |
Time (months)	n	Cholesterol (mmol/l)	Triglycerides (mmol/l)	Time (months)	n	Cholesterol (mmol/l)	Triglycerides (mmol/l)
$\geq$60	32	7.75	1.46	$\geq$60	9	7.23	1.26
36-59	35	7.52	1.26	36-59	36	6.84	1.24
24-35	33	7.29	1.36	24-35	34	7.07	1.24
12-23	46	7.44	1.36	12-23	38	6.84	1.11
6-11	27	7.05	1.29	6-11	13	6.89	1.01
0-5	31	6.92	1.22	1-5	15	6.99	0.94

When the women were re-studied six years later, information was obtained about the menopausal state of the women during the interval between the two studies. In this way it was known how long time remained to the menopause for those women who still had menstruations when the first study was performed during 1968-1969. Serum cholesterol values in relation to remaining premenopausal time are presented in the right part of Table 24.3. No association was found between cholesterol values and remaining premenopausal time.

Serum triglycerides   Similarly as for serum cholesterol, serum triglyceride values were higher in 50-year old postmenopausal women than in those 50-year old women who still menstruated (Table 24.2), and there was a tendency towards higher values among those who had had their menopause earliest (left part of Table 24.3). In the group of 50-year old women who still menstruated, those who had their menopause soon after the first population study had the lowest triglyceride values (right part of Table 24.3). It thus seemed that there was a fall in triglyceride values during the years just prior to the menopause.

Blood pressure   As seen from Table 24.2 systolic blood pressure was significantly higher in premenopausal 50-year old women than in postmenopausal women of the same age. Although significant, the difference was rather small, only 5 mm Hg for the mean values of systolic blood pressure, and no difference was found for the diastolic blood pressure.

Smoking habits   Table 24.4 shows the number of smokers in premenopausal and postmenopausal 50-year old women. There were significantly more smokers in the postmenopausal group of women. There was also a tendency towards heavier smoking among the postmenopausal smoking women. Thus 21 of 84 postmenopausal smokers (25 percent) consumed $\geq$15 cigarettes per day compared to 8 of 44 premenopausal smokers (18 percent). This difference was, however, not statistically significant.

Table 24.4   Number of smokers in premenopausal and postmenopausal 50-year old women

	n	%
Premenopausal women	44/175	25
Postmenopausal women	84/173	49

Smoking was not a consequence of the menopause, as only two of the postmenopausal 50-year old women had started smoking during the last 10 years preceeding the examination (2 percent) compared to five in the premenopausal group of women (11 percent). The tendency was thus the opposite. It seemed that the postmenopausal women had been smokers for a longer period than the premenopausal women. The earlier menopause in smoking women was found to be related to smoking and not vice versa.

Discussion

According to our results from a case control study and from a prospective study and according to the results from most other investigators, there is an association between precocious menopause and ischaemic heart disease. It seems that much of this overrepresentation of coronary heart disease in women with early menopause may be explained by an increased number of risk factors for coronary heart disease in these women. Serum cholesterol values in the present study were thus higher in women with early menopause than in women of the same age who still menstruated. However, high serum cholesterol values do not seem to be a very important risk factor for coronary heart disease in women (Epstein 1967, Kannel and Castelli 1972, Bengtsson 1973). Serum triglyceride values were also higher in postmenopausal women, and high serum triglyceride values seem to be a more important risk factor for coronary heart disease in women (Kannel and Castelli 1972, Bengtsson 1973). The higher lipid values in postmenopausal women might partly explain a higher incidence of coronary heart disease in these women.

The results from the studies of arterial blood pressure were opposite to those found for serum lipids. Systolic blood pressure was higher in still menstruating women than in postmenopausal women, while no difference was found for diastolic blood pressure. Blood pressure seems to be an important risk factor for coronary heart disease in women (Bengtsson, 1973, Bengtsson, 1977), but the difference between premenopausal and postmenopausal women in blood pressure was probably too small to be of clinical importance. The expected effect from the blood pressure would thus otherwise reduce the difference in occurrence of coronary heart disease between premenopausal and postmenopausal women.

Smoking seems to be another important risk factor for coronary heart disease, especially for myocardial infarction (Bengtsson 1973). There was also a striking difference in smoking habits between premenopausal and postmenopausal 50-year old women as found in the present study. The great majority of women with myocardial infarction in our case control study were smokers (Bengtsson 1973). Table 24.5 shows the number of women who had their menopause at the age of 45 years or earlier in the total series of women with myocardial infarction in the case control study and in the reference group. Separately the corresponding figures are presented when only smokers in the same study are included. It is seen that when the comparison is confined to smokers, part of the difference in prevalence of early menopause between women with myocardial infarction and women in the population sample disappears. It thus seems probable that the high number of smokers among the postmenopausal women might explain part of the increased incidence of myocardial infarction in these women.

Table 24.5 Number of women who had their menopause at the age of 45 years or earlier in women with myocardial infarction and in a reference group of women in the population sample of similar age (figures presented for the total groups and separately for the smokers)

	Women with myocardial infarction		Women in the reference group	
	n	%	n	%
Total group	10.46	22	67/578	12
Confined to smokers	8/37	22	32/216	15

Abstract

Results from our previous studies and from other investigations indicate that there is an increased incidence of myocardial infarction in women with early menopause. We have tried to find out whether such an increased incidence can be ascribed to the menopause *per se* or to differences between women with early and women with late menopause in risk factors for myocardial infarction. It was found that blood lipids were higher in women with early menopause than in women of the same age with late menopause. A tendency to the opposite direction was found for blood pressure. Smoking was more common in women with early menopause. The smoking women had been smokers for many years and did thus not start smoking at the time of the menopause. As smoking is an important risk factor for myocardial infarction in women it seemed from the present study that the increased number of smokers among women with early menopause can explain part of the increased incidence of myocardial infarction in women with early menopause.

References

Bengtsson, C. (1973) Ischaemic heart disease in women. A study based on a randomized population sample of women and women with myocardial infarction in Göteborg, Sweden. *Acta Medica Scandinavica,* suppl. **549.**

Bengtsson, C. (1977) Arterial hypertension as a risk factor for ischemic heart disease in women – results from a retrospective and from a prospective study. *Acta Medica Scandinavica,* suppl. **602,** 44-47.

Bengtsson, B., Blohmé, G., Hallberg, L., Hällström, T., Isaksson, B., Korsan-Bengtsen, K., Rybo, G., Tibblin, E., Tibblin, G. & Westerberg, H. (1973) The study of women in Gothenburg 1968-1969 – a population study. General design, purpose and sampling results. *Acta Medica Scandinavica,* **193,** 311-318.

Blanc, J.-J., Boschat, J., Morin, I.-F., Clavier, J. & Penther, T. (1977) Menopause and myocardial infarction. *American Journal of Obstetrics and Gynecology,* **127,** 353-355.

Epstein, F.H. (1967) Some uses of prospective observations in the Tecumseh Community Health Study. *Proceedings of the Royal Society of Medicine,* **60,** 56-60.

Kannel, W.B. & Castelli, W.P. (1972) The Framingham study of coronary disease in women. *Medical Times (N.Y.),* **100,** 173-195.

Kannel, W.B., Hjortland, M.C., McNamara, P.M. & Gordon, T. (1976) Menopause and risk of cardiovascular disease. The Framingham study. *Annals of Internal Medicine,* **85,** 447-542.

Levine, J.B. & Zak, B. (1964) Automated determination of serum total cholesterol. *Clinica Chimica Acta,* **10,** 381-384.

Loftland Jr, H.B. (1964) A semiautomated procedure for the determination of triglycerides in serum. *Analytical Biochemistry,* **9,** 393-400.

Oliver, M.F. & Boyd, G.S. (1959) Effect of bilateral ovariectomy on coronary disease and serum lipid level. *Lancet,* **II,** 690-694.

Rose, G.A. (1962) The diagnosis of ischaemic heart pain and intermittent claudication in field surveys. *Bulletin of the World Health Organization,* **27,** 645-658.

Discussion 6C

Mitchell (Nottingham) Were any of your 50 year old pre-menopausal women still on the pill? Could this have influenced the lipid results?

Bengtsson   No definitely not. None of the group aged 50 were on oral contraceptives. We can show that, independent of the menopause, serum cholesterol rose with age. At the age of 46, there was no difference in serum triglycerides between pre- and post-menopausal women, but serum cholesterol was higher in post menopausal women.

Hazzard (Seattle)   I am going to ask a difficult question. Is there any association between a late menopause and increased longevity, in general? It would appear to me that smoking may be accelerating ageing in general and that the menopause may be an index of ageing.

Bengtsson   I would not like to comment.

Vessey (Oxford)   Perhaps we could try and use this information in health education, and tell women that cigarette smoking is knocking out their sexual function earlier. Of course, they may prefer to have an early menopause.

General discussion

Gordon (Bethesda)   I want to ask Dr. Morris a question about the difference between those with chest pain who apparently had coronary heart disease, and those who did not. You pointed out that there was quite a lot of hypertension in both. Does this not imply that hypertension is associated with chest pain through other mechanisms besides coronary atherosclerosis?

Morris (Atlanta)   Yes, the blood pressure is elevated in both groups and they had pain typical of angina pectoris. But in some, coronary arteriograms are clear, although this does not mean that they do not have some type of smaller vessel disease. There was no difference incidentally, between blacks and whites.

Kitchin (Edinburgh)   What proportion were these patients with normal coronary arteries of the total group studied with angina pectoris? Did you find a higher prevalence of hypertension in the group with normal coronary arteries than those with atheroma? Thirdly, what was the long term outcome of these cases?

Morris (Atlanta)   There were 34 patients with significant coronary obstruction. The pain sounds like it, but not all of them had ischaemic heart disease or even angina pectoris. We have insufficient long term follow up yet to answer your other question.

Vessey (Oxford)   Can Dr. Oliver say how common in a general population would be a positive family history of CHD? Would those with CHD under 45 have up to a 50 percent chance of having a positive family history of CHD?

Oliver (Edinburgh)   I cannot comment on this with any accuracy. I do not know how to score family history accurately.

Slack (London) I think the only right way to think about this is to realise that cholesterol and blood pressure change with age and sex, so the family has variations with age and sex. The risks are different for men and women, and they have changed appreciably over the last 30 years. A coronary in a man at the age of 50 in 1940 is probably equivalent now to a coronary in a man aged 40 in 1970. So, in looking at family histories, we have to make a rather complicated adjustment as to which year the coronary took place in relation to the risk in that year and the sex.

Fulton (Glasgow) In Dr. Morris' series there was quite a large number of women with myocardial infarction. How many had coronary angiograms, how many had occlusions and what percent had clear coronary arteries?

Morris (Atlanta) Of the 28 total patients, coronary angiograms were done on 15. There was only one who had a normal coronary arteriogram.

Fulton (Glasgow) You made the point that various predictive indices or markers were often absent where there was one vessel disease, but invariably present in multi-vessel disease. Does this in any way relate, do you think, to chronicity of the disease process? I feel that it is probable that one vessel disease is more liable to have had a shorter period of evolution, whereas multivessel disease probably implies a much longer process.

Morris (Atlanta) I think the point is correct.

Short (Edinburgh) Listening to the discussions over the last three days, it has struck me that nobody has really addressed themselves to the central issue of why there should be this spectacular sex difference in the incidence of coronary heart disease during the reproductive years. We are so concerned with the aetiology of the disease process itself that we have lost sight of its biological significance to the species. So let us consider for a moment what possible adaptive significance there could be in the selective increase in mortality of men.

In polygynous animal communities there is good evidence to show that although the secondary sex ratio at birth almost invariably approaches equality, there is a preferential mortality of males after birth, so that the tertiary sex ratio at the time of sexual maturity is biased in favour of females. This mortality is probably hormonally induced; for example, male mortality may be increased as a result of testosterone-induced patterns of behaviour, such as increased aggressiveness. From the point of view of the species, it is clearly advantageous to have fewer surplus males around, utilising scarce resources; the greater the degree of polygamy, the more unequal the tertiary sex ratio can afford to be.

So what of our own species? I have reviewed elsewhere some of the anatomical and anthropological evidence which points to the fact that we are basically a polygynous species, although this may often take the form of serial monogamy rather than the commoner harem-type of polygamous situation (Short, R.V. (1978) *Advances in the Study of Animal Behaviour,* in press). Therefore, perhaps we should expect to find a skewed tertiary sex ratio, with a preferential mortality of males during the early years. If we accept Darwin's concept of Sexual Selection, we should also expect to find that this mortality was related to lack of 'fitness' in the most general sense of the word, and that it was hormonally related. The evidence, such as it is, does indeed show that male eunuchs have a significantly greater life expectancy that intact men (Hamilton, J.B. and Mestler, G.E. (1969) *J. Gerontol,* **24**, 395-411). If there is an underlying endocrine aetiology to coronary heart disease, we must be careful how we tamper with our hormone levels. The development of male con-traceptives that use exogenous androgens to suppress spermatogenesis might produce aggressive individuals; but at least, they would die young!

SESSION 7 Future recommendations

Chairman: M.F. Oliver

25. Future recommendations

W. SOMERVILLE

My remit was to draw up a number of recommendations based on our discussions over the past two days. The main objective of our deliberations was to identify young women who are at risk of developing angina pectoris (AP) or acute myocardial infarction (AMI) some time in the future. The strategy was to review a number of series of coronary heart disease (CHD) in young women, examining closely the genetic influences and risk indicators. We discussed in some depth the influence of smoking, the oral contraceptive (OC), blood pressure, lipids and diabetes. We reviewed the present knowledge of sex hormone production in women and in men, the immunological mechanisms involved in CHD and particularly in relation to the OC and the arteriographic pattern and histology of the diseased coronary arterial wall in young women.

How are vulnerable young women to be recognised? Mass screening is out of the question. One approach is by primary prevention techniques whereby the children of CHD patients are routinely examined. Another is via pre-employment physical examinations. A number of them will present in pregnancy or suspected pregnancy, or when applying for the OC. Family history provides one of the few clues; Dr. Joan Slack underlined the significance of CHD in a parent under the age of 50, while disease in both parents is an even stronger marker. A few will be picked up from a family history of hypertension or diabetes. Professor Beaumont and his colleagues may well have developed another clue in coronary-prone women taking the OC, with their discovery of circulating anti-ethinyl oestradiol antibodies; the risk of developing obstructive atherosclerotic lesions is associated with these antibodies which may develop in more than 10 percent of OC-users.

Advice to a young woman with these markers — certainly family history and possibly antibodies — should follow these lines:-
1. She should be a life-long non-smoker;
2. She should never take the OC, even the 30 ugm. oestrogen variety;
3. A resting blood pressure should never be allowed to exceed 145/90:
4. Her carbohydrate tolerance should be investigated for the earliest threat of diabetes;
5. A fasting cholesterol and triglyceride measurement should be made and if an unequivocal hyperlipidaemia is discovered, it should be corrected;
6. She should never get fat;
7. The prime diet advice should be aimed at obesity.

Excepting the few with hyperlipidaemia, young women should be told that if the body weight is correct, so is the diet. There is no proof of the protective value of diet manipulation in young women in this category without hyperlipidaemia. What else can be done to identify and protect the vulnerable young woman? Routine exercise stress ECGs in women are a particularly weak indicator of CHD and the suggestion of a routine exercise test is not practical.

Type A personality identication has little to recommend it in young women. Even allowing for the fact that a high percentage of them have superficial Type A characteristics, we have no methods available of changing her to Type B, even if that were shown to be desirable.

These recommendations centre around the importance of family history as a coronary marker. To make best use of this knowledge, a vulnerable young woman should be advised not to beget a child by a man with a family history of CHD, hypertension or diabetes.

The coronary artery anatomy of vulnerable women is the ultimate determinant of CHD. At present, certain constraints limit the use of coronary arteriography, particularly mortality and morbidity, however, miniscule. In the future, when the coronary arteries can be visualised more effectively and safely, all young women at risk will have their coronary arteries surveyed for the earliest appearances of atheromatous plaques.

Discussion 7

Jarrett (London) The relationship between obesity and cholesterol levels is very slender. Surely it is cholesterol levels in girls not obesity that determine those very much at risk of coronary heart disease. At this young age, treatment is most likely to be effective. At the ages of 40 and 50 we may be wasting our time with cholesterol estimations as there is little chance of altering the established disease. At the age of 20, you may have a reasonable chance of altering the natural history.

Somerville I would immediately concede that the relationship between obesity and hypercholesterolaemia is slender. I think that if one were to pick up hypercholesterolaemia by a chance encounter, then you should treat it. You should consider the patient as a special individual who has a strong marker of hyperlipidaemia. However, how does one manage those patients who have a cholesterol level slightly above normal? There will be many, and the number of those with real hyperlipidaemia will be very few.

Jarrett (London) I am not talking about hyperlipidaemia. I am saying that the normal blood cholesterol level in a 20 year old girl is not 250 but 150 mg/100 ml.

Somerville Are you suggesting that all women whose blood cholesterol is above 150 mg/100 ml should have a special diet?

Jarrett (London) I suggest that if anybody were found with a value of 200 mg/100 ml or above, at the age of 20, they should be advised about the nature of their diet.

Gresham (Cambridge) I have two points. First of all, if someone is at the right weight, they are not taking in a large amount of calories as fat, unless they are eating a perverse diet. My other point is that it is more practical to persuade patients to 'keep their weight down' rather than place them on exotic diets.

Jarrett (London) There are a number of surveys now which show that there is an inverse relationship between calorie intake and obesity. The thin person, in general, is eating more calories, whether from carbohydrates or fat, than a fat person. The reason for this is that the thin person is able to expend the excess energy.

Gordon (Bethesda) There is little association between obesity and serum cholesterol levels, but there is a strong association between obesity with triglycerides and with HDL. There is now substantial evidence that you can modify the level of both those lipids, as well as cholesterol for that matter, by weight change.

Hazzard (Seattle) I entirely agree. However, how do you advise the young fat woman? Should she lose weight or not? The answer is dependent on whether or not her blood pressure is satisfactory, whether or not she has a diabetic diathesis and whether or not she has a hyperlipidaemia. In other words obesity *per se* may not be a risk factor, but if she has other risk factors, reduction of weight is perhaps the best and most direct way of reducing those risks.

Singh (Birmingham) Dr. Jarrett, is it not true serum cholesterol levels only fall in an obese person if there is weight reduction?

Jarrett (London) I do not think weight reduction is a very impressive means of reducing serum cholesterol. If intense weight reduction is achieved mainly by carbo- hydrate restriction, there is not a very impressive fall in level of cholesterol. If weight reduction is by fat restriction then there may be.

Mitchell (Nottingham) I had always thought that there was a very close association between obesity and triglyceride levels. However, we have had the opportunity of looking at 40 women who were so fat that they are being assessed for ileal by-pass. In all of those women, except one, the serum triglyceride levels were normal and their body weight was enormous. This directly conflicts with what I had in my mind. While we are talking about obesity I think it is worth mentioning that there are several varieties of types of obesity. The gynoid or hyper-gynoid obesity, where most of the fat occurs from the waist down is usually not associated with any meta- bolic abnormality. The android type, where the fat is located in the upper half of the body, is associated almost invariably with hyperlipidaemia, with glucose in tolerance and insulin resistance. The same is true in men, although the gynoid type of obesity in men is rare, and most men either have global obesity or android-type obesity. The most critical measurement of all in obesity is the existence of insulin resistance. In my experience, this is the most useful of all the biochemical predictors of atherogenesis.

Bengtsson (Goteborg) It is important to remember that there are few smokers who are really obese.

Potts (London) I would like to ask Dr. Somerville how he would manage a woman who had been taking the pill for a couple of years, with no history of any risk factors, but her blood pressure slowly creeps up. At what level would be recommend withdrawing the pill and would he make that level different from a woman of 25 and a woman of 35?

Somerville   Changes in blood pressure should be taken more seriously and a higher degree of responsibility attached to them in the 25-year old people than the 35-year old. My own experience is that it is pretty hopeless trying to control blood pressure successfully in the person who has pill-induced hypertension by any means other than withdrawing the pill.

Potts (London) How would you define that level of blood pressure?

Somerville   A fixed blood pressure reading of 150/90 is grossly abnormal in a girl of 25.

Potts (London) Supposing one has a woman of 40 on the 'pill' with no family history and no risk factors, but you have the capacity to do what you call 'a simple lipid study'. What exactly would you include? At what levels would you stop giving her the pill?

Somerville   I would prefer to hand that problem to a person like Dr. Oliver.

Oliver (Edinburgh) I suggest the following for a simple lipid screen. Take a fasting blood specimen and let it stand for a period of about 3 hours allowing clot retraction to take place. If the plasma is clear, you can practically be sure that it is unnecessary to make any triglyceride estimation. You can then send the specimen to the laboratory for serum cholesterol analysis. If this is abnormal further investigations may be indicated. Not everybody here will agree about this, but it is at least simple.

Mann (Oxford) I think the age limits which Dr. Potts notes are very important as we cannot go around studying everyone about to go on the pill. It is significant that more deaths occur in those over the age of 35 taking the pill and perhaps we should lay down even more clear guidelines for the older woman, be she 35 or 40. I think in addition to having initial tests, as described, it is also very important to have follow-up tests done, because an initial lipid measurement may be unpredictive as to subsequent events. If we are going to select out a group of women for special care, it should be the older pill user. In so doing, we have to concede that there are very young pill users who develop a thrombotic episode, but perhaps at the moment we cannot predict those at risk.

Marquis (Edinburgh)   What are the arguments against a woman of 35 or 40 being sterilised rather than using the contraceptive pill?

Baird (Edinburgh)   I think it is very difficult to generalise. The obstetricians are at present conducting a survey on the morbidity or mortality associated with laparoscopic sterilisation. First we must establish this.

Loudon (Edinburgh)   We have to take into consideration the fact that some women do not wish to be sterilised.

Bonnar (Dublin)   There is another worrying point in that most studies on sterilisation in this age group have indicated that between 30 and 50 percent subsequently come for hysterectomy. In fact, many gynaecologists faced with this problem in a woman of 35 or over would probably prefer to do a hysterectomy and this would without doubt carry a higher morbidity than the routine sterilisation procedure.

Baird (Edinburgh)   Many women come to hysterectomy following sterilisation because they have stopped the oral contraceptive pill. We tend to forget that those who are taking the pill have a reduced risk of having a hysterectomy.

Loudon (Edinburgh)   I would like advice as to which pill you would advise particularly in those who are 'borderline'. Professor Wynn talked earlier about insulin resistance on the 30 microgram pill, but he was talking only of Ovran 30.

Wynn (London)   Unfortunately, the 150 microgram norgestrel pill combined with 30 micrograms of oestrogen produces as much insulin resistance as the pill with 250 micrograms of norgestrel. I personally do not think we have a safe oral contraceptive formulation at the moment. However, new formulations are being rapidly introduced and appropriate investigations may show one which is metabolically apparently safer than others. We are still in a situation where we cannot make a definitive statement as to which is the safest pill although we can definitely say from a metabolic point of view that no contraceptive pill should contain more than 50 micrograms of oestrogen. When that dose is lowered there are still metabolic disturbances which over a long period of time are likely to have deleterious effects.

Jarrett (London)   There are some unpublished prospective studies in men which have shown no relationship between insulin levels and CHD incidence. We know that obesity, which is also associated with high insulin levels, is not in itself associated with CHD.

Closing comments about future studies

M. F. OLIVER

This meeting has shown many problems which merit further study.

First, what is the nature of the sensitivity or resistance to arterial disease within the hereditary pattern that has been so clearly described by Dr Joan Slack? Do genetic factors operate through identifiable abnormalities, such as hyperlipidaemia, hypertension and diabetes, in conjunction with environmental risk factors — or through independent as yet unmeasured influences?

Second, the identification of anti-oestrogen antibodies in the sera of a small proportion of oral contraceptive users needs confirmation and consolidation. If these women develop a thrombotic vasculitis, can such tests be used for discriminate screening to identify the vulnerable?

Third, once again we seem to have no definite views about the ways oral contraceptives affect coagulation mechanisms. One of the problems is that many of the coagulation tests are *in vitro* tests and there are tremendous difficulties in translating these results, even in the best circumstances, to the *in vivo* situation. We are dealing with a thrombotic condition, venous and arterial, and this is obviously an area which needs further attention.

Fourth, we have no clear knowledge about the safety or otherwise of the 30 microgram oral contraceptive. Dr Mann has made it very clear that all the figures we have been considering with regard to vascular risk relate to pills containing 50 micrograms or more of oestrogen. This risk may not be relevant to the lower dose pill. It is urgent that studies are established to settle this point.

Finally, there is the problem of oestrogen replacement therapy. This may be more important than anything else we have been discussing, if we are to follow the prescribing habits of practitioners in the west coast of North America. Professor Doll said he could not see any basis for a controlled trial which he would accept because of the prior selection of women for oestrogen replacement therapy. There is difficulty also in interpreting the data as to whether oestrogen is protecting or aggravating, and this appears to be a further area of urgent consideration.

Conversion Table—old to new units

	Old units	New units	Conversion factors (Old to new units)
Androstenedione	mg/1	umol/1	3.45
Cholesterol	mg/100 ml	mmol/1	0.0259
Dehydroepiandrosterone	mg/1	umol/1	3.47
Fibrinogen	g/100 ml	g/l	10
Glucose	mg/100 ml	mmol/l	0.0555
Oestradiol	ug/l	nmol/l	3.67
Oestrogen	ug/l	nmol/l	3.70 (as oestrone)
Oestrone	ug/l	nmol/l	3.70
Progesterone	ug/l	nmol/l	3.18
Pyruvate	mg/100 ml	umol/l	115
Testosterone	ug/l	nmol/l	3.47
Triglycerides	mg/100 ml	mmol/l	0.011

Index